MILADY STANDARD
NATURAL HAIR CARE
AND BRAIDING

Diane Carol Bailey

⚡ Cengage

Australia • Brazil • Canada • Mexico • Singapore • United Kingdom • United States

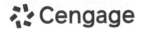

Milady Standard Natural Hair Care and Braiding
Diane Carol Bailey

Editorial Contributions: Diane Da Costa,
  Anu Prestonia and Tulani Kinard

Executive Director, Milady: Sandra Bruce

Senior Product Manager: Martine Edwards

Content Developer: Maria Moffre-Barnes

Product Assistant: Sarah Prediletto

Director, Marketing & Training: Gerard McAvey

Associate Marketing Manager:
  Matthew McGuire

Senior Production Director: Wendy Troeger

Production Manager: Sherondra Thedford

Senior Content Project Manager:
  Nina Tucciarelli

Senior Art Director: Benj Gleeksman

Cover image: © Vasilchenko Nikita/Shutterstock

For product information and technology assistance, contact us at
Cengage Customer & Sales Support, 1-800-354-9706
For permission to use material from this text or product,
submit all requests online at **www.cengage.com/permissions**
Further permissions questions can be emailed to
permissionrequest@cengage.com

Library of Congress Control Number: 2013938409

ISBN-13: 978-1-133-69368-0

ISBN-10: 1-133-69368-7

Cengage
200 Pier 4 Boulevard
Boston, MA 02210
USA

Cengage is a leading provider of customized learning solutions with office locations around the globe, including Singapore, the United Kingdom, Australia, Mexico, Brazil, and Japan. Locate your local office at
www.cengage.com/global

To learn more about Cengage platforms and services, register or access your online learning solution, or purchase materials for your course, visit **www.cengage.com.**

Printed at CLDPC, USA, 04-23

Table of Contents

Procedures at a Glance

Preface

You are about to begin a journey into a career that can be filled with success and personal satisfaction. The need for natural stylists continues to grow in new and exciting ways, providing numerous opportunities for personal triumph in a variety of career paths.

As your school experience begins, consider how you will approach your course of study through attitude, study skills and habits, and perseverance—especially when the going gets tough. Stay focused on your goal: to become a natural hair care stylist and embark on your career. Never hesitate to talk to your instructor should any problems arise that might prevent you from reaching your destination.

Features of This Edition

This edition includes many features and learning tools that will help you master key concepts and techniques.

Why Study This?

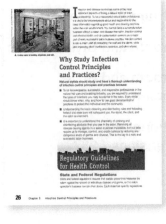

Milady knows, understands, and appreciates how excited students are to delve into the newest and most exciting products and equipment, and we recognize that students can sometimes feel restless spending time learning the basics of the profession. To help you understand why you are learning each chapter's material and to help you see the role it will play in your future career as a natural stylist, Milady has added this new section to each chapter. This section includes three or four bullet points that tell you why the material is important and how you will use the material in your professional career.

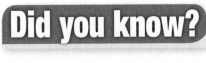

This feature provides interesting information that will enhance your understanding of the material in the text and call attention to a special point.

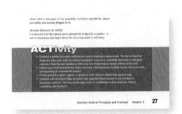

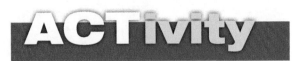

Activity boxes describe hands-on classroom exercises that will help you understand the concepts explained in the text.

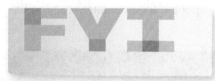

Web Resources provide you with Web addresses where you can find more information on a topic and references to additional sites for more information.

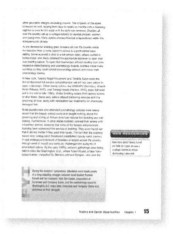

FYIs offer important, interesting information related to the content. Often, **FYI** boxes direct you to a Web site or other resource for further information.

CAUTION

Some information is so critical for your safety and the safety of your clients that it deserves special attention. The text directs you to this information in the **CAUTION** boxes found in the margins.

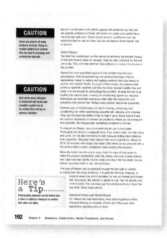

Here's a Tip.......

These helpful tips draw attention to situations that might arise and provide quick ways of doing things. Look for these tips throughout the text.

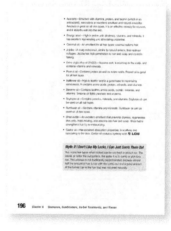

Myth

This feature will bring light to current and past misconceptions and untruths related to natural hair care and its practice.

Educational Chapter Formatting

Each chapter of *Milady Standard Natural Hair Care and Braiding* includes specialized formatting and strategies for the presentation of material to enhance your experience while working with the chapter and to facilitate the learning process.

Learning Objectives

At the beginning of each chapter is a list of learning objectives that tell you what important information you will be expected to know after studying the chapter.

Learning Objectives

After completing this chapter, you should be able to:

☑ **LO1** Name and describe the structures of the hair root.

☑ **LO2** List and describe the layers of the hair shaft.

☑ **LO3** Discuss the qualities and characteristics of the varying hair textures.

☑ **LO4** List the different factors to consider during hair analysis.

☑ **LO5** Describe the three growth phases of hair.

Throughout the chapter, you will see a special icon that indicates you have finished reading the material that corresponds to each of these Learning Objectives. ☑ **LO**

Key Terms

The words you will need to know in a chapter are given at the beginning in a list of Key Terms. When the word is discussed for the first time within the chapter, it appears in **boldface** type. If the word is difficult to pronounce, a phonetic pronunciation follows it in parentheses.

Key Terms

Page number indicates where in the chapter the term is used.

braid designer p. 18	cultural aesthetic p. 20	natural hair care license p. 19	natural hair textures p. 17
braid stylist p. 18	holistic approach p. 19	natural hairstyles p. 12	tignon p. 6
braid technician p. 18	master braider p. 18	natural hair stylist p. 3	transitioning p. 16
cosmetology p. 3	natural hair care p. 3		

Procedures

All step-by-step procedures offer clear, easy-to-understand directions and multiple photographs for learning the techniques. At the beginning of each procedure, you will find a list of the needed implements, materials, and supplies along with any preparation that must be completed before the procedure begins.

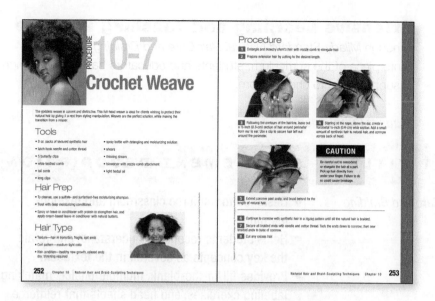

All of the procedures appear in a special **Procedures** section at the end of the chapter.

Review Questions

Each chapter ends with questions designed to test your understanding of the chapter's content. Your instructor may ask you to write the answers to these questions as an assignment or to answer them orally in class. If you have trouble answering a chapter review question, go back to the chapter to review the material and then try again.

Review Questions

1. Why is it imperative for natural hair stylists to understand hair typing and hair texture?
2. What follicle shapes produce coily and curly hair fibers?
3. What are the three growth phases of hair, and how long does each one last?
4. According to the text, is hair physically alive? Define keratinization.
5. Name two parts of the hair structure. What part of the structure does the natural stylist manipulate?
6. Where is the dermal papilla located, and what is its function?

Marginal Glossary

All key terms and their definitions are included in the **marginal glossary** in the chapter.

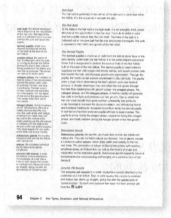

Extensive Learning and Teaching Package

Although *Milady Standard Natural Hair Care and Braiding* is the centerpiece of the curriculum, students and educators have a wide range of supplements to choose from.

Student Supplements

SUPPLEMENT TITLE	SUPPLEMENT DESCRIPTION
Milady Standard Natural Hair Care and Braiding Student Workbook	• Designed to reinforce classroom and textbook learning. • Helps students recognize, understand, and retain the key concepts as covered in the textbook. • Provides fill-in-the-blank, multiple-choice, matching, labeling exercises, and head sheets that reinforce practical applications.

Educator Supplements

Milady proudly offers a full range of innovative products created especially for natural hair care and braiding educators to make classroom preparation and presentation easy, effective, and enjoyable.

SUPPLEMENT TITLE	SUPPLEMENT DESCRIPTION
Instructor Resource on CD for Milady Standard Natural Hair Care and Braiding	• This is the primary instructor resource to *Milady Standard Natural Hair Care and Braiding*. • This resource contains lesson plans complete with classroom handouts and PowerPoint slides for each chapter. • Computerized test bank. • Step-by-step head sheets for nine procedures.
DVD Series for Milady Standard Natural Hair Care and Braiding	• The DVD Series for *Milady Standard Natural Hair Care and Braiding* features demonstrations covering both practical and theory information from the text. The video will provide the viewer with procedural tips and helpful reminders to better prepare for career success. With two hours of content, this resource will enhance the classroom experience for your students.

Thank you for choosing Milady as your Total Learning Solutions Provider. For additional information on the above resources or to place an order, please contact your Milady Sales Representative or visit us online at www.milady.cengage.com.

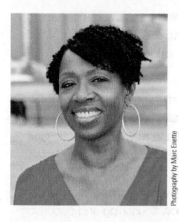

Photography by Marc Enette

Diane C. Bailey

Diane C. Bailey is the former president and art director of **Tendrils Hair Spa**, a comprehensive natural hair care salon. As a salon entrepreneur, she created a venue that addressed the needs of clients seeking natural hair care services. A native of Brooklyn, New York, she established Tendrils in 1987 in her Fort Green/Clinton Hill community. Known as a celebrity stylist, Ms. Bailey has styled Beyonce Knowles, Lauren Hill, Terry McMillan, and Iyanla Vanzant.

Honored as a "Master Pioneer" and "trailblazer" of the natural hair care industry with over 25 years of experience, Ms. Bailey has positioned herself as an innovator and standard bearer for natural hair care. She has influenced the creation of new textured hair fibers and hair styling techniques and has developed semantics, systems, and procedures that have been groundbreaking throughout the industry. Ms. Bailey has previously authored three books: *Natural Hair Care and Braiding, Braiding—Easy Styles for Everyone,* and *Basic Care for Naturally Textured Hair: Cultivating Curly, Coily, and Kinky Hair*. Ms. Bailey also contributed to multiple editions of *Milady Standard Cosmetology*. Ms. Bailey is currently a natural beauty consultant for Shea Moisture/Nubian Heritage of Sundial Brands and Design Essentials Natural by McBride Research Laboratories; she has developed workshops that feature both product lines and demonstrate natural hair, locks, and protective and transitional styling techniques.

Ms. Bailey co-produced a one-day event with A Tribe Called Curl and Mane Moves titled *Super Natural: Celebrating Coils, Kinks and Curls* which promoted natural hair care workshops, a hair show, product demonstrations, and giveaways for the natural hair care community.

Ms. Bailey was the keynote speaker for the 2010 Barbering and Cosmetology Summit in Milwaukee, Wisconsin. As an expert in her field, she is often requested to be a guest and motivational speaker throughout the country.

As an adjunct professor, Ms. Bailey taught and wrote the curriculum for "Fundamentals of Braiding" at Medgar Evers College for the adult education program, in the City University of New York.

Appointed by the New York Secretary of State, Diane Bailey served five years on the New York State Appearance Enhancement Advisory Committee. She was the first African American to be appointed to the committee in 1992. She co-founded The International Braiders Network (IBN), a professional trade association that promoted the cultural, historical, and technical aspects of braiding, locking, and natural hair care. It advocated for the inclusion of African-textured hair and styling within the traditional cosmetology industry. Ms. Bailey assisted New York state in establishing a natural hair care braiding license—one of the first licenses of its kind in the United States. As the treasurer and events coordinator of the Natural Hair and Braiders Association (NHBA), Ms. Bailey developed workshops specifically for the natural beauty industry.

Ms. Bailey was featured in the *Essence Total Makeover* book. Her most recent feature was in *Self Seduction by Essence's* beauty director, Mikki Taylor. Ms. Bailey has been published and featured on YouTube, and television, radio, newspapers, and popular magazines including *Essence, Heart & Soul, Source, Allure, Modern Salon, Braids and Beauty, The New York Times, Newsday, Daily News,* and *The Amsterdam News*.

Tulani Kinard

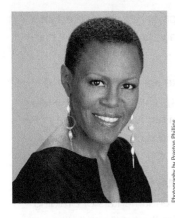

Photography by Preston Phillips

Tulani Kinard is an artistic pioneer whose innovations are known across various creative platforms. She is highly respected in the natural hair care field for her critical role in fundamentally changing the industry and improving its best practices for people of African descent. With civil rights attorney Esmeralda Simmons, Kinard wrote the language for legislation, sponsored by New York State Senator Velmanette Montgomery, that created the first natural hair care license in the United States. She is also the best-selling author of *No Lye—The African American Woman's Guide to Natural Hair Care* (St. Martin's Press), a groundbreaking "how-to" book for natural hair care and braiding.

Tulani's Regal Movement was the first comprehensive natural hair care salon in Brooklyn, New York. Based on her preeminence in the field, Tulani co-created the first symposium to discuss the art of braiding and its historical and contemporary relevance in African American culture. The symposium, curated by Dr. Bernice Johnson Reagon, was the first of its kind to be showcased at the Smithsonian Institute in Washington, D.C. Tulani also co-founded The International Braiders Network (IBN) and has served as president of the National Braiders Guild. These two organizations provide annual platforms in various cities for natural hair stylists to gather and share techniques in celebration of the art of braiding.

As a master braider, Tulani has styled the heads of many celebrities, including Roberta Flack, Dianne Reeves, and Suzanne Douglass. In true innovative fashion, Tulani is credited for bringing to New York the micro cornrow braids featuring the beadwork of semiprecious stones and crystals. These popular and elaborate hairstyles were performed over several days. Tulani also created the salon-perfected hair product line, Nu Ade, which consists of nourishing oil treatments that cater to all hair textures. The products are sold in salons and online at mynuade.com.

Over the years, Tulani has mentored many young people in the art of braiding and natural hair care. Several of her students have established and maintained successful salons, including Nu Wave Kultural Kreations in New York and Essentials Beauty Spa in Maryland. Tulani reflects, "It's an honor to have provided the foundations for my students that are now flourishing and becoming leaders amongst their own generation of trailblazers."

Though Tulani continues to consult and mentor in the natural hair care field, her vision and reach have always been expansive. She is the former vocalist of the Grammy Award–winning ensemble Sweet Honey in Rock and the former musical director for Iyanla Vanzant, who has released two solo albums and performs regularly across the country. Tulani is ordained as an interfaith minister. She offers: "The common thread that runs through all my work in the creative and healing arts—be it the adornment of one's crown, the composition of a song, or the counseling of a soul in need—is my ability to inspire and help people rediscover their own power via their divine expressions."

Diane Da Costa

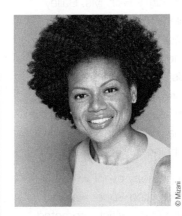

© Mizani

Diane Da Costa is a curly textured expert and author of *Textured Tresses, The Ultimate Guide to Maintaining and Styling Natural Hair* (Simon & Schuster, June 2004). Diane's philosophy is simple: Textured hair is gorgeous hair! With over 25 years in the beauty business, Diane has brought innovative curly styles to the forefront of today's multi-textured hair movement. A celebrity hair designer to the stars, she has had the pleasure of working with artists and celebrities, including seven-time Grammy winner Lauryn Hill and the Fugees, critically acclaimed actor Blair Underwood, rock star Lenny Kravitz, trumpeter and Grammy winner Roy Hargrove, heavyweight champion Lenox Lewis, jazz vocalist Dee Dee Bridgewater, jazz and rock drummer Cindy Blackman-Santana, *Legally Blonde, The Broadway Musical's* Amber Efe, MTV host and actress Julissa Bermudez, Les Nubian, vocalist Lizz Wright, Golden Globe winner S. Epatha Merkison, and many more.

Diane's cutting-edge styles have graced the pages of *The New York Times, EBONY, ESSENCE, British Elle, French Vogue, Heart & Soul, JUICY, The Source, In Style, Latin Girl, Latina.com, O Magazine, Rolling Stone, Sophisticates Black Hair, Vibe,* and *UPTOWN* magazines. Diane was a contributing stylist to the *ESSENCE Total Makeover* book and Harriette Cole's *Jumping the Broom.* She was also the first hair editor of *Honey* magazine.

Diane also opened Dyaspora Salon Spa, the first Aveda Concept salon in New York City, which was the leading textured hair care salon and spa in New York City during the 1990s. Diane is currently the owner and creative director of SimpleeBEAUTIFUL, a luxury beauty hairstyling and accessory boutique in Westchester, New York.

Diane is also the founder and principal executive of Beautiful Fund, LLC. Beautiful Fund, LLC, is a creative consulting and marketing firm that provides expert beauty and conceptual development, publicity and promotional branding, guest appearances, inspirational speaking, and educational development. She held the position of Creative Consultant, Multi-Textured Expert & Educator at MIZANI, whose parent company is L'Oreal. Diane was instrumental in developing the universal MIZANI Natural Curl Key, MIZANI True Textures for natural curls, and *MIZANI True Textures Professional Technical Guide for MIZANI Stylists.* Diane also exclusively designed the MIZANI true textures Styling Collection; a how-to, step-by-step guide for consumers and stylists. Diane's industry influence has led her to serve as a brand ambassador for top beauty brands including Aveda, McBride Industries (Design Essentials), Phyto, PhytoSpecific Hair Care, and Queen Helene's Royal Curl brand. Most recently, Diane

was named brand stylist for Carol's Daughter and was part of the expert panel behind the Carol's Daughter Transition Me Beautiful Contest. In this new role, Diane develops content for the Carol's Daughter Transitioning Movement Website, devoted to supporting the transitioning lifestyle.

"In my career I've been fortunate enough to see the growth and evolution of the curly textured hair industry. Consumers are eager for information about their hair, and beauty professionals are challenged now more than ever to have a thorough understanding of their client's individual needs. Education, skillful training and product knowledge will continue to be the critical elements to sustaining the natural hair care industry."
—Diane Da Costa

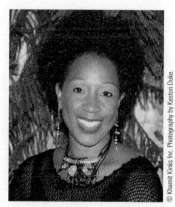
© Khamit Kinks Inc. Photography by Keston Duke.

Anu Prestonia

Anu began working in the natural hair care industry before it became a recognized industry. As a student she attended Howard University in Washington, D.C. To supplement her income, Anu began braiding hair during the summer school break. In the beginning she practiced a technique that originated in the Los Angeles area. This braiding style was that of micro braids adorned with micro beads. Because of her natural talent, Anu was immediately hired to braid hair and work in a popular salon in the Washington, D.C. area.

In 1989, after working in the Washington, D.C. area after college, Anu decided to open her own salon, Khamit Kinks, in Brooklyn, New York. In the early 1990s Anu participated in full stage and platform presentations at the Bronner Brothers Hair Shows. Always at the cutting edge of the industry, Anu's salon, Khamit Kinks, was one of the first to have a Web presence in the mid-1990s. The much lauded and easy-to-navigate Website khamitkinks.com is still in use today. In the past two decades, Khamit Kinks has introduced several styles into the natural hair care community. These styles include Casamas braids,

Senegalese twists, goddess braids, and other now well-known styles.

Over the years, Anu and her salon have attracted many celebrity clients. These clients include Oprah Winfrey, Stevie Wonder, Iman, Terry McMillan, Angela Bassett, Queen Latifa, Lenny Kraviz, Q-Tip, Solange Knowles, and Chrisette Michelle, to name a few. One of Anu's recent accomplishments is the launching of her extended line of natural and organically formulated products called Anu Essentials. This line includes natural products for hair care, skin care, and personal grooming.

Today, with the help of her longtime manager, Anu's job entails running the business through team management, training, and marketing by maintaining a presence across a number of social media platforms.

Acknowledgements

My sincere appreciation and thanks to my supportive and endearing style squad, my "dream team"—Susan Dutan, Alisha Richards, Carla Pinto, Nana Osei, and Robert Eastmond. You all are such a wonderful and cohesive unit and an extension of me. Also, to my former staff from Tendrils Hair Spa—Anita Brown, Wadiyah "Dee Dee" Musah—thank you for your support and the day-to-day teamwork exhibited by all of you. Many thanks to Debra Hare-Bey and Ida Harris for styling the models for the text. Your creative touch was truly appreciated.

To my family: with much love and gratitude to Soneni Smith, who helped me to refine my voice; to my sister, Susan Peterkin Bishop, who helps me to understand my voice; and to Kai Jackman, my daughter, who has my voice.

I am deeply grateful to my natural hair sisters and natural hair pioneers in the industry, Diane Da Costa, Tulani Kinard, and Anu Prestonia. I am honored to have your assistance in the revision of the book. Your brilliant talents have enriched this industry and left a legacy for future artists to hone their skills and to beautify the world of naturals.

A special thanks to Dr. Fran Bolton Cook: You are an excellent dermatologist, and your interview gave me so much insight on the complexities of the body and how it relates to skin and hair.

To my content developer Maria and my product manager, Martine: Thank you for your support in helping me through the hard times.

Finally, this acknowledgment would be incomplete without a thank-you to all my Tendrils clients, who have supported my vision for the natural hair industry; my journey continues.

Milady recognizes with gratitude and respects the professionals who have offered their time to contribute to this edition of *Milady Standard Natural Hair Care and Braiding* and extends an enormous thank-you to the following people:

Reviewers of *Milady Standard Natural Hair Care and Braiding*

David Jones, Lecturer at University at Albany-SUNY—New York

Jerry Tyler, Carlton Hair—California

Alicia George, Boys and Girls Club—New Jersey

Jeunesse D. Hall, Natural Roots by Jey—North Carolina

Candace J. Campbell, Glovers Beauty and Barber Shop—Georgia

Ida Harris, hotpeeznbutta.com—Georgia

Kenyada Jones, All Tressed Up—Virginia

Yolanda Matthews, The Cosmetology Connection & Consulting Services—Texas

A Special Thanks to Our Milady Team Support

Sarah Prediletto, Milady product assistant—Sarah has been with Milady since 2011. She has played an integral role in the development of the core book from the start. Without her diligence, hard work, and insight, we would be at a loss.

Alyssa Hardy, Milady content and development team intern (University at Albany; BA, English)—Alyssa has been with Milady since 2011. She has assisted in all aspects of the content development of *Milady Standard Natural Hair Care and Braiding*. She has worked tirelessly to ensure that the importance of this text is recognized and succeeds.

Photo Shoot Product Suppliers

Ouidad

McBride Research Laboratory (Design Essentials)

Karen's Body Beautiful

Burmax

Photography
Daesha Harris and Tom Dragonette of Visual Recollections

Photo Shoot Location
Milady offers special thanks to the Hair Design Institute of Brooklyn, and its schools in New York City, New York; West Palm Beach; and Orlando, Florida. Along with the school owner, directors, instructors, and students, the Hair Design Institute welcomed the Milady team to its schools in order to conduct this edition's photo shoot and were wholeheartedly kind, accommodating, and hospitable to all of our crew!

Technicians
Susan Dutan

Nana Osei

Carl Pinto

Robert Eastmond

Debra Hare-Bey

Ida Harris

Alisha Richards

Models
Frederique Monterio

Kisa Willis

Priscilla Dwomoh

Tighisti Amahazion

Barbara Lolo

Benita Ndiaye

Jessica Sills

Hephziba Jamie

Rachael Bolden-Kramer

Hope Blackstock

Raheemat Tikare

Veronika Payne

Irvana Moody

Kim V. Harris

Colin Moye

Teneil Nicole

Makeup
Timothy Johnson

History and Career Opportunities

Chapter Outline

- **Why Study Natural Hair Care and Braiding History and Career Opportunities?**

- **Brief History of Natural Hair Care and Braiding**

- **Career Paths for Natural Hair Stylists**

Learning Objectives

After completing this chapter, you should be able to:

☑ **LO1** Explain the origins of natural hair care and braiding.

☑ **LO2** Name the advancements made in black culture throughout the centuries.

☑ **LO3** List the career paths for natural hair stylists.

Key Terms

Page number indicates where in the chapter the term is used.

braid designer
p. 18

braid stylist
p. 18

braid technician
p. 18

cosmetology
p. 3

cultural aesthetic
p. 20

holistic approach
p. 19

master braider
p. 18

natural hair care
p. 3

**natural hair care
license**
p. 19

natural hairstyles
p. 12

natural hair stylist
p. 3

natural hair textures
p. 17

tignon
p. 6

transitioning
p. 16

Cosmetology is the art and science of beautifying and improving the skin, nails, and hair and includes the study of cosmetics and their applications. **Natural hair care** is under the umbrella of cosmetology. Natural hair care is the study and practice of chemically free hair styling that includes working with textured hair—braiding, extensions, twists, locks, and weaves. Its artistic goal is to create endless possibilities for those clients who desire to embrace, manage, and cultivate their natural textured hair. The natural hair care specialist, or **natural hair stylist**, is considered the trusted professional individual whom clients rely on to provide knowledgeable repeat services. Clients can now look and feel good without compromising the integrity of their hair with the use of heat or chemicals. As a professional natural hair stylist, you will be an authority in hair loss, scalp disorders, health/cleaning, decontamination, and proper hair tension. Professional natural hair stylists are generally proficient in aromatherapy, knowledgeable with botanicals, and understand the wellness approach to hair care.

Structurally and biochemically, all hair types are similar. The industry divides hair types into three ethnic groupings: European, Asian, and African. Biochemically, hair is the same for all racial groups. Structurally, they also are similar. All hair, regardless of texture, has the same basic parts: a *root*, a bulb, a follicle, a hair shaft, a cuticle, and a cortex, among other structural components. In textured hair, however, these basic components take on a different formation, and therefore it differs in its physical appearance and requires a special type of maintenance (refer to Chapter 5, "Hair Types, Structure, and Textural Differences"). The degree of texture is directly related to the development and shape of the follicle.

Many natural hairstyles worn today by women and men of color find their roots in ancient African culture. These are exciting times for a natural hair stylist, and many variations of natural hairstyles with an African cultural aesthetic are firmly grounded in the popular culture of the United States as well as the world. This chapter covers the historical origins that have shaped the trends, social standing, political awareness, and self-image of people of African descent throughout the world.

cosmetology the art and science of beautifying and improving the skin, nails, and hair; includes the study of cosmetics and their application.

natural hair care is under the umbrella of cosmetology. Natural hair care is the study and practice of chemically free hair styling that includes working with textured hair—braiding, extensions, twists, locks, and weaves.

natural hair stylist a person who advocates for the proper care of natural hair.

Why Study Natural Hair Care and Braiding History and Career Opportunities?

Natural hair stylists should study and have a thorough understanding of the history of natural hair care and braiding and the career opportunities available for these reasons:

- Many very old methods have evolved into techniques still used today. Studying the origin of these techniques can be useful in fully understanding how to use them today.

- Knowing the history of your profession can help you predict and understand upcoming trends.

- By learning about many possible career paths, you'll see the wide range of opportunities open to natural hair stylists.

Brief History of Natural Hair Care and Braiding

Africa (2630 BC)

North Africa and the Egyptians

The ancient Egyptians were among the first peoples to incorporate beauty methods into the culture. Their drawings were also among the earliest recorded imagery of natural hair care. In Saqqara, on the tip of the Nile Delta near Memphis, the capital of the Third Dynasty founded by Pharaoh Djoser, is the tomb of Akhethotep. An engraved image of a government official wearing braids, holding his staff and scepter of power, dated to the Third Dynasty (2630–2540 BC), was found in the tomb.[1] These pieces of the tomb, as well as many other engraved images that depict braided and locked hairstyles, are located in the Brooklyn Museum and the Metropolitan Museum of Art in New York **(Figure 1–1)**.

History, art, and culture tell us that throughout the continent of Africa, the adornment of the head commonly preceded major life transitions. Braided styles were used to symbolize a person's stature in the social hierarchy of the village, township, or region. Braided hair designs were a nonverbal traditional form of communication. Single women wore very different styles than married women and adolescent girls. Even pregnant women were afforded their own unique designs to usher in precious life. In Ancient Egypt, pregnant women knotted "their hair behind the head in a large bun or in numerous plaits, which would then hang down at either side of the head."[2] The most intricate designs were worn by the wives of rulers, married women, and head priests of spiritual cults. Married women have traditionally worn the most elaborately designed hair sculptures to mark the life-changing transition from their parent's home to that of their husband.

Central and West Africa

An exhibit at the New York Metropolitan Museum of Art entitled "Heroic Africans: Legendary Leaders, Iconic Sculptures" included many busts and full-sized sculptures of royalty and priests **(Figure 1–2)**. Their hairstyles told the story of their status in their respective communities from Kuba of the Democratic Republic of the Congo, the Chokwe of Angola and Zambia, and the Bangwa and Kom chiefdoms of the Cameroon grassfields. Sculptors from each of these regions used materials ranging from earth,

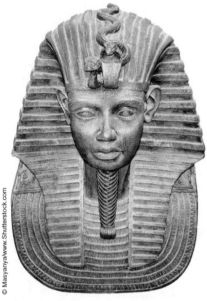

▲ Figure 1–1
The first recordings of natural hairstyles come from the ancient Egyptians.

clay, metal alloys, and wood to precious ivory. They used the materials to create captivating, energized, evocative, idealized, and enduring likenesses of their ancestors that otherwise would have been recorded only in the oral traditions. Especially notable are the sixteenth-century bronze busts of the royalty of Benin and their attendants with their hair braided in intricate multi-tiered sculptures.

Other nations represented in the exhibition were the ancient Yoruba of Ile-Ife and the Kingdom of Benin of Nigeria, the Akan of Ghana, the Luluwa, and the Hemba. These hair sculptures are the genesis of modern-day hair design of braids, Bantu knots, locks, coils, and lock extensions.

Southwest Africa

It is also important to note that in many African societies, teenage girls and boys underwent initiation rites as part of the journey to adulthood. The young Mbalantu women of Namibia have some of the most intricate hair designs that identified their pre- and post-induction status to the rest of the community.

It has always been clear from the earliest images of African people that their hair was a preeminent reflection of the state of their well-being and existence in the world. Adorning the head with elaborate hairstyles was and still is considered a sacred place in the African aesthetic. Many traditional African hairstyles photographed by anthropologist and art scholars from the 1930s and '40s depict life in rural areas, where hairstyles were created with natural fibers, clay, shells, and beads. These traditional African styles inspired the popular beaded braid styles of the 1960s, '70s and '80s in the United States. ☑ **LO1**

The New World (1600–1870): Era of American Slavery

The experiences of enslaved Africans in the New World were deeply degrading, a painful contrast to the beauty and spirituality that marked communal life on the mother continent. Women and men were made to feel subhuman in many ways. The description of their hair as "wool" served as validation to their enslavers that they were "animalistic," deserving the inhumane treatment that was inflicted on them daily. The hairstyles of enslaved Africans provided one marker of the process of cultural loss and adaptation: By the 1700s, many enslaved Africans fashioned their hairstyles after the popular European powdered wigs worn by white men and women of means and stature in the New World colonies.

Some enslaved Africans sought to emulate the look of the slave owner, and others took the style of the wigs and fashioned their own to create a new style with the texture and length of their own hair. These innovative

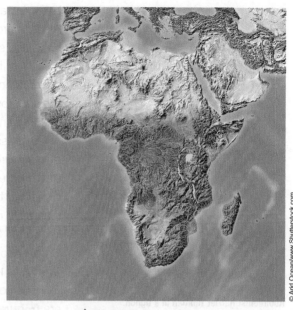
© Arid Ocean/www.Shutterstock.com

▲ Figure 1–2
Many of the natural hairstyles that are popular today have their roots in the continent of Africa.

Did you know?

Many women still choose to wear beaded hairstyles to stylize their braids for different occasions.

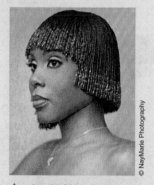
© NayMarie Photography

▲ micro braid bead adornment

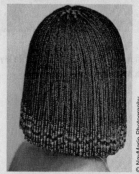
© NayMarie Photography

▲ micro braid bead adornment

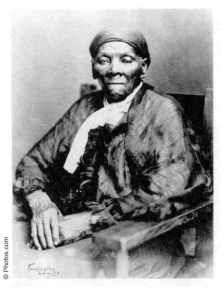

▲ Figure 1–3
Abolitionist Harriet Tubman in a tignon.

tignon a head scarf worn by Creole women.

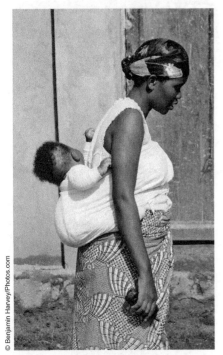

▲ Figure 1–4
Colorful tignons were a distinguishable style for American slaves.

hairstyles amazed and confused their slave owners. The styles enslaved Africans created to adorn their heads were evidence of their newfound pride and self-esteem, so much so that it became a reason for slave owners to inflict abuse and punishment. The enslaved Africans also understood that if you had any time at all to pay attention to your hair, then the slave owner would think you had too much idle time on your hands. The hair and fashion statements they wore were an important part of their self-expression and self-esteem as well as a potential threat to the slave owner. During the last years of slavery, it was not unusual for the wives of slave owners to cut off the hair of a young African girl or woman, especially if she had become the object of unwanted sexual advances from her slave master. In response to the increasing assertiveness of the slave population, in 1786 in New Orleans, the Spanish governor signed a law requiring Creole people of color and black women to wear their hair bound in a **tignon** or kerchief, as a badge of their lowly status in the colonial society.[3] Tignons could be seen on many of the American slaves into the late slave era **(Figure 1–3)**.

In the nineteenth century, partly because of their involvement in the textile industry, enslaved women were able to explore the creative possibilities of color and design for their head tie. They created an encoded cultural aesthetic of discordant color patterns and irregular patterns that differed from those of the dominant white society of that time **(Figure 1–4)**.

Reconstruction (1900–1920): Women in the Post-Slavery Era

Between the years of 1902 and 1920, three women made a permanent mark on the lives of African American women with their vision, courage, and tenacity to uplift themselves: Annie Pope Turnbo-Malone, Madam C. J. Walker, and Madame Sara Spencer Washington. During that time, nearly all Negro women were direct descendants of slaves and worked as domestic servants or in other laborious, unskilled fields. The desire to look and feel better, as well as escape degrading work, was foremost in the minds of many African American women. These inspiring women provided a way out of the crushing poverty by using the beauty culture to gain financial independence and success. With the help of these three women, this era marked the beginning of natural hair care as an American industry.

Annie Minerva Pope-Turnbo Malone

Annie Minerva Pope-Turnbo Malone was born on August 9, 1869, and is the first African American woman innovator. Pope-Turnbo Malone had a passion for styling and working with different textures of African American women's hair. Annie attended school in Illinois, where she apprenticed with her sister as a hairdresser. Annie rejected different forms of animal fat and "grease" that were used with hot rags to straighten the hair. These processes were unsuccessful and created damage and an unhealthy environment for the scalp. By 1889, Malone had developed her own scalp and hair products that she demonstrated and sold from a buggy throughout Illinois.

Pope-Turnbo Malone was a pioneering businesswoman who paved the way for many others to follow. During the early twentieth century, race improvement and positive self-image were seen as ways to increase social mobility. In 1902, Pope-Turnbo Malone named her hair care line Poro Products. By 1903, she trained women and men to sell her hair care system door to door. Pope-Turnbo Malone's Poro College and complex were located in St. Louis's upper-middle-class black neighborhood and included her business's office, manufacturing operations, and training center, as well as facilities for civic, religious, and social functions. The complex was valued at more than $1 million and included classrooms, barber shops, dining facilities, and laboratories as well as a theater, gymnasium, chapel, roof garden, and auditorium. The training center provided cosmetology and sales training for women interested in joining the Poro agent network. Instructors also taught students how to walk, talk, and behave in social situations. Many local and national organizations, including the National Negro Business League, were housed in the facility or used it for business functions.

By 1926, Pope-Turnbo Malone employed almost 200 people. She assisted with opening franchised locations in North and South America, Africa, and the Philippines, which employed a total of 75,000 women. In 1946, the facility was renamed in her honor as the Annie Malone Children and Family Center, and it still serves as a source of community support in the historic Ville neighborhood.[4]

Sarah Breedlove (Madam C. J. Walker)

In 1867, Sarah Breedlove was born in Delta, Louisiana. Her parents and elder siblings were slaves on a cotton plantation. She was one of six children and the first child born into freedom after the Civil War came to an end. Sarah (also known as Madam C. J. Walker) was hired by Pope-Turnbo Malone, and she became one of Annie's first sales agents—a position that likely gave her access to Pope-Turnbo Malone's formula. In 1905, she moved to Denver to sell Pope-Turnbo Malone's Wonderful Hair Grower.

In 1906, after marrying newspaper advertising salesman Charles Joseph Walker, Breedlove changed her name to Madam C. J. Walker. She followed the model of her former employer, Pope-Turnbo Malone, by creating a hair preparation cream, tonics to prevent hair loss, and tools

Did you know?

Annie Pope-Turnbo Malone created a line of hair care "treatments." In 1900, she patented the "hot comb" in the United States to straighten the hair texture and curl pattern of African Americans.

Did you know?

In 1845, Marcel Grateau, a Parisian hairdresser, invented the pressing comb and the curling iron to create curls and waves. "The Marcel iron" was named after Grateau. Today, people still widely use his technique and the Marcel irons.

WEB RESOURCES

Find out more about Annie Pope-Turnbo Malone at www.anniemalone.com

FYI

Annie Pope-Turnbo Malone was one of the first African American multimillionaires. By the late 1920s, her net worth was estimated at $14 million. She also donated money to charities and black colleges, such as Howard University and Tuskegee Institute, while serving as president of the St. Louis Colored Orphans Home.

to manage the hair. She also trained and employed thousands of African Americans in her door-to-door sales business. Madam Walker's strategic plan was to create awareness of self-empowerment among African Americans in order to facilitate their having their own businesses and to improve their economic standing. In countless speeches, she extolled the benefits of economic freedom for women who had long been financially dependent on men.

Madam Walker's genius was evident not only in her business model but also in the way she used slide shows, newspaper articles, speeches, and a magazine entitled *Woman's Voice* to market her beliefs, biographical background, and lifestyle. The magazine, funded by the Walker Company, was one of the few publications at the time that was controlled and edited by African American women. The magazine became an important media arm to aid Madam Walker's efforts to organize women's political groups with the ultimate aim of empowering African American women **(Figure 1–5)**.

The greater impact of Walker's legacy continues to be revealed as her business model inspires each generation of African American entrepreneurs in the now multibillion-dollar black hair care industry to create their own economic wealth and freedom. Her strategy provided an initial blueprint to develop and manufacture hair care products as well as educate and train employees.

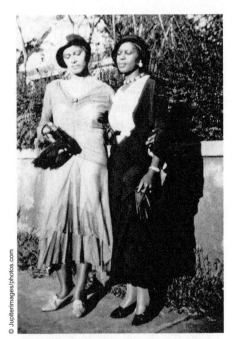

▲ Figure 1–5
By the 1920s, African American women gained confidence to style themselves in the latest fashion trends.

WEB RESOURCES

Visit Madam C. J. Walker's Website at www.madamcjwalker.com

Sarah Spencer

Sarah Spencer was born in 1889 in Beckley, Virginia. She graduated from Norfolk Mission College, and in 1913 she decided to enter the beauty profession despite her family's objections. She was inspired by the successes of Madam C. J. Walker and Annie Pope-Turnbo Malone's in the manufacturing and door-to-door sales of their products. To prepare for her new business venture, Sarah studied cosmetology in Philadelphia. Her strong interest in chemistry product development led her to take additional courses in chemistry at Columbia University in New York. In 1916 Sarah moved to Atlantic City, New Jersey, where she began to experiment with ingredients. She later was granted a patent for and developed the Apex system, a new system of straightening the hair of black women. Sarah opened a small beauty parlor using the name Madame Sarah Spencer

FYI

Madam Walker has been listed in past editions of the *Guinness Book of World Records* as the first self-made American woman millionaire who neither inherited nor married into her money. Although it is impossible to document the exact figures of Walker's net worth, at the time of her death her estate had an estimated value of $600,000 to $700,000 (equivalent to approximately $6 million to $7 million in today's dollars). During the final year of her life, her company—the Madam C. J. Walker Manufacturing Company—reported total sales of more than $500,000, making the value of her company several times that amount. The combined value of her business and personal assets (real estate, furnishings, jewelry, etc.) was well over $1,000,000.

You can read more about Madam C. J. Walker in the book entitled, *On Her Own Ground: The Life and Times of Madam C. J. Walker*, by A'Lelia Bundles.[5]

Washington. During the day, she worked in the salon and taught students the trade. In the evenings, she sold her products door to door throughout the city.

In 1919, Spencer founded Apex News and Hair Company, the largest New Jersey black-owned business and one of the nation's leading black manufacturing companies. Apex maintained a lab and school in Atlantic City as well as an office in New York City. Eventually, her beauty colleges were located in 12 states and had 35,000 agents all over the world. In 1946, she had 200 employees and the company was worth $500,000. Sarah Spencer was one of the first African American millionaires. She was awarded a medallion at the 1939 World's Fair as one of the "Most Distinguished Businesswomen" in the country and one of ten top businesswomen in the world. She loved her community and was a great philanthropist.[6]

The Jim Crow Era (1930s–1960s)

As the African American beauty industry grew, so too did the white beauty industry in America, which was threatening to the less affluent African American beauty business. For this reason, before the 1940s integration was not a desired social change among African American beauticians and product manufacturers. From their perspective, integration served to keep economic stability within their communities.

Straightening Out

Although African Americans had made great entrepreneurial strides in the beauty industry, they still struggled with the deeply imbedded belief that their hair was not "good hair" and needed to be fixed. As far back as 1856, *Urban Legend* has an article stating that in New York, a free black man named Hodges attempted to straighten another black man's hair in a public demonstration. Unfortunately, the demonstration went awry and caused the man's hair to come out immediately after the application.[7]

In the 1880s, the hot comb was in full circulation and was manufactured for white women in Sears and Bloomingdales catalogs. In 1900, Annie Pope-Turnbo Malone patented modifications to the hot comb for tightly coiled hair, and Madam C. J. Walker further improved the device and made it popular. Contrary to popular belief, Madam Walker did not invent perms and did not use the words *hair straightener* in her advertisements.[8] Until 1930, most of hair-straightening techniques were performed with thermal heat and used the hot combs or hot rods developed by Marjorie Joyner of the Walker Company (patented in 1928).

The first relatively safe lye hair straightener was developed in 1909 by Garrett Augustus Morgan Sr. He had a tailor shop in Cleveland and discovered that the liquid he used to prevent the needles from scorching the fabric as it was sewed in the machine could also straighten the woolly fiber of fabric. He further tested it successfully on a neighbor's Airedale dog[9] and on his own hair. When he was satisfied with the results, he created a cream that straightened tightly coiled hair. As a result,

Did you know?

Sara Spencer owned Apex Publishing Company, which published *Apex News* for beauticians and sales agents, as well as Apex Laboratories, Apex Drug Company, and Apex Beauty College. Spencer also owned 12 beauty schools in the United States and franchised schools overseas in the Caribbean and South Africa. Three thousand students graduated from her schools every year and went on to become licensed beauticians.

Did you know?

THE JIM CROW ERA
As the African American beauty industry grew, so too did the white beauty industry in America. The sale of hair products flourished and became extremely lucrative for both the white and African American product manufacturers. Due to segregation, white manufacturers were unaware of the millions of dollars that were being generated by the seemingly less affluent African American beauty product manufacturers. For this reason, before the 1940s integration was not a desired social change among African American product manufacturers. From their perspective, segregation served to keep economic stability within their communities.

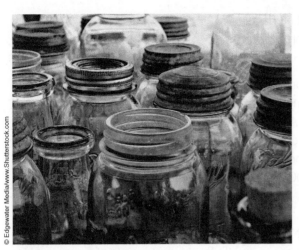

▲ Figure 1–6
Those who couldn't afford professional straightening often created their own dangerous relaxers in mason jars.

G. A. Morgan Hair Refining Company began operations in 1910. From this preparation, Morgan created a long line of hair products, such that a few years later, he claimed to offer "the only complete line of hair preparations in the world." The natural texture, the wave, the curl, and the coil were the main impetus for African Americans to achieve straightened hair at almost any cost.

In the 1930s, the conk lye-based relaxer was popular. Perhaps the most famous experience was chronicled by Malcolm X in his autobiography. He described the recipe for his first "conk" as follows: Combine Red Devil lye, two eggs, and two mashed white potatoes in a mason jar. Vaseline was applied to protect the scalp, and at the end of treatment, the mixture was rinsed off with soap and water **(Figure 1–6)**.[10] By 1940, this crude and dangerous mixture had been improved with chemical-based hair straighteners, better known as relaxers and commonly referred to as perms. Hair straighteners were applied in salons for those who could afford them.

By the late 1940s and into the 1950s, home kits were invented. They became very popular for African American women. Yet, the potential for hair damage was underscored even in advertisements for the products. Lustersilk, one of the most popular brands of that era, stated in a print ad, "Product is covered by Products Liability Insurance."[11]

In 1954, George E. Johnson founded Johnson Products and developed Ultra Wave, a permanent relaxer for men. Several years later, he developed Ultra Sheen, a relaxer for women. In 1971, Johnson Products became the first African American–owned company to be listed on the American Stock Exchange. Over the years many more relaxers were created, culminating in the 1970s and 1980s with the Jheri Curl, texturizers marketed mainly to men, and new and improved no-lye relaxers.

Activism vs. Segregation

By the late 1940s two salons, one in Washington, D.C. and the other in Harlem, New York, were known epicenters of the beauty culture business. Both owners were outspoken in their views about the racial divide and servicing clientele that were multiracial. In 1946, *Ebony* magazine observed that Rose Morgan, a popular successful Harlem beautician, "has been conducting a one-woman campaign against the notion widely held among Negros that negroid hair is inferior." In 1946, a similar statement was made by the sister of a Washington D.C. stylist, to a reporter for the *Baltimore Afro-American:* "The secret of (The Cardozo Salon) success is that (the sisters) realize colored people have far better hair than they ever thought they had."[12]

African American beauticians of this era were politically astute and an active voice for equality within their industry. They organized and became a powerful voice in the process of determining labor and education standards for beauticians and the regulation of state cosmetology boards across the country. Rose Morgan was appointed to the New York board in 1947, and Elizabeth Cardozo Barker was appointed to the District of Columbia's board of cosmetology. They were instrumental in raising beauty school standards, promoting better wages and working conditions for beauticians, and rooting out segregation.[13]

The Civil Rights and Black Power Movements (1960s–1980s)

The Afro

Recognition of African Americans' natural beauty was slow in coming. Those who dared to wear their hair naturally were often met with harsh criticism and backlash from community leaders and family members. An established standard of beauty with very specific parameters of skin tone, facial features, and hair textures had been carefully crafted and successfully promoted since the beginning of the twentieth century. At this time, advertisements promoted beauty products or hair grooming of African Americans wearing their hair only in straight, permanently relaxed, and thermally pressed styles. Those women who attempted to wear their hair naturally were often artists who had no reason other than their own personal convictions to do so. Most artists were not politically motivated by racial pride. For the younger generation, however, their hairstyles became the ultimate political statement.

In 1943, Annabelle Baker, a Hampton Institute art student, became one of the brave few who decided to wear her hair naturally. Appreciating the beauty of her natural hair, Baker confessed to a growing "regard for bone structure, skin tone and texture." The reaction of Hampton's Dean of Women, Flemmie Kittrell, was insensitive and immediate. Baker had been invited to a conference at Wellesley College in Massachusetts. She was initially told that her hair made her "unacceptable" to represent Hampton at the conference. After considerable debate, she was allowed to attend the conference. At Wellesley, Baker encountered criticism in her dorm room from "two strikingly beautiful Negro co-eds with hair that flowed into long page boys." "They told me that I should be ashamed to be seen with my hair in its natural state." Upon returning home to Hampton, Baker became the subject of repeated disciplinary actions. Life became difficult for her, and Baker contended that her hair caused her to be targeted.

As the civil rights movement grew in the early 1960s, college students all across the country began wearing their hair in Afros **(Figure 1–7)**. Many women on campuses faced the same disapproval that Baker received 20 years earlier, especially on conservative black college campuses in the South. African Americans who decided to wear their hair naturally were met with "have you gone crazy?" comments from their peers; to "disapproving stares" at school, in the workplace, and at houses of worship and family gatherings. Many, emboldened by a sense of pride, chose to ignore the looks and comments and brave the disapproval. They now experienced

In the early 1950s, the great African American dancer Ruth Beckford wore an Afro. Later in the decade, prominent singers such as Miriam Makeba, Odetta, and Nina Simone, as well as dancers Katherine Dunham and Pearl Primus, all wore Afros.

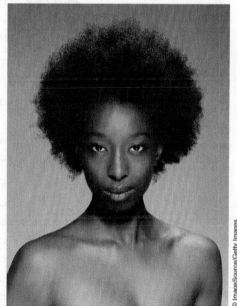

© ImageSource/Getty Images

▲ Figure 1–7
Many African Americans began to embrace their natural hair, which gave rise to the Afro.

relief from chemicals on the hair and scalp and extreme heat from thermal straightening processes, the economic stress of the professional services, and the all-day trips to the beauty salon. For some, it was as simple as embracing black consciousness and confronting the socio-political reality of the times.

By the early 1970s, African American salons could no longer resist the trend and began creating markets to service the Afro-style client. According to Rose Morgan, the sale of Afro wigs helped to revitalize waning businesses. A newfound "black is beautiful" consciousness took hold in the African American community, sparking a global fashion revolution that was in sync with an era marked not only by the civil rights movement in the United States. Women who wore Afros quickly encouraged each other and family members to follow suit in the name of racial pride and black unity. In the 10-year period from 1965 to 1975, black people around the globe embraced a new aesthetic inspired by African Americans and the black power movement.

What was once categorized as a fad by those unwilling to acknowledge the beginnings of a huge shift in salon services was now a viable new way of life for many African Americans. This was an exciting and creative landscape. A new era of discovery was emerging, similar to the creative energy of the revolution in African American hairstyles that was launched nearly a century before by such visionaries as Annie Pope-Turnbo Malone and Madam C. J. Walker. New techniques were created by amateurs and professional stylists alike to accommodate the newly rediscovered hair textures. Tightly coiled hair needed to be braided before going to bed: loosely coiled hair needed to be twisted, and curly/coiled hair needed to be braided and then twisted. The combinations were endless. Experimentation determined the end result and the person's final preference. Afros were usually braided into cornrows or sectioned into individual small plaits or twisted and then taken out in the morning. Then, they were combed out with a new device called the pick.

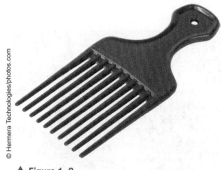

▲ Figure 1–8
The pick created an extreme look in the Afro.

The original pick was a 5-inch (12.5 cm) comb base with ten 5- to 6-inch (15-cm) steel wires protruding from its base. The pick was used to comb out the hair by lifting the hair from the scalp and pulling the hair up. When used with the Afro pick, this technique helped to make the hair stand up all over the head. Over time, many different types of picks were created for daily and decorative use **(Figure 1–8)**.

For the first time in history, all natural hair types and lengths were celebrated. Never before had men, women, and children adopted the same hairstyle simultaneously. Photos featuring multiple generations of family members, all wearing the same **natural hairstyles**, became common. Older women and men were sporting silver Afros, both short and long. Long hair no longer hung down; it now stood up and out. As more women embraced the look, the opposition grew, especially among white Americans who exerted authoritative power in the workplace by enforcing dress codes that had not existed before the Afro.

natural hairstyles chemically free hairstyles that include naturally curly hair and textured styles, like braids, extensions, twists, locks, coils, and weaves.

African American Hair Companies

African American beauty product companies worked feverishly to keep up with the demand for the new products that were being developed to aid in the styling of the Afro. Johnson Products, Soft Sheen, and Pro Line developed products for Afro grooming. For the first time in the history of advertising, images of African Americans wearing their natural hair were commonly seen in print media and television. Johnson Products exclusively sponsored *Soul Train*, a popular dance program featuring top African American music recording artists. All the *Soul Train* dancers featured on the show had some type of natural style, which helped to sell the advertised products. You might think that Johnson Products and other black-owned product companies were enjoying a financial boom with these new products that serviced a global market for natural styles. However, this was not the case.

Since the 1950s, African American beauty products companies began to feel the financial effects of white-owned companies cutting into their market share. By the mid-1980s, large companies such as Albert Culver and Revlon were actively challenging the smaller black-owned firms in an all-out war for their market share. In 1986, according to *Newsweek* magazine, white-owned companies were muscling minority firms out of the black hair care industry's $1 billion market. Irving Bottner, president of Revlon's professional products division, said, "In the next couple of years, black-owned businesses will disappear. They'll all be sold to the white companies." Bottner also implied that his firm could make better products for black people than some black-owned companies. "We are accused of taking business away from the black companies, but black consumers buy quality products. Too often, their black brothers didn't do them any good." Revlon later apologized for Bottner's controversial remarks,[14] but the damage had already been done. Bottner's remarks sparked outrage throughout the African American community. The community proceeded to organize a boycott against Revlon and every white-owned cosmetic company. African Americans were further outraged when they discovered that black product companies were, in fact, owned by white-owned companies that understood how to appeal to their racial pride. These companies were catering to African Americans with products for their Afros by using the word *African*, or the red, black, and green colors of the African nationalist flag. These companies established brand names, such as "African Pride," "Dark and Lovely" and "Right On." African American consumers were dismayed

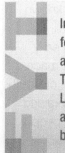

In 1981, eleven companies owned by African Americans founded the American Health and Beauty Aids Institute (AHBAI), a trade organization to ensure the survival of their businesses. The association also developed a brand symbol, the "Proud Lady," that could be placed on products and member's product advertisements to indicate that products were manufactured by black-owned companies.

Did you know?

In 1971, African American television news reporter Melba Tolliver was assigned to cover the wedding of President Nixon's daughter, Patricia, at the White House. Before Tolliver went to Washington, she decided to "go natural" and wear her hair in an Afro. Upon her return, the WABC news director in New York told her, "I hate your hair; you've got to change it. And you know what, you no longer look feminine." Management threatened to keep her off the air if she didn't change her hair back to a straight style or wear a hat or scarf. Newspapers publicized the controversy and began calling the station, including the news director. Many viewers wrote letters in support of Tolliver's right to wear her hair as she pleased, even if no one liked it. The incident proved to be bad publicity for the station, which had to back down and put Tolliver back on the air. It was a defining moment in television history as African Americans grappled with defining themselves.

when informed in a 1993 brand awareness study that brands like African Pride, Dark and Lovely, Let's Jam, and TCB were made by white-owned companies; further, 79 percent said it was important to purchase products made by black-owned companies in the future.[15]

The New Cultural Aesthetic (1980s)

As the popularity of the Afro began declining in the 1980s, three styles became the natural choice for African American men and women. The Afro transitioned to a much shorter cut and became an acceptable conservative style for women and a look most men embraced **(Figure 1–9)**. At the same time, braided hairstyles became a styling option, much more than just a look worn for a cultural occasion. The growing popularity of braiding came at a good time. As black women more commonly styled their hair at home, many began to see more chemical damage to their hair after using home kits. A solution needed to be found.

The art of braiding can be traced back centuries to its roots in Africa. Historically, every country in Africa has a form of braiding incorporated into its standard of beauty for men and women. Throughout the African American hair experience, braiding has been used as a restorative technique for the health and well-being of the hair. Until the 1960s, braiding was performed in the privacy of the home and not worn as an adult style. In the twentieth century in the United States, young girls always had their hair braided until a "coming of age" ushering in the straightening comb or a permanent relaxer for the accepted standard of beauty for African American women. Yet, mainstream acceptance of braided hairstyles was in many respects a natural outgrowth of the Afro during the 1960s, along with the celebration of cultural authenticity. Grounded in this newfound cultural awareness and the predominant natural beauty aesthetic, braided hairstyles became an option for African American women of college age as well as those younger than 35 years of age **(Figure 1–10)**.

For those who wanted an alternative to the Afro and hair straightening, braids became the perfect option. Braids served as a protective hairstyle that could be worn to work and maintained for weeks when done professionally. Most styles during the early 1970s incorporated synthetic and human hair fibers used as protective additions to increase styling options and the longevity of the style. These hair fibers gave support to cornrows—braids that lie close to the scalp—while other braids, known as single, individual, or box braids, hung from the scalp from small, symmetrically parted sections. Simple styles prevalent during the early 1960s gradually gave way to intricate, sophisticated designs that made room for a new standard of beauty. Longevity and the restoration of health to the hair shaft became one of the primary selling points of the braided styles. With a creative fire that seemed ancestrally infused, black people adorned their natural braided styles (without synthetic fiber extensions) with beads, thread-wrapping, and double-strand twisted hair with and without synthetic extensions. Braids were styled into French rolls and

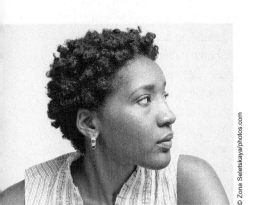

▲ **Figure 1–9**
The shorter, conservative Afro became popular in the 1980s, giving women the opportunity to experiment with different styles like the Knot Out.

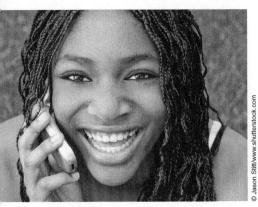

▲ **Figure 1–10**
For a time, braids were appropriate only for women and girls under 35.

other geometric designs simulating crowns. The longevity of the styles increased as well, ranging from days to weeks to months with a cleansing regimen to care for the scalp until the style was removed. Braiders all over the country set up a cottage industry to service children, women, and young men. Many stylists attained financial independence within this entrepreneurial climate.

As the demand for braiding grew, braiders all over the country made the transition from a home-based business to a professional salon setting. Some acquired a chair in a full-service salon, others worked in barbershops, and many obtained the appropriate licensure to open their own braiding salons. To open their businesses without scrutiny from their respective state licensing and cosmetology boards, braiders made many sacrifices so they could attend cosmetology schools and obtain their cosmetology license.

In New York, Tulani's Regal Movement and Tendrils Salon were the first professional full-service comprehensive natural hair care salons to open in Brooklyn. Other trendy salons, like KINNAPS (Brooklyn), Khamit Kinks (Tribeca, NYC), and Turning Heads (Harlem, NYC), soon followed suit in the mid to late 1980s. Unlike braiding salons that opened before or after them, these early salons offered barbering services and the grooming of locs, along with restorative hair treatments for chemically damaged hair.

Braid practitioners who attended cosmetology schools were keenly aware that the beauty school curriculum taught nothing about the grooming and styling of African American natural hair braiding and hair locking. Furthermore, in other states braiders opened their salons with a business license, knowing that none of the beauty enhancement licensing laws addressed the service of braiding. They soon found out that it did not matter if they paid their taxes. The fact that the braiding salons were unregulated threatened established beauty salon owners. A vast underground network of braiders emerged across the country through word of mouth and seriously challenged the authority of established salons. By the early 1980s, network gatherings were being held in cities like Washington, D.C., where Tulani Kinard, a New York–based braider, consulted Dr. Bernice Johnson Reagon, who was the

WEB RESOURCES

Read more about Pamela Ferrell and Talib Din Uqdah at www.ij .org/legal-barriers-to-african -hairbraiding-nationwide

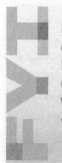

During the braiders' symposium, attendees were made aware of a long-standing struggle between local braider Pamela Ferrell and her husband, Talib Din-Uqdah, proprietors of Cornrows and Company Salon, and the cosmetology board in Washington, D.C. Years later, Cornrows and Company Salon was victorious in their struggle.

In the 1980s, there was still discrimination in the workplace. Even though braiding had become socially acceptable and far removed from the charged politics of the 1960s and early 1970s, many employers still discriminated against black employees who wore braided hairstyles. College graduates were warned against wearing braided styles when entering the corporate workforce. In 1987, Cheryl Tatum, an employee of the Hyatt Regency in Chrystal City, Virginia, faced the threat of losing her job because she wore a braided cornrow hairstyle to work. According to Tatum, her manger told her, "I can't understand why you would want to wear your hair like that anyway. What would our guests think if we allowed you to all wear your hair like that?" After refusing to take the braids out, Cheryl was forced to resign from her position. She then sought legal recourse and was victorious. In a rare defeat for employers who try to dictate their workers' appearances, the Equal Employment Opportunity Commission ruled that Hyatt hotels engaged in racial discrimination by prohibiting black women from wearing their hair in cornrows.

program director of the folk life division at the Smithsonian. The two would work together to curate a symposium for scholars and braiders. Experts attended the symposium from all over the country. Dr. Rosalind Jeffries, a noted historian in African culture, gave the keynote address.

The next braiders' network conference was organized by Hiddekel Burkes, founder of the National Braider's Guild and master braider from Chicago. The conference was held in Washington, D.C. Again, braiders traveled from all over the United States and the Caribbean to learn from the most skilled among them and to establish the best practices, techniques, and a governing structure for the guild.

Locs (1990s)

After the controversy over braiding began to die down, in the early 1990s another natural hairstyle began gaining popularity. Many men and women of African descent were wearing newly formed locs or mature locs—hair that is three to four years old, often grown down to the shoulders. This natural hairstyle is considered a long-term commitment, because many people wear their locked style for 5 to 10 years or more. Locs can be styled like braids or as natural hair in its loose state. They can be colored, bleached, or rolled on rods and rollers; they can be crimped with cornrows and flat-twist sets and wrapped with thread. In the early 1990s locs became very popular, to the point where the grooming, styling, and maintenance of locs now make up as much as 50 percent of the natural hair care salon business **(Figure 1–11)**. Mature locs cannot be combed out, but they can be picked apart with a thin implement, like a needle. Most people will opt to cut them off and start again. The average growth time for locs to reach the shoulder blade is three to four years. Those who want longer locs might grow them for a lifetime.

Transitioning (2000s–present)

By the year 2000, African American women had attained a newfound awareness of their natural beauty. **Transitioning**, the process that involves growing out the hair while going from chemically relaxed hair to natural, is a conscious approach to stop relaxing and to refrain from using harsh chemicals or extreme heat to reduce and modify the client's natural

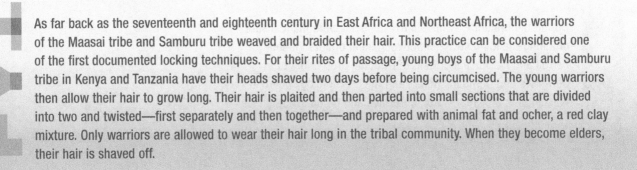

As far back as the seventeenth and eighteenth century in East Africa and Northeast Africa, the warriors of the Maasai tribe and Samburu tribe weaved and braided their hair. This practice can be considered one of the first documented locking techniques. For their rites of passage, young boys of the Maasai and Samburu tribe in Kenya and Tanzania have their heads shaved two days before being circumcised. The young warriors then allow their hair to grow long. Their hair is plaited and then parted into small sections that are divided into two and twisted—first separately and then together—and prepared with animal fat and ocher, a red clay mixture. Only warriors are allowed to wear their hair long in the tribal community. When they become elders, their hair is shaved off.

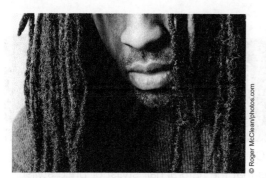

▲ Figure 1–11
Locs were a very popular hairstyle in the 1990s.

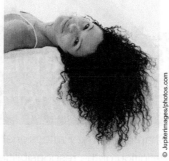

▲ Figure 1–12
Today women are embracing their natural hair like never before.

WEB RESOURCES

In the Caribbean, singer, activist, and cultural icon Bob Marley greatly popularized locs in the 1970s. You can read about his historical background and input at www.bobmarley.com.

virgin hair texture. Blogs devoted to natural hairstyles were becoming very popular. Millions of men and women with the desire to learn about their natural hair were ready to listen to a familiar voice over the Internet and build a global community of support. The hair crisis women once suffered in the privacy of their bathroom mirror was now being shared on YouTube, where members of the "transitioning" community could respond and offer advice. No one was crying out, "Too much information!" Various questions were being asked, and a group of people with similar issues were able to e-mail, blog, send instant messages, and use Facebook and MySpace together.

Some of the earliest blogs and Websites in the 2000s, which provided a virtual space for sharing, were Motown Girl, Nappturality, Natural Chica, Natural Roots Magazine, naturallycurly.com, Afrobella, and many more. As part of the global Internet revolution, these sites have become very profitable through the sale of advertisements. They also have received many awards from professional blogging organizations, become key stakeholders in online fashion trend marketing groups, and sponsored major meet-up events and conferences.

Women are now falling in love with their natural hair like never before. Their desire for more education on products, tools, hair accessories, shampoos, conditioners, hair oils, and conditioning treatments have reached unheard-of levels. Meet-ups are happening all over the world and focusing on **natural hair textures**. Time and distance are no longer obstacles. Classes are streamed over the Internet, discussion groups are teleconferenced over the phone, and smart phones record spontaneous experiences with images of natural hair **(Figure 1–12)**. ☑ **LO2**

transitioning (going natural) process that involves growing out the hair while going from chemically relaxed hair to natural. It is a conscious approach to stop relaxing or refrain from using harsh chemicals or extreme heat to reduce or modify the client's natural, virgin hair texture.

natural hair textures virgin hair that is a non-chemical curly hair pattern described as wavy, curly, coily and highly textured hair.

WEB RESOURCES

Learn more about Websites and hair care companies dedicated to natural curly hair.

www.naturallycurly.com

www.carolsdaughter.com

www.janecartersolutions.com

www.missjessies.com

www.mynuade.com

FYI

In 2010, CurlyNikki.com was sold to naturallycurly.com for an undisclosed amount and has become one of the leading blogging Websites.

From the late 1990s until today, companies like Carol's Daughter, Jane Carter Solutions, Nu Adé, and Miss Jessie's, which first developed their products in home kitchens, are now considered major manufacturers.

Career Paths for Natural Hair Stylists

Chapter 4, "The Professional Consultation" will give you a detailed definition of the responsibilities that the natural hair stylist or braid stylist has to the client. This textbook offers the following professional job descriptions, which will help define the hierarchy of training and skills within this growing industry.

braid technician an entry-level position—an assistant or apprentice in the specialty of braiding. The braid technician is in the process of acquiring technical skills and perfecting various braiding techniques.

braid stylist one who has been trained and has adequate technical skills for braiding styles. The braid stylist is knowledgeable in hair loss, scalp disorders, health/cleaning and disinfection, proper hair tension, and interpersonal skills; he or she understands the holistic relationship between the client and the stylist.

braid designer one who is proficient and highly skilled in the art form of braiding; has more than just the technical skills and can incorporate skills into advanced techniques, such as creating and developing new styles. A braid designer is well-versed in client/stylist holistic relations and interpersonal communication satisfaction.

master braider one who has a technical, artistic, historical, and intellectual knowledge of the industry of braiding and natural hair care. The master braider is proficient in creating, designing, and teaching various braid styles; can demonstrate principal skills with a minimum of 10 and up to 15 techniques; is a chief authority in hair loss, scalp disorder, health/cleaning and disinfection, proper hair tension, and client–stylist holistic relations and interpersonal communications.

- **Braid Technician.** This is an entry-level position—an assistant or apprentice in the specialty of braiding. The braid technician is in the process of acquiring technical skills and perfecting various braiding techniques.

- **Braid Stylist.** One who has been trained and has adequate technical skills for braiding styles. The braid stylist is knowledgeable in hair loss, scalp disorders, health/cleaning and disinfection, proper hair tension, and interpersonal skills, he or she understands the holistic relationship between the client and the stylist.

- **Braid Designer.** One who is proficient and highly skilled in the art form of braiding; has more than just the technical skills and can incorporate skills into advanced techniques, creating and developing new styles. A braid designer is well versed in client/stylist holistic relations and interpersonal communication satisfaction.

- **Master Braider.** One who has a technical, artistic, historical, and intellectual knowledge of the industry of braiding and natural hair care. The master braider is proficient in creating, designing, and teaching various braid styles; can demonstrate principal skills with a minimum of ten to fifteen techniques; is a chief authority in hair loss, scalp disorder, health/cleaning and disinfection, proper hair tension, and client–stylist holistic relations and interpersonal communications. Usually, the master braider has at least ten years of professional experience and several (at least two) years of teaching or training experience. ☑ **LO3**

Rules and State Regulations

Virgin hair has not been chemically altered in texture, color, or volume. Virgin hair is not straightened or altered by excessive heat, electric curling, or other thermal service. If the hair has been altered chemically, new hair can begin to grow back within one to two months. However, depending on the desired length, the hair may require six months to a year to grow into its natural state.

It is important to note that as states begin to adopt natural hair care licensing, the rules and regulations governing the license may allow services that contradict and confuse what natural hair should represent **(Figure 1–13)**. Clients will often believe that if it does not involve a chemical application, then it is a natural service. For example, the New York State **natural hair care license** allows natural hair to be thermally altered, but restricts a natural stylist from coloring natural hair. Clients in New York may not be aware that although thermal pressing is in the stylist's scope of practice, it may not align with the true definition of "natural hair care."

Many cosmetologists, natural hair care specialists, and master braiders have chosen to step outside that definition and redefine the word *beautiful* based on our cultural aesthetics. Through the practice of natural hair styling, the word *beautiful* has been redefined to include the look of true beauty—embracing different hair types, textures, lengths, shapes, and silhouettes; and caring for natural hair, whether it is wavy, curly, coily, or tightly coiled. True beauty is not forced or contrived; rather, it complements, creates balance, and leaves us with the feeling of well-being.

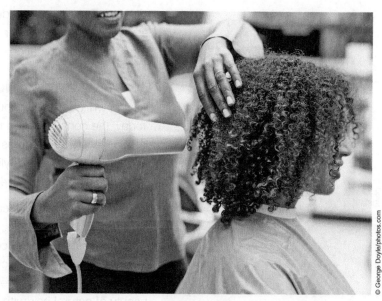

▲ Figure 1–13
There are very specific regulations for being a licensed natural hair stylist.

The Holistic Approach to Natural Hair Care Services

Natural hair care truly has evolved. It has grown into a major product industry, filling the demand for products and services that replenish and provide a therapeutic and healthy balance to hair care. The **holistic approach** to hair care embraces the use of therapies that considered the body and the mind as an integrated whole. It encompasses many integrated health practices that have existed for hundreds of years. Practitioners use essential oils, aromatherapy, and massage practices. They also use herbal nutrients, vitamin supplements, and customized botanical hair recipes, as well as chemically free hair care regimens that are earth friendly and renewable. This nurturing approach to hair care creates balance for the client and works to create *beauty wellness*—an integrated beauty and an effective way to maintain a healthy body and mind. Natural hair care respects the body by using products and services that keep the entire body whole and healthy. This holistic approach not only benefits the body and mind, but also respects the environment.

Many of the products used for textured or natural hairstyles eagerly promote their products as containing no sulfates, paraben, silicone, or petrochemicals and being free from animal testing. It is so important for people to limit their exposure to harmful chemicals—to create a gentle balance that promotes healing for healthy hair and scalp. We are exposed to hundreds of chemicals every day in our air, water, food, and

Did you know?

The first license for natural hair care and braiding was adopted In New York State on July 5, 1994. It included a one-year grandfather clause for licensing existing braiders and anyone who could show proficiency in the art.

natural hair care license state-recognized regulations for natural hair care and braiding. Not all states require licensing.

holistic approach refers to the complete wellness of the entire body.

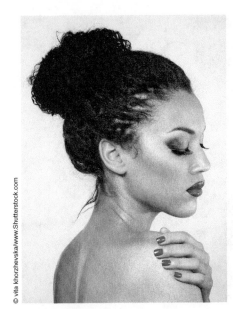

▲ Figure 1–14
The cultural aesthetic comes in many forms.

cultural aesthetic the styles and trends that are specific to a culture.

clothing. The more we reduce the impact of chemicals on our bodies and environment, the healthier we become each day, and the cleaner the earth is for the next generation.

Market and Industry Influences

As you will learn throughout this book, not all textures are the same. Today, the consumer and professional industry understand how important it is to identify the degrees of all textures—wave, curl, or coil formations—and the grooming and styling differences that are necessary to work with textured hair **(Figure 1–14)**.

Natural hair care and African braiding is a significant cultural art form appreciated by all people. Textured hair and African braid styles are now being integrated into the contemporary beauty enhancement industry's diverse approach to hair care. Natural hair stylists who are proficient in particular techniques were asked to submit their work and share the beauty of natural hair with readers. They produced textured and braided styles for high fashion, casual, and career looks. This **cultural aesthetic** is appreciated in other ethnic communities and is a standard of beauty inspired by that group's beliefs, customs, behavior, and technical skills. Self-affirmed and empowered clients, both men and women who are comfortable wearing culturally relevant styles, also benefit from developing a cultural aesthetic.

The Effect of Social Media

Social media has had the largest impact on the natural hair care industry. Those who regularly write and talk about curly, textured hair have become nearly a cult. When two or more women with natural hair get together, they automatically discuss their hair. Facebook, natural hair blogs, Websites, meet-ups, short films, e-books, certificate classes, and how-to DVDs all help support the consumer base that is taking this wonderful journey into natural hair. Social media has changed the face of many industries, and natural hair is no exception. Although most of the information is enlightening, informative, and entertaining, it is consumer based and product motivated. That may be good for the product manufacturers and blog sites, but the commercialism factor can promote misinformation in attempting to make profits. New standards of beauty are emerging. New language and semantics are being used to connect people to their hair. New natural and curly hair products are the latest rage—all to help clients embrace their wavy, curly, coily, and tightly coiled hair curl patterns **(Figure 1–15)**.

The desire for maintaining or transitioning to natural curly hair really is a revolution, and we as stylists must be a major part of this movement. As professionals, we must be the authority in the industry; we must know the science of natural hair care and styling and the ingredients of all hair care products. As the authority in natural hair care and braiding, natural hair

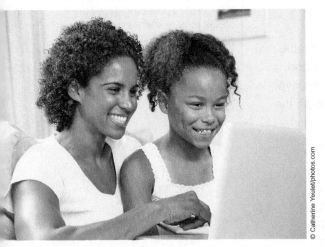

▲ Figure 1–15
Social media can encourage different generations to take pride in their natural hair.

care specialists and master braiders are knowledgeable in more than one hair type, texture, or product line. Be open to all hair types and textures; understand the benefits and features of products that you can use in the salon and recommend to the client.

Dispelling the Myths of Natural Textured Hair

Thanks to a long list of misconceptions, untruths, and misleading information, people in the African American community have been deterred and discouraged from truly embracing their natural hair. Society has sent the message that straight, long, blond hair is the preferred look. Some believe that natural textured hair, which has a tight curl or coily pattern, is "bad hair"; but hair that is long, straight, and silky is "good hair" or "beautiful hair." For decades, African Americans believed that their hair was ugly or bad and that the only way to make their hair fit this culture's beauty standards and make it good was to change or remove the natural texture. Unfortunately, men and women of color still believe these myths. Our hair has always been a mystery—a dark and gloomy subject. In the past, the cosmetology industry and hair care product companies did not teach the features, benefits, and hair care procedures of our textured tresses.

As professionals, we are here to remove the myths, provide excellent salon service, and educate the client about home care regimens. The myths and facts discussed throughout this textbook will shine a bright light on the subject and remove some of the negative images people of color have adopted regarding textured hair and natural hair care.

Review Questions

1. What are the origins of natural hair care and braiding?
2. What are some of the advancements made in natural hair care and braiding in the last three centuries?
3. What are some of the career opportunities for licensed natural hair technicians?

Chapter References

1. Sertima, I. (1976). *They came before Columbus.* New York: Random House.
2. Romant, B. (1978). *Life in Egypt in ancient times.* Genève: Minerva.
3. French Creole | Origins of the Tignon. (n.d.). Welcome to Frenchcreoles.com. Retrieved November 26, 2012, from www.frenchcreoles.com/ArtTheater/tignon
4. Bundles, A. (2001). *On her own ground: The life and times of Madam C.J. Walker.* New York: Scribner.
5. *On Her Own Ground: The Life and Times of Madam C. J. Walker* by A'Lelia Bundles.
6. Claiborne, C. (1946). "She Can Write a Check for Seven Figures." *The Afro-American Newspaper* (6):29.
7. Sinclair, A. (1993). "Black Hair and the Cultural/Political Movement." *New York Amsterdam News.* 84 (6):26.
8. 2006, Madam C. J. Walker official Website www.madamcjwalker.com/faqs/#10
9. Sherrow, V. (2006) *Encyclopedia of hair: A cultural history.* Westport, CT: Greenwood.
10. My First Conk. (n.d.). Scribd. Retrieved November 26, 2012, from www.scribd.com/doc/29978/My-First-Conk
11. Witkowski, T. H. (2001). Milestones in marketing history: Proceedings of the 10th Conference on Historical Analysis and Research in Marketing (CHARM), John W. Hartman Center for Sales, Advertising & Marketing History, Duke University, Durham, North Carolina, May 17–20, 2001. Long Beach, CA: Association for Historical Research in Marketing.
12. Page, C. (1986). "Dueling For Dollars In Hair Wars." *Chicago Tribune.* Featured Articles from the Chicago Tribune. Retrieved November 29, 2012, from articles.chicagotribune.com/1986-11-05/news/8603230291 _1_black-consumers-black-owned-black-companies
13. Witkowski, T. H. (2001). New hair freedom? Milestones in marketing history: Proceedings of the 10th Conference on Historical Analysis and Research in Marketing (CHARM), John W. Hartman Center for Sales, Advertising & Marketing History, Duke University, Durham, North Carolina, May 17–20, 2001 (p. 35). Long Beach, CA: Association for Historical Research in Marketing.
14. American Health & Beauty Aid Institute. (n.d.). American Health & Beauty Aid Institute. Retrieved November 26, 2012, from www.ahbai.org
15. Schachter, J. (1988). EEOC Says Hyatt Showed Bias in Its Ban on Cornrows. *Los Angeles Times.* Featured Articles from the Los Angeles Times. Retrieved November 29, 2012, from articles.latimes.com/1988 -05-17/business/fi-2915_1_hyatt-hotels

CHAPTER 2

Infection Control Principles and Practices

Chapter Outline

- Why Study Infection Control Principles and Practices?

- Regulatory Guidelines for Health Control

- Infectious Diseases

- Principles of Prevention and Infection Control

- How to Use Antiseptics and Disinfectants

- Universal Precautions

- Salon Wellness: Professional Salon Image

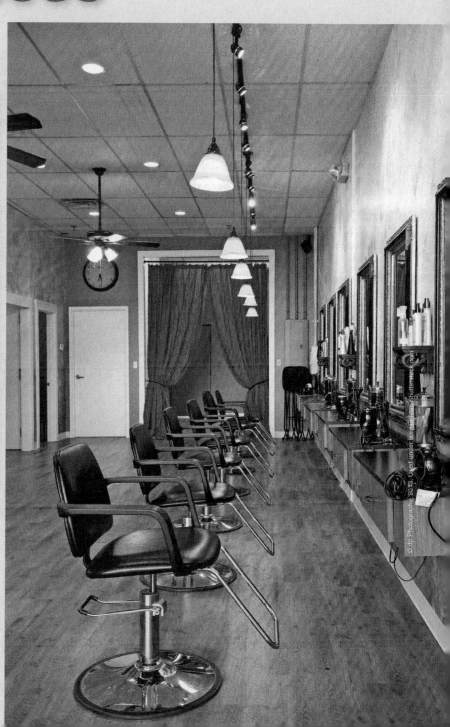

© db Photography 2013. Used under license from Shutterstock.com

Learning Objectives

After completing this chapter, you should be able to:

☑ **LO1** Understand the state laws and rules regarding infection control.

☑ **LO2** List the types of bacteria and their classifications.

☑ **LO3** Explain how bloodborne pathogens are transmitted.

☑ **LO4** Explain the differences between cleaning, disinfecting, and sterilizing.

☑ **LO5** Discuss Universal Precautions.

Key Terms

Page number indicates where in the chapter the term is used.

acquired immunodeficiency syndrome (AIDS)
p. 37

allergy
p. 41

antibiotics
p. 31

antiseptics
p. 42

artificially acquired immunity
p. 39

asymptomatic
p. 49

bacilli
p. 32

bacteria
p. 27

binary fission
p. 32

bleach
p. 45

cilia
p. 32

cleaning
p. 30

cocci
p. 32

contagious
p. 33

decontamination
p. 30

diplococci
p. 32

disinfectants
p. 29

disinfection
p. 30

efficacy
p. 44

exposure incident
p. 49

flagella
p. 32

fungi
p. 37

hepatitis
p. 35

hepatitis A
p. 36

hepatitis B
p. 36

hepatitis C
p. 36

hepatitis D
p. 37

hospital disinfectants
p. 29

human immunodeficiency virus (HIV)
p. 37

immune system
p. 39

immunization
p. 36

inflammation
p. 32

methicillin-resistant staphylococcus aureus (MRSA)
p. 33

microorganisms
p. 30

mildew
p. 37

multiuse
p. 47

naturally acquired immunity
p. 39

nonpathogenic bacteria
p. 31

nonporous surfaces
p. 29

Occupational Safety and Health Administration (OSHA)
p. 27

parasites
p. 38

pathogenic bacteria
p. 31

pediculosis capitis
p. 38

phenolic disinfectants
p. 45

porous
p. 47

quaternary ammonium compounds
p. 45

Safety Data Sheets (SDS)
p. 27

scabies
p. 39

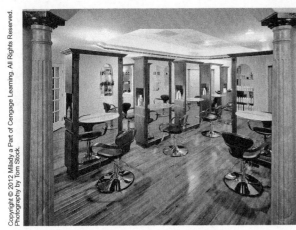

▲ A clean salon is inviting, organized, and safe.

Infection and disease control are some of the most important aspects of being a natural stylist or salon professional. To be a successful natural salon professional, it is vital to be knowledgeable about and responsible for the basic information regarding good health and cleaning practices within the work environment. You cannot have a successful salon business without a clean and disease-free salon. Infection control and effective health and decontamination systems are a major part of every successful salon business practice. Infection control is also a major part of protecting the staff and the clients, while also improving client confidence, retention, and client referral.

Why Study Infection Control Principles and Practices?

Natural stylists should study and have a thorough understanding of infection control principles and practices because:

■ To be knowledgeable, successful, and responsible professionals in the natural hair care and braiding industry, you are required to understand the types of infections you may encounter in the salon. Every stylist should know when, why, and how to use good decontamination practices to protect the individual and the community.

■ Understanding the basic cleaning and disinfecting rules and following federal and state laws will safeguard you, the stylist, the client, and the salon environment.

■ It is important to understand the chemistry of cleaning and disinfecting products that you use in the salon. Removing all disease-causing agents in a salon is almost impossible, but our jobs require us to manage, control, and create balance by reducing any dangerous levels of germs and disease. This is the key to a safe and successful salon business.

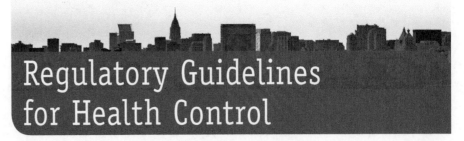

Regulatory Guidelines for Health Control

State and Federal Regulations

State and federal regulations require that certain preventive measures be taken against the spread of infectious disease and germs, or the salon operator's business can be shut down. Each state has specific regulations that address the responsibilities of the salon owner as well as the renter of a salon booth or chair. These regulations are standardized health and sanitary codes that all natural hair care specialists, braiders, locticians, and barbers must comply with. Keep the regulations handy and refer to them often. Be sure to check for changes and updates with your state regulatory agency.

Occupational Safety and Health Administration (OSHA)

The federal agency that monitors safety and health standards in the workplace is the **Occupational Safety and Health Administration (OSHA)**. As part of the U.S. Department of Labor, OSHA was developed to regulate, protect, and inform employees about exposure to potential hazards or toxic materials in the work environment. OSHA focuses its safety and health concerns on the work environment and employee protection. The primary functions of OSHA are to regulate, monitor, and ensure employee safety from toxic materials used in the work area and reduce exposure to infectious diseases. The braid stylist is vulnerable to daily exposure to **bacteria** and infection. Although natural stylists do not use chemicals to alter hair textures, other chemicals in the salon—such as antiseptics, cleansers, disinfectants, styling aids, shampoos, and conditioners—are used, and these products have guidelines. OSHA also sets standards for mixing, storing, and disposing of chemicals and hazardous products. It is the stylist's responsibility to be aware of product contents to protect themselves and their clients. Since 1970, all chemical manufacturers and importers must analyze and communicate any potential hazards associated with their products. When that information is finalized, **Safety Data Sheets (SDS)** are developed to accompany the product, which informs the buyer of any potentially hazardous ingredients, usage, and safety precautions **(Figure 2–1)**.

Develop Systems for Safety

It is important for the natural salon professional to develop a system—a set of procedures that help reduce the risk of exposure to infectious

Occupational Safety and Health Administration (OSHA) a federal agency created as part of the U.S. Department of Labor to regulate and enforce safety and health standards to protect employees in the workplace.

bacteria; singular, bacterium one-celled microorganisms that have both plant and animal characteristics. Some are harmful; some are harmless.

Safety Data Sheets (SDS) information compiled by the manufacturer about product safety, including the names of hazardous ingredients, safe handling and use procedures, precautions to reduce the risk of accidental harm or overexposure, and flammability warnings.

ACTivity

- Establish a written procedure outlining your salon's employee exposure plan. This plan or checklist states the daily steps taken to minimize employees' exposure to potentially hazardous or infectious materials. Keep the plan updated to reflect any new technological changes offered by the state.
- Enforce good work practices that reduce exposure: cleaning hands, handling laundry, sterilizing tools, and disposing of contaminated material.
- Provide protective gloves, gowns, or aprons for each stylist to protect their physical body.
- Establish post-procedure steps for stylists who may have been exposed to any infectious or hazardous materials. This may include steps such as confidential medical evaluation, testing, counseling, and treatment.

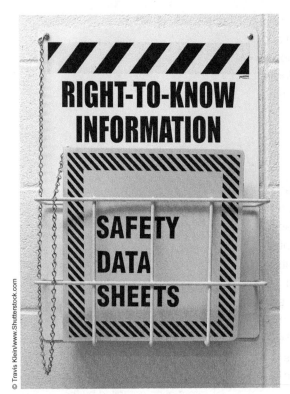

© Travis Klein/www.Shutterstock.com

▲ Figure 2–1
Learn and read the Safety Data Sheets.

diseases and hazardous product ingredients. The system must be uncomplicated, concise, and follow state procedures. There should be a written plan or checklist of procedures that ensures safety and that emphasizes a responsibility to protect and provide services with integrity. The following sections will help you to develop a safety checklist.

Safety Data Sheets (SDS)

Safety Data Sheets (SDS) (formerly known as Material Safety Data Sheets) contain manufacturer's information about product safety. This includes names of hazardous ingredients along with specific codes, the physical and chemical characteristics of the product, proper handling procedures, precautions to reduce risk, procedures in case of accidents or overexposure, and warnings about flammability or explosion. The SDS also provides information on how to dispose of the product in a way that is environmentally safe as well as medical or first-aid information. Federal and state laws require salons to obtain SDS from the product manufacturers and/or distributors for each professional product that is used. SDS often can be downloaded from the product manufacturer's or the distributor's Website.

Not having SDS available poses a health risk to anyone exposed to hazardous materials and violates federal and state regulations. Salons and schools are subject to inspection by the Occupational Safety and Health Administration (OSHA) and state boards of beauty enhancement. Both require that the SDS be kept available at all times during salon business hours. Both the OSHA and the state board inspectors can issue fines for not having the SDS available. It is important for every employee to read the SDS information whether they use the product or not.

Organize Your Salon's SDS

Develop a system to organize the SDS, and keep a record that each employee has read and is knowledgeable about the usage and disposal of all hair products, disinfectants, sanitizers, or other solvents used in the salon. SDS sheets can be downloaded from the manufacturer's Website and placed in three-ring binders to give everyone easy access. Mark the book in bright colors, and write "SDS" on the front and sides so that employees can easily recognize it. Place SDS binders near the front desk and at the back bar. Every time a new product arrives in the salon, add it to the SDS binder. After reading the materials in the SDS binder, each employee must sign and acknowledge that they have read the information.

Environmental Protection Agency (EPA)

The Environmental Protection Agency (EPA) sets high standards for manufacturers of products that claim to kill germs, fungi, or viruses. All disinfectants must be registered with the EPA. An EPA registration number is given to products that have the highest level of germicidal, fungicidal, or virucidal **disinfectants**. Disinfectants are chemical products that kill all bacteria, fungi (but not spores), and viruses on working surfaces. Household disinfectants will not kill the various bacteria you will be exposed to when in the salon.

Two Types of EPA Disinfectants

Two types of EPA disinfectants are specifically produced to be effective in a work environment and kill bacterial organisms.

- **Hospital disinfectants** are effective for killing bacteria in blood or bloody fluids on implements and surfaces. These chemical agents are used to destroy most bacteria and viruses that cause disease. They are not to be used on skin. Disinfectants are to be used on **nonporous surfaces** in the salon (that is, service equipment, implements, furnishings, floors, walls, and communication equipment).

- **Tuberculocidal disinfectants** are chemical agents that are known to kill the bacteria that cause tuberculosis—a bacterial disease that is transmitted through sneezing and coughing. These bacteria and spores, which are much harder to destroy, create sores. Tuberculocidal disinfectants are extremely powerful and must be used with extreme caution. These agents can be harmful to salon tools and equipment. Check in your state to determine that the products you choose comply with state requirements and are EPA approved. Follow the product label instructions for mixing and surface application to comply with state laws. You can be held responsible if a lawsuit is brought against your workplace.

State Compliance

Every state has regulatory agencies that exist to protect the salon industry, the consumer's safety, and the health and well-being of the community. State regulatory agencies include the licensing department, state board of natural hair styling, and health departments. These regulatory agencies develop and enforce rules and procedures that all natural hair care professionals must follow. The state agencies enforce the rules or regulations with salon inspections and the investigations of consumer complaints. Penalties vary from state to state and include warning notices, fines, probation, and suspension or revocations of licenses. Following the regulations is vital to a salon's success and reputation as well as to client safety.

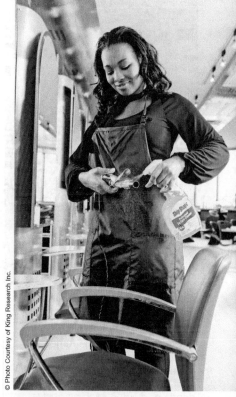

© Photo Courtesy of King Research Inc.

▲ Stylist cleaning tools.

disinfectants chemical products that destroy all bacteria, fungi, and viruses (but not spores) on surfaces.

hospital disinfectants disinfectants that are effective for cleaning blood and body fluids.

nonporous surfaces surfaces that are made or constructed of a material that has no pores or openings and cannot absorb liquids.

tuberculocidal disinfectants disinfectants that kill the bacteria that causes tuberculosis.

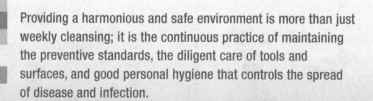

FYI

Providing a harmonious and safe environment is more than just weekly cleansing; it is the continuous practice of maintaining the preventive standards, the diligent care of tools and surfaces, and good personal hygiene that controls the spread of disease and infection.

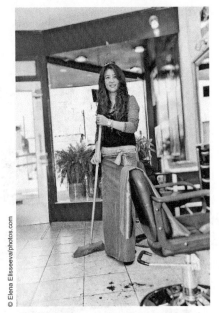

▲ Clean salon, removing hair with broom and dust pan.

decontamination the removal of blood or other potentially infectious materials from the surface of an item and the removal of visible debris or residue such as dust, hair, and skin.

cleaning a mechanical process (scrubbing) using soap and water or detergent and water to remove all visible dirt, debris, and many disease-causing germs. Cleaning also removes invisible debris that interferes with disinfection. Cleaning is what natural stylists are required to do before disinfecting.

disinfection a chemical process that uses specific products to destroy harmful organisms (except bacterial spores) on environmental surfaces.

sterilization the process that completely destroys all microbial life, including spores.

microorganisms any organism of microscopic or sub-microscopic size.

Everything in the salon has a working surface: the tables, counters, chairs, floors, shelves, mirrors, tools, and implements. All surfaces, especially tool surfaces, must be kept free from contaminants, such as dirt, oils, debris, and micropathogens. You are decontaminating your salon by removing these disease-causing substances. **Decontamination** of tools and surfaces is maintained on three levels: **cleaning**, **disinfection**, and **sterilization**. ☑ **LO1**

Infectious Diseases

Bacteria

Bacteria are tiny, one-celled **microorganisms** that have both vegetable and animal characteristics. They can exist nearly anywhere: in water and air, on clothing, beneath nails and on skin, in body fluids, and on surfaces. They are so small you can see them only with a microscope. Bacteria, also known as germs, are especially numerous in dust, dirt, garbage, decayed matter, and diseased tissues **(Figure 2–2a, b, c, d)**.

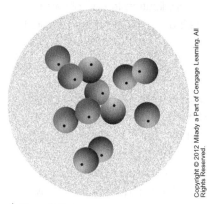

▲ Figure 2–2a
Cocci.

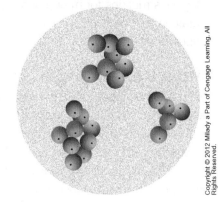

▲ Figure 2–2b
Staphylococci.

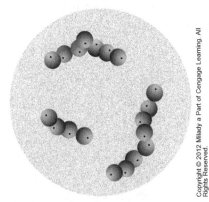

▲ Figure 2–2c
Streptococci.

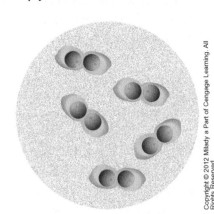

▲ Figure 2–2d
Diplococci.

Types of Bacteria

The earth has thousands of different types of bacteria. However, they fall into two primary categories: nonpathogenic and pathogenic.

Nonpathogenic bacteria are harmless organisms that do not cause disease, but have useful functions—like yogurt, cheese, and some medicines. Healthy bacteria like probiotics help the body digest food, and **antibiotics** help the body fight infection. Nonpathogenic bacteria help stimulate the immune system. They can inhibit the growth of microorganisms or destroy them.

Pathogenic bacteria are harmful organisms that cause infection and disease when they enter the body. When we are cleaning our salons, we are trying to reduce and prevent the spread of these organisms. While in school, you must learn and understand the importance of infection control practices to ensure that you maintain the same high standards when starting your career.

Table 2–1 summarizes the different types of pathogens, including their terms and definitions.

nonpathogenic bacteria harmless microorganisms that may perform useful functions and are safe to come in contact with because they do not cause disease or harm.

antibiotics a medicine (such as penicillin or its derivatives) that inhibits the growth of or destroys microorganisms.

pathogenic bacteria harmful microorganisms that can cause disease and infection in humans when they invade the body.

CAUSES OF DISEASE	
TERM	**DEFINITION**
BACTERIA	One-celled microorganisms having both plant and animal characteristics. Some are harmful and some are harmless.
DIRECT TRANSMISSION	Transmission of blood or body fluids through touching (including shaking hands), kissing, coughing, sneezing, and talking.
INDIRECT TRANSMISSION	Transmission of blood or body fluids through contact with an intermediate contaminated object, such as a razor, extractor, nipper, or an environmental surface.
INFECTION	Invasion of body tissues by disease-causing pathogens.
GERMS	Nonscientific synonym for disease-producing organisms.
MICROORGANISM	Any organism of microscopic to sub-microscopic size.
PARASITES	Organisms that grow, feed, and shelter on or in another organism (referred to as the host), while contributing nothing to the survival of that organism. Parasites must have a host to survive.
TOXINS	Various poisonous substances produced by some microorganisms (bacteria and viruses).
VIRUS	A parasitic sub-microscopic particle that infects and resides in cells of biological organisms. A virus is capable of replication only through taking over the host cell's reproductive function.

Table 2–1 Causes of Disease.

cocci round-shaped organisms that appear singly or in groups. The three types are staphylococci, streptococci, and diplococci.

staphylococci pus-forming bacteria that grow in clusters like a bunch of grapes. They cause abscesses, pustules, and boils.

streptococci pus-forming bacteria arranged in curved lines resembling a string of beads. They cause infections such as strep throat and blood poisoning.

diplococci spherical bacteria that grow in pairs and cause diseases such as pneumonia.

bacilli short, rod-shaped bacteria. They are the most common bacteria and produce diseases such as tetanus (lockjaw), typhoid fever, tuberculosis, and diphtheria.

spirilla a bacterium with a rigid spiral structure, found in stagnant water and sometimes causing disease.

flagella one to eight long, slender, hairlike extensions used by bacilli and spirilla for locomotion (moving about); may also be called cilia.

cilia hundreds of slender, hairlike extensions used by bacilli and spirilla for locomotion (moving about).

binary fission the division of bacteria cells into two new cells called daughter cells.

spore a tiny, typically one-celled reproductive unit capable of giving rise to a new individual without sexual fusion; characteristic of lower plants, fungi, and protozoans.

inflammation a condition in which the body reacts to injury, irritation, or infection and is characterized by swelling, redness, and heat or fever and pain.

methicillin-resistant staphylococcus aureus (MRSA) a type of infectious bacteria that is highly resistant to conventional treatments such as antibiotics.

contagious disease (communicable disease) disease that is spread from one person to another person. Some of the most contagious diseases are the common cold, ringworm, conjunctivitis (pinkeye), viral infections, and natural nail or toe and foot infections.

Classifications of Pathogenic Bacteria

Bacteria have three distinct shapes that help to identify them. Pathogenic bacteria are classified as follows.

1. **Cocci** are round-shaped organisms that appear singly or in the following groups:

    a. **Staphylococci**—pus-forming organisms that grow in bunches or clusters. They cause abscesses, pustules, and boils.

    b. **Streptococci**—pus-forming organisms that grow in chains. They cause infections such as strep throat and blood poisoning.

    c. **Diplococci**—organisms that grow in pairs and cause pneumonia.

2. **Bacilli**—short, rod-shaped organisms. They are the most common bacteria and produce diseases such as tetanus (lockjaw), influenza, typhoid fever, tuberculosis, and diphtheria.

3. **Spirilla**—curved or corkscrew-shaped organisms. They are subdivided into several groups. Of chief importance to us is the treponemapallida, which causes syphilis.

Movement of Bacteria

When bacteria are alive, the organisms move in different ways. Cocci rarely show active self-movement or motility. They are transmitted through the air, in dust, or in the substance they settle in. Bacilli and spirilla both have self-movement and use hairlike projections, known as **flagella** or **cilia**, for locomotion (moving about). A whiplike motion of these hairs propels bacteria about in liquid.

Bacterial Growth and Reproduction

Bacteria have a life cycle. They manufacture their own food from the surrounding environment, whether they are inside or outside the body. They give off waste products, grow, and reproduce. The life cycle of bacteria consists of the active stage or the inactive (spore-forming) stage.

Active-stage bacteria grow and reproduce; they multiply in warm, dark places with sufficient food. Once they reach their largest size, they divide into two cells; this process is also known as **binary fission**. The cells can multiply every 20 to 60 minutes, and some bacteria can grow even faster. The pathogen staphylococcus can increase its cell division every 27 to 30 minutes. When conditions become unfavorable, bacteria either die or become inactive.

In the inactive or spore-forming stage, **spores** may form on certain bacteria to withstand unfavorable conditions such as cold, heat, and dryness. They can be blown about and are not harmed while in this stage. When conditions are favorable, the bacteria spores grow, reproduce, and change into the active phase.

Bacterial Infections

No infection can take place without the presence of pathogenic bacteria. An infection occurs when the body is unable to cope with the bacteria and their harmful toxins. A local infection is indicated by a boil or pimple that contains pus. There may be **inflammation**, a condition in which the body reacts to injury, irritation, or infection and is characterized by swelling, redness, heat or fever, and pain.

The presence of pus is a sign of bacterial infection. Bacteria, waste matter, decayed tissue, body cells, and living and dead blood cells are all found in pus. Staphylococci are the most common pus-forming bacteria, and are generally carried by one-third of the population. "Staph" as it is often called, can be picked up on doorknobs, phone handles, work surfaces, unsterilized tools, and implements, as well as by skin-to-skin contact. A general infection results when the bloodstream carries the bacteria and their toxins to all parts of the body. Staph infections are the most common complaint in the salon. Staph is responsible for food poisoning, toxic shock syndrome, and a wide range of other diseases. One staph bacterial infection that is extremely resistant to antibiotics is **methicillin-resistant staphylococcus aureus (MRSA)**. MRSA was generally found in people with weakened immune systems. Currently, it has been found in perfectly healthy people. Some people just carry the bacteria around with them without knowing; they have no symptoms, but they are infecting others. MRSA first appears as a skin infection in the form of pimples, rashes, or boils that are resistant to treatment. If not properly treated, MRSA can go throughout the entire body and cause death. It is vital to clean and disinfect all tools, implements, and the salon environment to reduce the impact of these resistant bacteria on the community. ☑ **LO2**

A disease becomes **contagious**, or **communicable**, when it spreads from one person to another by contact. Some of the most common contagious diseases that prevent a stylist from working are tuberculosis, common cold, ringworm, scabies, head lice, and viral infections.

The chief sources of contagion are unclean hands and implements. Contagious diseases can also be spread by open sores, pus, mouth and nose discharges, shared drinking cups, telephone receivers, and towels. Uncovered coughing or sneezing and spitting in public also spread germs.

Infections can be prevented and controlled through personal hygiene and environmental cleaning.

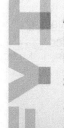

A disease results when bacteria is carried throughout the body. It becomes communicable or contagious when it spreads from one person to another.

Some common contagious diseases are:

- Tuberculosis
- Common cold
- Ringworm
- Viral infections
- Head lice
- MRSA
- HPV

CAUTION

As a professional natural stylist, you are not required to perform any hair services on any client who has visible signs of scalp infections, open cuts or sores, rashes, abrasions, bleeding wounds, or inflammation. The natural hair care specialist is required only to work on healthy hair and scalp. If a client comes into the salon, you are required to inform the client that you see an open cut, pimple, or infection and then refer the client to a physician. As salon professionals, we are not permitted to treat infectious diseases or extremely contagious disorders. Always be professional and compassionate about the client's need for privacy in the salon.

CAUTION

Contagious diseases caused by parasites should never be treated in a school or salon. A disease becomes communicable or contagious when it spreads from one person to another.

TERMS RELATED TO DISEASE

TERM	DEFINITION
ALLERGY	Reaction due to extreme sensitivity to certain foods, chemicals, or other normally harmless substances.
CONTAGIOUS DISEASE	Also known as *communicable disease*; disease that is spread from one person to another person. Some of the more contagious diseases are the common cold, ringworm, conjunctivitis (pinkeye), viral infections, and natural nail or toe and foot infections.
CONTAMINATION	The presence, or the reasonably anticipated presence, of blood or other potentially infectious materials on an item's surface or visible debris or residues such as dust, hair, and skin.
DECONTAMINATION	The removal of blood or other potentially infectious materials on an item's surface and the removal of visible debris or residue such as dust, hair, and skin.
DIAGNOSIS	Determination of the nature of a disease from its symptoms and/or diagnostic tests. Federal regulations prohibit salon professionals from performing a diagnosis.
DISEASE	An abnormal condition of all or part of the body, or its systems or organs, that makes the body incapable of carrying on normal function.
EXPOSURE INCIDENT	Contact with nonintact (broken) skin, blood, body fluid, or other potentially infectious materials that is the result of the performance of an employee's duties.
INFECTIOUS DISEASE	Disease caused by pathogenic (harmful) microorganisms that enter the body. An infectious disease may or may not be spread from one person to another person.
INFLAMMATION	Condition in which the body reacts to injury, irritation, or infection. An inflammation is characterized by redness, heat, pain, and swelling.
OCCUPATIONAL DISEASE	Illnesses resulting from conditions associated with employment, such as prolonged and repeated overexposure to certain products or ingredients.
PARASITIC DISEASE	Disease caused by parasites, such as lice and mites.
PATHOGENIC DISEASE	Disease produced by organisms, including bacteria, viruses, fungi, and parasites.
SYSTEMIC DISEASE	Disease that affects the body as a whole, often due to under-functioning or over-functioning internal glands or organs. This disease is carried through the blood stream or the lymphatic system.

Table 2–2 Terms Related to Disease.

Viruses

A **virus** is a submicroscopic parasitic agent that is infectious and can live only within other living bacteria, plant, or animal cells. Viruses need a host cell in order to live. Outside the host cells, viruses do not function; they are alive but stay dormant until they find a host **(Figure 2–3)**. Viruses are about a thousand times smaller than bacteria. Viruses live only by taking over host cells and becoming a part of them, but bacteria can live and reproduce on their own.

Viruses are everywhere in our living environment, just waiting to find a host. They can enter the body through the nose, mouth, an open scar, or body fluids. Once inside the body, they find a host cell to infect. Influenza is the cold and flu virus that attacks cells in the respiratory or digestive systems and enters through the mouth, nose, or stomach. The human immunodeficiency virus (HIV), which causes AIDS, attacks the T cells of our immune system. Other viruses that infect humans are measles, mumps, chicken pox, hepatitis, smallpox, human papilloma (warts), H1N1, and polio.

Generally, bacteria can be treated with antibiotics, but viruses are not affected by antibiotics. Viruses are difficult to diminish without harming the body's own cells or immunity process. Health authorities recommend vaccination to prevent some viruses from growing in the body. Not all viruses have vaccinations. Hepatitis A and B have vaccines, and they are recommended for people who are in direct contact with the public. Consult with your doctor before getting any vaccinations.

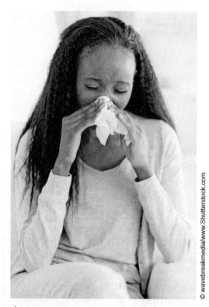

▲ Figure 2–3
Woman with a virus.

virus a parasitic, sub-microscopic particle that infects and resides in cells of biological organisms. A virus can replicate only by taking over the host cell's reproductive functions.

Bloodborne Pathogens

Bloodborne pathogens are disease-causing microorganisms in human blood and other body fluids. They include hepatitis B (HBV), hepatitis C (HCV) and HIV. Bloodborne pathogens can be transferred in the salon when the microorganisms enter the body through breaks in the skin inadvertently caused by haircutting, nipping with clippers, burns from chemicals, waxing, facial treatments, tweezing, or shaving. Although the natural stylist may not provide these services, it is important to know that the client may have a history of these services and may already have been exposed to bloodborne pathogens. Use great care to avoid cutting or damaging the client's skin during any services. Avoid any transfer of body fluids from anyone. Stylists and clients exposed to viral microorganisms like HIV are at risk for life-threatening illness and death. This is why you are required to disinfect and cleanse all tools and surfaces after every service. ☑ **LO3**

Hepatitis Viral Infections

Hepatitis is a bloodborne virus that causes disease and can damage the liver. In general, it is difficult to contract hepatitis. However, hepatitis is easier to contract than HIV, because hepatitis can be present in all

hepatitis a bloodborne virus characterized by inflammation of the liver, which causes disease and can damage the liver.

body fluids of those who are infected. Also unlike HIV, hepatitis can live on a surface outside the body for a long time. For this reason, it is vital to thoroughly clean and disinfect all surfaces that contact a client.

Some of the most common hepatitis varieties that are of concern in the salon are hepatitis A, hepatitis B, hepatitis C, and hepatitis D. Hepatitis B is the most difficult type to kill on a surface, so check the label of the disinfectant you use to be sure that the product is effective against hepatitis B. Hepatitis B and C are spread from person to person through blood and, less often, through other body fluids such as semen and vaginal secretions.

Hepatitis A   **Hepatitis A** is generally contracted from eating food contaminated with the virus, usually through fecal material and poor infection control practices. (Think of a restaurant worker who used the restroom but did not wash her hands before returning to prepare the next menu item.) It is also the type of hepatitis associated with eating raw shellfish. This form of hepatitis used to be called infectious hepatitis.[1]

Hepatitis B   **Hepatitis B (HBV)**, or serum hepatitis, is a more serious infection and is often spread by body fluids or sexual contact. Symptoms may last for months or even be nonexistent. Some hepatitis B patients can develop chronic hepatitis infection without an acute stage. Some people recover from it; however, some develop permanent liver damage, and about 10 percent become carriers. Liver cancer is known to occur in long-term carriers after 30 or more years of living with the virus. A vaccine series is available for hepatitis B, and **immunization**, the act of making a human unsusceptible to a pathogen, is highly recommended for those whose work may expose them to risk of infection.

Hepatitis C   **Hepatitis C (HCV)** symptoms are similar to those of hepatitis B, and it is sometimes associated with HIV infection. Hepatitis C is most often the type of hepatitis infection people acquire from blood transfusions and intravenous drug use. Even with current blood-screening technology, the risk of HCV infection from a

hepatitis A a bloodborne virus that causes diseases and can damage the liver.

hepatitis B (HBV; serum hepatitis) a more serious infection that is often spread by body fluids or sexual contact.

immunization the act of making a human unsusceptible to a pathogen.

hepatitis C (HCV) a virus whose symptoms are similar to those of hepatitis B and that is sometimes associated with HIV infection. Hepatitis C is most often the type of hepatitis infection people acquire from blood transfusions and intravenous drug use.

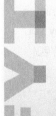

The main sources for spreading diseases are as follows:

- Unclean hands, surfaces, and implements
- Open sores
- Pus
- Mouth and nose discharges
- Common use of silverware, cups, or towels
- Unprotected and uncovered coughing or sneezing
- Spitting

transfusion is approximately 1 in 10,000. It can also be transmitted through injuries involving broken skin and through sexual contact.[2] Hepatitis C patients develop the chronic form, which can occur without a preceding acute stage.

Hepatitis D (HDV)   **Hepatitis D (HDV)** can develop only in people who have the hepatitis B virus. This finding reinforces the need for immunization. HDV is a serious viral infection that is much more likely than other types of hepatitis to cause permanent liver damage. Thus it is all the more imperative for people at risk of exposure to blood or other potentially infectious materials (OPIM) to seek the vaccination series.[3]

HIV/AIDS

Human immunodeficiency virus (HIV) is the bloodborne virus that causes **acquired immunodeficiency syndrome (AIDS)**. HIV weakens the body's immune system and its ability to fight infections and cancer. HIV is spread through contact with infected blood, body fluids, secretions, excretions (except sweat), mucous membranes, and nonintact skin. The virus that causes HIV is spread mainly through the sharing of needles by intravenous (IV) drug users and by unprotected sexual contact. HIV is considered to be a sexually transmitted disease (STD), because it can be contracted and spread through unprotected sex. Less commonly, HIV is spread through accidents with needles in health-care settings. The virus is less likely to enter the bloodstream through cuts and sores. A person can be infected with HIV for many years without having symptoms, but testing can determine whether a person is infected within 6 months after exposure to the virus. Sometimes, people who are HIV-positive have never been tested and do not know they have the potential to infect other people. A person cannot get HIV from bug bites, public baths, swimming pools or whirlpools, touching, holding hands, kissing, sharing a drink, or using a public telephone. There is no documentation that any one person has ever been infected with HIV at a hair salon. However, if a person with HIV is cut, the tool is contaminated and must be cleaned and disinfected. Continuing to use a contaminated implement without cleaning and disinfecting it puts you and others in the salon at risk of infection.

Fungi/Fungus

Fungi are microscopic plant parasites that include molds, mildews, and yeasts. They can produce contagious diseases, such as ringworm. **Mildew**, another fungus, affects plants or grows on inanimate objects but does not cause human infections in the salon **(Figure 2–4)**.

Tinea is the technical term for ringworm. It is characterized by itching, scales, and sometimes by painful circular lesions. Several patches may be present at one time. Tinea is caused by a fungal organism and not a parasite, as the old-fashioned term ringworm seems to suggest.

hepatitis D (HDV) a virus that can develop only in people who have the hepatitis B virus.

human immunodeficiency virus (HIV) a virus that causes acquired immunodeficiency syndrome (AIDS).

acquired immunodeficiency syndrome (AIDS) a disease that breaks down the body's immune system. AIDS is caused by the human immunodeficiency virus (HIV).

fungi microscopic plant parasites, including molds, mildews, and yeasts; fungi can produce contagious diseases, such as ringworm.

mildew a type of fungus that affects plants or grows on inanimate objects but does not cause human infections in the salon.

tinea technical term for ring worm, a contagious condition caused by fungal infection and not a parasite, characterized by itching, scales, and sometimes painful lesions.

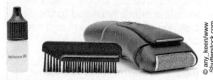

▲ Figure 2–4
Disinfect electrical tools.

tinea capitis a fungal infection of the scalp characterized by red papules, or spots, at the openings of the hair follicles.

tinea favosa (tinea favus) an infection characterized by dry, sulfur-yellow, cuplike crusts, called scutula, on the scalp.

scutula dry, sulfur-yellow, cuplike crusts on the scalp that have a distinctive odor.

tinea barbae the most frequently encountered fungal infection resulting from hair services; also known as barber's itch. Tinea barbae is a superficial fungal infection that commonly affects the skin. It is primarily limited to the bearded areas of the face and neck or around the scalp.

parasites organisms that grow, feed, and shelter on or in another organism referred to as the host, while contributing nothing to that organism's survival. Parasites must have a host to survive.

All forms of tinea are contagious and can be easily transmitted from one person to another. Infected skin scales or hairs that contain the fungi are known to spread the disease. Bathtubs, swimming pools, and uncleaned personal articles are also sources of transmission. Practicing approved cleaning and disinfection procedures will help prevent the spread of this disease in the salon.

Tinea capitis is another type of fungal infection characterized by red papules, or spots, at the opening of the hair follicles. The patches spread, and the hair becomes brittle. Hair often breaks off, leaving only a stump, or the hair may be shed from the enlarged open follicle.

Tinea favosa, also known as tinea favus, is characterized by dry, sulfur-yellow, cuplike crusts on the scalp called **scutula**. Scutula has a distinctive odor. Scars from tinea favosa are bald patches that may be either pink or white and shiny.

Tinea barbae, the most frequently encountered fungal infection resulting from hair services, is also known as barber's itch. Tinea barbae is a superficial fungal infection that commonly affects the skin. It is primarily limited to the bearded areas of the face and neck or around the scalp. This infection occurs almost exclusively in older adolescent and adult males. A person with tinea barbae may have deep, inflamed or noninflamed patches of skin on the face or the nape of the neck.[4] By practicing excellent cleaning and disinfection procedures, people can greatly reduce the transmission of this superficial fungus. Natural stylists who use clippers or blades must reduce all risks of transmitting diseases by removing all hair clippings and debris from clippers with compressed air, using clipper disinfectant sprays, removing nonelectrical parts, and cleaning and disinfecting properly. Always read and then refer to manufacturer's directions for cleaning and storing **(Figure 2–5)**.

Parasites

Parasites are living organisms that feed, grow, and thrive on or in a host organism. Parasites need host organisms to survive. Parasites live inside and on living plants, animals, and humans. Internal parasites are found in our food and water as well as in improperly cooked fish and meat. External parasites that affect humans include ticks, mites, and fleas.

Pediculosis Capitis

Pediculosis capitis is the infestation of the hair and scalp with head lice **(Figure 2–6)**. As these parasites feed on the scalp, it begins to itch. If the scalp is scratched, it can cause an infection. Head lice are transmitted from one person to another by contact with infested hats, combs, brushes, and other personal articles. You can distinguish head lice from dandruff flakes by looking closely at the scalp with a magnifying glass.

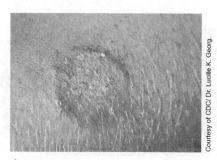

▲ Figure 2–5
Ringworm.

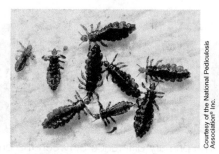

▲ Figure 2–6
Head lice.

Properly practicing state-board–approved cleaning and disinfection procedures will prevent the spread of this infestation. Several nonprescription medications are available.

You should not perform a service on anyone who has head lice. A client with this condition must be referred to a physician or a pharmacist.[5]

It is your responsibility to maintain a healthy environment for yourself, staff, and clients. Always practice state procedures for cleansing and disinfecting tools, chairs, and the entire salon environment.

Scabies

Scabies, another contagious skin disease, is caused by the itch mite. Severe itching occurs when the mites feed and burrow under the skin. The skin becomes inflamed with blisters and pustules (pimples with pus) from this infestation. Extreme itching creates infection.

Practicing extreme care to clean and disinfect all tools. All surfaces, towels, head rests, capes, chairs, and equipment must be properly treated with an EPA-registered disinfectant. You are not required to perform a service on anyone who has any contagious disorders. As a professional, gently and discreetly tell the client your concerns and refer him to a physician.

Immunity

Immunity is the ability to neutralize pathogens that have gained entrance to the body and to protect the body against infection or illness. The **immune system** is an incredible protection mechanism. The immune system is made up of white blood cells, proteins, tissues, and organs that defend the body against millions of bacteria, microbes, viruses, toxins, and parasites. Immunity against disease can be natural or acquired and is a sign of good health. **Naturally acquired immunity** is partly inherited and partly developed through healthy living. An example of naturally acquired immunity is the transfer of antibodies in the placenta from mother to fetus during pregnancy and after birth from breast milk. **Artificially acquired immunity** is immunity that the body develops after overcoming a disease, receiving inoculation (such as flu vaccinations), or having exposure to natural allergens such as pollen, cat dander, and ragweed.

pediculosis capitis (head lice), infestation of the hair and scalp with head lice.

scabies a contagious skin disease that is caused by the itch mite, which burrows under the skin.

immune system protects the body from disease by developing immunities and destroying disease-causing toxins and bacteria.

naturally acquired immunity an immunity that is partly inherited and partly developed through healthy living.

artificially acquired immunity immunity that the body develops after overcoming a disease, receiving inoculation (such as flu vaccinations), or having exposure to natural allergens such as pollen, cat dander, and ragweed.

Principles of Prevention and Control

The primary difference between the professional and nonprofessional natural stylist is in the high standards of health and decontamination systems maintained in the salon. An orderly and clean hair salon offers a harmonious, safe environment for the client. It is paramount for natural hair care specialists to keep the salon environment free from dirt, dust, oils, infectious diseases, and germs. It is the natural stylist's responsibility to clients and coworkers to ensure their safety. Providing a harmonious and safe environment involves more than just weekly cleaning. It is the continuous practice of preventive procedures, the expedient cleaning and care of tools and equipment surfaces, and the personal hygiene that minimizes and controls the spread of infection.

If a client or coworker becomes seriously ill due to inadequate care of tools or an unsafe work environment, the salon owner can be held liable and the business may be irreparably damaged. If clients lose confidence in the safety of the salon, they will not return for future services. As a salon entrepreneur, you must realize that it is good business to have a safe, harmonious working environment. It is also the law.

Salon Wellness: Principles of Prevention

The most well-designed salon can lose its attractiveness if it is not routinely going through a decontamination process. To decontaminate is to reduce or prevent the spread of diseases caused by infectious germs in the work environment. Decontamination is important for preventing exposure to blood, infectious materials, dust, dirt, and other contaminates and pathogens in the salon environment. There are two methods of decontamination:

- **Decontamination method 1: Cleaning and Disinfecting**—cleaning with a detergent and then disinfecting with an EPA-approved disinfectant.

- **Decontamination method 2: Cleaning and Sterilizing**—cleaning with a detergent and then sterilizing through heat and pressure in an autoclave (kills spore-forming bacteria on implements).

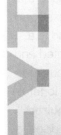

FYI

It is good business practice to have a safe and harmonious working environment. It is paramount to ensure that the salon is free from dirt, germs, and infectious diseases. A clean and safe salon environment builds confidence in the clients and is necessary for keeping their business.

Decontamination Method 1

Decontamination method 1 involves two steps: cleaning and disinfecting. Remember that when you clean, you must remove all visible dirt and debris from tools, implements, and equipment by washing with liquid soap and warm water and by using a clean and disinfected nail brush to scrub any grooved or hinged portions of the item.

A surface is properly cleaned when the number of contaminants on the surface is greatly reduced. By reducing the contaminants, you reduce the risk of infection. The vast majority of contaminants and pathogens can be removed from the surfaces of tools and implements through proper cleaning. This is why cleaning is an important part of disinfecting tools and equipment. A surface must be properly cleaned before it can be properly disinfected. Using a disinfectant without cleaning first is like using mouthwash without brushing your teeth—it just does not work properly!

Cleaned surfaces can still harbor small amounts of pathogens, but the presence of fewer pathogens means infections are less likely to be spread. Putting antiseptics on your skin or washing your hands with soap and water will drastically lower the number of pathogens on your hands. However, it does not clean them properly. The proper cleaning of the hands requires rubbing hands together and using liquid soap, warm running water, a nail brush, and a clean towel. (See Procedure 2–1, Proper Hand Washing, later in this chapter.) Do not underestimate the importance of proper cleaning and hand washing. They are the most powerful and important ways to prevent the spread of infection.

There are three ways to clean your tools or implements:

- Wash with soap and warm water. Then scrub with a clean and properly disinfected nail brush.

- Use an ultrasonic unit.

- Use a cleaning solvent.

The second step of decontamination method 1 is disinfection. Remember that disinfection is the process that eliminates most, but not necessarily all, microorganisms on nonliving surfaces. This process is not effective against bacterial spores. In the salon setting, disinfection is extremely effective in controlling microorganisms on surfaces, such as shears, nippers, and other multiuse tools and equipment (multiuse and single-use tools are discussed later in this chapter). Any disinfectant used in the salon should carry an Environmental Protection Agency (EPA) registration number, and the label should clearly state the specific organisms the solution is effective in killing when used according to the label instructions.

Remember that disinfectants are products that destroy all bacteria, fungi, and viruses (but not spores) on surfaces. Disinfectants are not for use on human skin, hair, or nails. Never use disinfectants as hand cleaners, because this can cause skin irritation and **allergy**, a reaction due to extreme sensitivity to certain foods, chemicals, or other normally harmless substances.

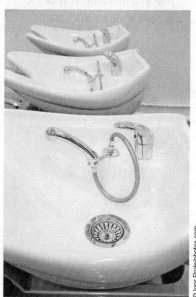

CAUTION

Disinfectants are pesticides and can be harmful if absorbed through the skin. All disinfectants clearly state on the label that you should avoid skin contact. This means avoiding contact with your skin, as well as, the client's. Do not put your fingers directly into any disinfecting solution. Disinfectants are pesticides and can be harmful if absorbed through the skin. If you mix a disinfectant in a container that is not labeled by the manufacturer, the container must be properly labeled with the contents and the date it was mixed. All concentrated disinfectants must be diluted exactly as instructed by the manufacturer on the container's label.

▲ Clean shampoo bowls.

allergy a reaction due to extreme sensitivity to certain foods, chemicals, or other normally harmless substances.

Decontamination Method 2

Decontamination method 2 also has two steps: cleaning and sterilizing. The word *sterilize* is often used incorrectly. Sterilization is the process that completely destroys all microbial life, including spores.

Sterilization is the highest form of decontamination. Under most circumstances, a natural stylist is not required to perform sterilization procedures; however, you will need to understand how to use and practice sterilization. The sterilization process actually kills germs, including the most resistant form of bacterial spores. To sterilize tools and implements, a sterilizing chamber—such as a high-pressure steam autoclave—is used. The steam autoclave (often seen in dentists' offices, doctors' offices, or nail salons) works like a pressure cooker. Simply exposing instruments to steam is not enough. To be effective against disease-causing pathogens, the steam must be pressurized in an autoclave so the steam penetrates the outer coats of the spore-forming bacteria. Dry-heat forms of sterilization are less efficient and require longer times at higher temperatures. Dry-heat sterilization is not recommended for use in salons.

Most people without medical training do not understand how to use an autoclave. For example, dirty implements cannot be properly sterilized without first being properly cleaned. Autoclaves need regular maintenance and testing to ensure they are in good working order. Color indicator strips on autoclave bags can provide false readings, so do not rely on them to determine whether instruments have been sterilized. These strips are only an indication, not verification that the autoclave is working.

The Centers for Disease Control and Prevention (CDC) requires that autoclaves be tested weekly to ensure they are properly sterilizing implements. The accepted method is called a spore test. Sealed packages containing test organisms are subjected to a typical sterilization cycle and then sent to a contract laboratory that specializes in testing autoclave performance. Other regular maintenance is also required to ensure the autoclave reaches the correct temperature and pressure. Keep in mind that when an autoclave does not reach the intended temperature for killing microorganisms, it may instead create a warm, moist place where pathogenic organisms can grow and thrive. Salons should always follow the autoclave manufacturer's recommended schedule for cleaning, changing the water, arranging service visits, replacing parts, and doing any required maintenance.

How to Use Antiseptics and Disinfectants

Antiseptics

Antiseptics are germicides that are safe to use on the skin, scalp, and hair. Antiseptics can reduce and kill bacteria on the skin and are regulated by the

---

> ## CAUTION
>
> Do not combine disinfectants. Read and follow directions carefully. For any disinfectant to work properly, it is important that you measure or dilute it according to instructions.

antiseptics substances that prevent the growth of disease-causing microorganisms.

Food and Drug Administration (FDA). Liquid antiseptic soaps are excellent for cleaning visible dirt and oils and removing bacteria. For minor cuts and burns, antiseptic creams, gels, or liquids should be used to protect from infection. Antiseptics usually contain alcohol or benzalkonium chloride, which is not as drying as alcohol. Other types of antiseptics include witch hazel and hydrogen peroxide. When using commercial antiseptic creams or gels, look for the active ingredients. Such creams as Bacitracin® or Neonycen® can prevent infection and aid the healing process. After applying any ointments or liquids to clean cuts or burns, cover with a bandage. First-aid kits are available with various types of antiseptics. Always follow the product label directions.

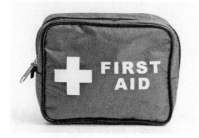
▲ First-aid kit.

Natural Antiseptics

Every natural hair care salon should also have first-aid staples on hand. Aloe vera gel and tea tree oil should always be on the shelf. Aloe vera gel can be found bottled or in its most natural plant state. The plant is a native of Africa and the Mediterranean region. It has been used for hundreds of years in those areas **(Figure 2–7)**.

- The aloe plant is characterized by its long, tapered, thick green leaves. When the leaves are broken, they exude a light emulsive sap that can be applied externally to cuts and burns. The gel directly soothes itching and burning once it is applied. It aids in the regeneration of new tissue when scarring and normal pigmentation has been affected. Adding benzoin tincture to aloe vera can make an antiseptic solution that prevents blistering.

- Tea tree oil is known as the "medicine kit in a bottle." This oil is a native of Australia. Tea tree oil is a clear, aromatic oil that increases the healing process. It soothes insect bites, herpes sores, cuts, burns, and fungal infections. This antiseptic oil increases the process of healing burns or cuts because it escalates skin regeneration. Normal pigmentation loss can return if used consistently. Tea tree oil is also effective on itchy scalps and dandruff.

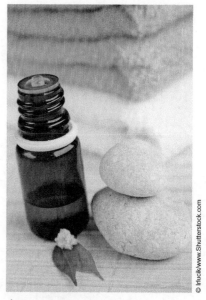
▲ Figure 2–7
Tea tree oil is a natural antiseptic.

The natural stylist should have both ethyl (grain) and isopropyl alcohol available for use in the salon, although they are not specifically designed to disinfect professional tools. The EPA recognizes these alcohols as adequate disinfectants that will stop the spread of bacteria. However, the use of alcohols has some disadvantages. They are extremely flammable, evaporate quickly, and are slow-acting, less effective disinfectants. Alcohols corrode tools and make sharp edges become dull. The vapor formed upon evaporation can cause headaches and nausea in high concentrations or after prolonged exposure. Alcohols work more effectively as antiseptics. When considering any antiseptic for use in the salon, check and abide by all state and federal regulations for its use.

Choosing and Using Disinfectants

Every stylist in the salon must read, understand, and follow the manufacturer's instructions when using disinfectants. Not all disinfectants are made alike. Some can be used directly from the bottle; others must be diluted for effectiveness. If the word *concentrate* is on the label, then you need to know the mixing ratio to dilute the detergent. Many disinfectants are already mixed and require no mixing or diluting. All EPA-registered disinfectants will specify how long the nonporous surface or tool must stay in contact with the disinfectant in order for the solution to be most effective. This contact time will vary from product to product and must be followed. Disinfectants provide **efficacy** claims on every label. Efficacy claims state the ability of the product to provide the effect displayed on its label—in other words, to be effective according to the label instructions.

Natural hair care is a specialty service. It is important to select the appropriate disinfectants suited for this specialty. The following items will help you decide which disinfectants best suit your salon:

- The product must be EPA approved.

- The product must be environmentally friendly or safe to be disposed of without upsetting the ecological balance in the community.

- The disinfectant must be nontoxic without fumes.

- The product must maintain its effectiveness while in storage.

- The disinfectant should be cost effective.

- The product must be noncorrosive to the plumbing system.

- The product have several retail and manufacturing sources available for reorders.

- The product must maintain efficacy in the presence of bioburden, which is the number of viable organisms in or on an object or surface or the organic material on the surface of an object before decontamination or sterilization.

- The product should not require frequent changing (at least a week or more, not daily).

- The product must be inexpensive.

- The product must include strips for checking effectiveness.

Salons pose a lower infection risk when compared to hospitals. For this reason, hospitals must meet much stricter infection control standards. They often use disinfectants that are too dangerous for the salon environment. Even though salons pose a lower risk of spreading certain types of infections, it is still very important to clean and then disinfect all tools, implements, surfaces, and equipment correctly. When salon implements accidentally contact blood, body fluids, or unhealthy conditions, they should be properly cleaned and then completely immersed in an EPA-registered hospital disinfectant solution that shows effectiveness against HIV, hepatitis, and tuberculosis. They also can be immersed in a 10 percent bleach solution. Always wear gloves and follow the proper Universal Precautions protocol for cleaning up after an exposure incident (Universal Precautions are described later in this chapter).

efficacy to be effective according to the label instructions.

Proper Disinfection

The correct disinfecting procedures involve specific steps. It is a state requirement to cleanse and disinfect all tools, implements, equipment, and surfaces. Implements must be thoroughly cleaned of all visible matter or residue before being placed in disinfectant solution. This is because residue will interfere with the disinfectant and prevent proper disinfection. Properly cleaned implements and tools, free from all visible debris, must be completely immersed in disinfectant solution. Complete immersion means there is enough liquid in the container to cover all surfaces of the item being disinfected, including the handles, for 10 minutes or for the time recommended by the manufacturer **(Figure 2–8)**.

Types of Disinfectants

Not all disinfectants are made equal. Disinfectants differ based on how they are used; some are exclusively for tools and implements, others are for nonporous surfaces, and still others are for glass and metals. Be aware of the disinfectant specifically for salon use. This subsection describes the disinfectants that are appropriate for salon use.

Quaternary ammonium compounds also known as quats (KWATZ)—are good cleaning solutions for implements and tools. Quats are effective disinfectants when used properly in the salon. The most advanced formulations are called multiple quats. Multiple quats contain sophisticated blends of quats that work together to dramatically increase the effectiveness of these disinfectants. Quats solutions require that the tools and implements are submerged for 10 minutes to be effective. They also have been formulated with anti-rust ingredients to avoid dulling or damaging tools. Remove tools from the solution after the specified period and then rinse (if required), dry, and store them in a clean, covered container.

Phenolic disinfectants are powerful tuberculocidal disinfectants. They are a form of formaldehyde, have a very high pH, and can damage the skin and eyes. Phenolic disinfectants can be harmful to the environment if put down the drain. They have been used reliably over the years to disinfect salon tools; however, they do have drawbacks. Phenol can damage plastic and rubber and can cause certain metals to rust.

Bleach, 5.25 sodium hypochlorite (i.e., household bleach), is a very effective disinfectant that can be used throughout the salon. Bleach can be corrosive and damaging to metals and plastics and can cause skin irritation and eye damage. Its fumes can cause lung damage, so be sure to follow manufacturer's instructions on use.

- To be effective, the bleach must contain at least 5 percent sodium hypochlorite and must be diluted properly to a 10 percent solution consisting of nine parts water to one part bleach.

- Store the bleach solution away from heat and light.

- Mix a fresh bleach solution every 24 hours or whenever the solution has been contaminated.

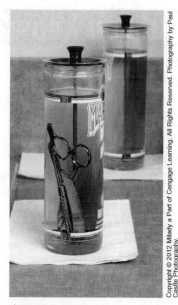

▲ Figure 2–8
Completely immerse tools in disinfectant.

quaternary ammonium compounds (quats) disinfectants that are very effective when used properly in the salon.

phenolic disinfectants powerful tuberculocidal disinfectants. They are a form of formaldehyde, have a very high pH, and can damage the skin and eyes. Phenolic disinfectants can be harmful to the environment if put down the drain. They have been used reliably over the years to disinfect salon tools; however, they do have drawbacks. Phenol can damage plastic and rubber and can cause certain metals to rust.

bleach a chemical (typically a solution of sodium hypochlorite or hydrogen peroxide) used to whiten or sterilize materials.

WARNING!

Phenolics are known carcinogens. Never use them to disinfect equipment. Take extra care to avoid contacting skin with phenolic disinfectants.

- After mixing the bleach solution, date the container to ensure that the solution is not saved from one day to the next. Wear gloves when making solutions.

- Be very careful of fumes, because bleach can be very irritating to the eyes, lungs, and skin.

Disinfect or Dispose?

How can you tell which items in the salon can be disinfected and reused? Salons use two types of items: multiuse (reusable) items, and single-use (disposable) items.

Safety Tips for Disinfectants

Always

- Keep an SDS on hand for the disinfectant(s) you use.

- Wear gloves and safety glasses when mixing disinfectants.

- Avoid skin and eye contact.

- Add disinfectant to water when diluting (rather than adding water to a disinfectant) to prevent foaming, which can result in an incorrect mixing ratio.

- Use tongs, gloves, or a draining basket to remove implements from disinfectants.

- Keep disinfectants out of reach of children.

- Carefully measure and use disinfectant products according to label instructions.

- Follow the manufacturer's instructions for mixing, using, and disposing of disinfectants.

- Carefully follow the manufacturer's directions for when to replace the disinfectant solution to ensure the healthiest conditions for you and your client. Replace the disinfectant solution every day—more often if the solution becomes soiled or contaminated.

Never

- Let quats, phenols, bleach, or any other disinfectant come in contact with your skin. If you do get disinfectants on your skin, immediately wash the area with liquid soap and warm water. Then rinse the area and dry it thoroughly.

- Place any disinfectant or other product in an unmarked container. All containers should be labeled. Jars or containers used to disinfect implements are often incorrectly called wet sanitizers. The purpose of disinfectant containers is to disinfect, not to clean. Disinfectant containers must be covered, but not airtight. Remember to clean the container every day and to wear gloves when you do. Always follow the manufacturer's label instructions for disinfecting products.

Multiuse, also known as reusable, items can be cleaned, disinfected, and used on more than one person, even if the item is accidentally exposed to blood or body fluid. These items must have a hard, nonporous surface. Multiuse items include shears, combs, and rollers.

Single-use, also known as disposable, items cannot be used more than once. These items cannot be properly cleaned so that all visible residues are removed—or they are damaged or contaminated by cleaning and disinfecting. Single-use items include tissues, paper towels, and neck strips. Single-use items must be thrown out after each use.

Porous items are made or constructed of a material that has pores or openings. These items are absorbent. Some porous items can be safely cleaned, disinfected, and used again. Examples of porous items are towels and linens.

If a porous item contacts broken skin, blood, or body fluid, it must be discarded immediately. Do not try to disinfect the item. If you are not sure whether an item can be safely cleaned, disinfected, and used again, throw it out.

Keeping a Logbook

Salons should always follow manufacturers' recommended schedules for cleaning and disinfecting tools and implements, regular service visits for equipment, and replacing parts when needed. Although your state may not require you to keep a logbook of all equipment usage, cleaning, disinfecting, testing, and maintenance, it may be advisable to keep one. Showing your logbook to clients provides them with peace of mind and confidence in your ability to protect them from infection and disease.

Disinfecting Nonelectrical Tools and Implements

State rules require that all multiuse tools and implements must be cleaned and disinfected before and after every service—even when they are used on the same person. Mix all disinfectants according to the manufacturer's directions, and always add the disinfectant to the water, not the water to the disinfectant.

Disinfecting Electrical Tools and Equipment

Hair clippers and other types of electrical equipment have contact points that cannot be immersed in liquid. These devices should be cleaned and disinfected using an EPA-registered disinfectant designed for use on them. Follow the procedures recommended by the disinfectant manufacturer for preparing the solution, and follow the item's manufacturer directions for cleaning and disinfecting the device.

Disinfecting Work Surfaces

Before beginning every client service, all work surfaces must be cleaned and disinfected. Be sure to clean and disinfect tables, styling stations, shampoo sinks, chairs, arm rests, and any other surface that a customer's skin may have touched. Clean doorknobs and handles daily to minimize the transfer of germs to your hands.

multiuse (reusable) items that can be cleaned, disinfected, and used on more than one person even if the item is accidentally exposed to blood or body fluid.

single-use (disposable) items that cannot be used more than once.

porous an item that is made or constructed of a material that has pores or openings. These items are absorbent.

CAUTION

When consulting with a new client, it is recommended that you wear gloves to protect you and your client in case a scalp disorder is revealed. Conducting a thorough hair and scalp analysis is important to determine the client's needs and to find any disorders or open sores.

Cleaning Towels, Linens, and Capes

Clean towels, linens, and capes must be used for each client. A towel, linen, or cape that has been used on a client must not be used again until it has been properly laundered. To clean towels, linens, and capes, launder according to the label directions. Be sure that towels, linens, and capes are thoroughly dried. Items that are not dry may grow mildew and bacteria. Store soiled linens and towels in covered or closed containers, away from clean linens and towels, even if your state regulatory agency does not require you to. Whenever possible, use disposable towels, especially in restrooms. Do not allow capes that are used for cutting, shampooing, and chemical services to touch the client's skin. Use disposable neck strips or towels. If a cape accidentally touches skin, do not use the cape again until it has been laundered.

Hand Washing

Properly washing your hands is one of the most important actions you can take to prevent spreading germs from one person to another. Proper hand washing removes germs from the folds and grooves of the skin and from under the free edges of the nail plates by lifting and rinsing germs and contaminants from the surface.

You should wash your hands thoroughly before and after each service. Follow the hand-washing procedure in this chapter, and if you perform nail services, be sure that your clients first wash their hands using a clean and disinfected nail brush before their service begins.

Antimicrobial and antibacterial soaps can dry the skin, and medical studies suggest that they are no more effective than regular soaps or detergents. Therefore, it is recommended that you minimize the use of antimicrobial and antibacterial soaps. Repeated hand washing can also dry the skin, so using a moisturizing hand lotion after washing is a good practice. Be sure the hand lotion is in a pump container, not a jar.

Avoid using very hot water to wash your hands, because this is another practice that can damage the skin. Remember: You must wash your

Did you know?

Salons have many tools and surfaces that require disinfection. Commonly used tools that require disinfection are:	Surfaces to consider cleansing and disinfecting are:	Other tools to remember to clean include:
• combs • brushes • scissors • razors	• tops of tables or counters • telephone receivers • doorknobs • cabinet handles • mirrors • cash registers	• mixing utensils • pins • clips and curlers • hair dryers • chairs • fans and humidifiers

hands thoroughly before and after each service, so do all you can to reduce any irritation that may occur. ☑ **LO4**

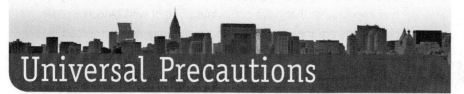
Universal Precautions

Universal Precautions are the guidelines issued by the Centers for Disease Control and Prevention (CDC) and OSHA. These guidelines require everyone to assume that all human blood and body fluids are infectious and contain bloodborne pathogens. This means that you should treat every client with the highest standards for their safety and your protection from disease. Universal means "all," without exception. You cannot look at a person and determine if a person is infected with HIV or hepatitis. These bloodborne pathogens are in most cases **asymptomatic**, which means that the person shows no signs or symptoms of infection. Taking precautions with all clients lessens your chances for exposure. Always dispose of razors and blades in the disposal box, especially if they have been in contact with blood from shaving or razor cuts. ☑ **LO5**

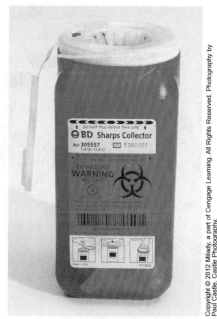

▲ **Dispose of blades in disposal box.**

An Exposure Incident: Contact with Blood or Body Fluid

You should never perform a service on any client who comes into the salon with an open wound or an abrasion. Sometimes accidents happen while a service is being performed in the salon, however.

An **exposure incident** is contact with nonintact (broken) skin, blood, body fluid, or other potentially infectious materials resulting from the performance of an employee's duties. Should the client suffer a cut or abrasion that bleeds during a service, follow these steps for the client's safety, as well as your own:

1. Stop the service.

2. Put on gloves to protect yourself from contact with the client's blood.

3. Stop the bleeding by applying pressure to the area with a clean cotton ball or piece of gauze.

4. When bleeding has stopped, clean the injured area with an antiseptic wipe. Every salon must have a first-aid kit.

5. Bandage the cut with an adhesive bandage.

6. Clean and disinfect your workstation or styling station by using an EPA-registered disinfectant designed for cleaning blood and body fluids.

7. Discard all single-use contaminated objects such as wipes or cotton balls by double-bagging (place the waste in a plastic bag and then in

Universal Precautions a set of guidelines published by OSHA that require the employer and the employee to assume that all human blood and body fluids are infectious for bloodborne pathogens.

asymptomatic showing no symptoms or signs of infection.

exposure incident contact with nonintact (broken) skin, blood, body fluid, or other potentially infectious materials that results from the performance of an employee's duties.

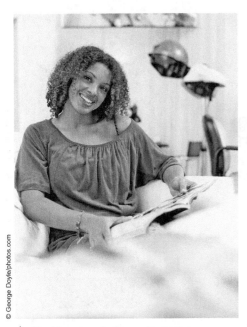

© George Doyle/photos.com

▲ **Client in a clean, inviting, natural salon.**

a trash bag). Place a biohazard sticker (red or orange) on the bag, and deposit the bag into a container for contaminated waste. Deposit sharp disposables in a sharps box.

8. Before removing your gloves, make sure that all multiuse tools and implements that have come into contact with blood or other body fluids are thoroughly cleaned and completely immersed in an EPA-registered disinfectant solution designed for cleaning blood and body fluids, or in a 10 percent bleach solution for at least 10 minutes, or for the time recommended by the product manufacturer. Be sure not to touch other work surfaces in the salon, such as faucets and counters. If you do, these areas must also be properly cleaned and disinfected. Remember: Blood may carry pathogens, so you should never touch an open sore or a wound.

9. Remove your gloves and seal them in the double bag along with the other contaminated items for disposal. Thoroughly wash your hands, and clean under the free edges of your nails with soap and warm water before returning to the service.

10. Recommend that the client see a physician if any signs of redness, swelling, pain, or irritation develop.

Professional Salon Image

As a natural hair care salon professional, you have many responsibilities. However, the most important responsibility is protecting and safeguarding your clients' health and safety. It is vital for you to practice all precautions daily. Do not skip steps in trying to save money or product. Cleaning and disinfecting in the salon are a part of your professional business image as well as a requirement of the state regulations. Remember: If you do not protect your client, you will be liable.

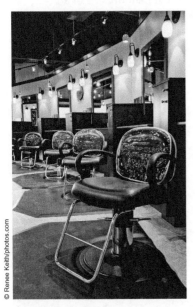

© Renee Keith/photos.com

▲ **Figure 2–9**
Salon wellness depends on salon cleanliness.

Salon Wellness: Professional Salon Image

Salon wellness is the general guide to keeping the salon environment balanced, harmonious, safe, and clean. Providing a harmonious, disease-free, balanced environment involves more than just weekly cleansing. It is a continuous practice of maintaining the preventive standards with clean tools and surfaces as well as ensuring personal hygiene that controls the spread of disease and infection **(Figure 2–9)**.

Be sure that your salon routinely follows these guidelines for cleaning and disinfecting:

• Keep floors and workstations dust-free. Sweep hair off the floor after every client. Mop floors and vacuum carpets every day.

• Control dust, hair, and other debris.

- Cover and empty your facility's garbage receptacles every day. High-traffic salons should remove trash several times each day.

- Empty waste receptacles on salon floor regularly throughout the day. A metal waste receptacle with a self-closing lid works best.

- Keep floors free of debris and unused working materials. When working with hair extensions, do not allow hair to accumulate on the floor or obstruct passageways in the work space.

- Regularly clean air conditioner filters, fans, and ventilators.

- Keep all work areas well lit.

- Clean and disinfect restroom surfaces, including door handles.

- Provide toilet tissue, paper towels, liquid soap, properly disinfected soft-bristle nail brushes, and a container for used brushes in the restroom.

- Do not allow the salon to be used for cooking or living purposes.

- Clean and disinfect all work surfaces after every client.

- Make sure all containers are properly marked and properly stored.

- Never place any tools or implements in your mouth or pockets.

- Properly clean and disinfect all multiuse tools before reusing them.

- Store clean and disinfected tools in a clean, covered container. Clean drawers may be used for storage if only clean items are stored in the drawers. Always isolate used implements from disinfected implements.

- Have clean, disposable paper towels for each client.

- Always properly wash your hands before and after each service.

- Use clean linens and disposable towels on clients. Keep soiled linens separate from clean linens. Use single-use neck strips or clean towels to avoid skin contact with shampoo capes and cutting or chemical protection gowns. If a cape touched the client's skin, do not reuse that cape until it is properly laundered.

- Keep floors in good condition. Clean floors with detergents daily and after any spills to prevent clients from slipping.

- Vacuum carpets and doormats.

- Remove dust, debris, and oil from all surfaces, including dryer hoods, ceiling corners, walls, shelves, and baseboards.

- Plumbing fixtures for wash basins, toilets, and shampoo sinks must be maintained and kept in good condition. These plumbing fixtures are also inspected for compliance with state and local codes.

- Bathrooms must be cleaned daily or more often for high-traffic salons. Every employee is responsible for the cleanliness of any bathroom area used and that all surfaces are kept in order.

- Bathrooms should always be equipped with an ample supply of paper towels, toilet tissue, and a pump-type antiseptic liquid soap. Avoid using bar soaps in the salon.

- Bathroom handles should be regularly wiped or sprayed with a disinfectant.

- After using the restroom and between client services, hands must be scrubbed with an antiseptic (germicide) liquid soap for several minutes. Waterless hand sanitizers contain antiseptics. Sinks and neck rests must be cleaned after every service with disinfectant wipes or disinfectant spray. All sinks should have hot and cold running water and drain properly.

- Never eat or drink while you service a client. Take a break between braiding sessions for relaxing and eating.

- Cooking is prohibited in a working salon.

- Keep refrigerated foods separate from salon products. Some natural oils and herbal solutions should be kept in a cool place; however, never store them with food.

- Natural stylists must wear clean, ironed clothing without tears and holes or uniforms and smocks to protect from dirt and hair clippings.

- Stylists must wear shoes. Shoes should have the appropriate support for services that require stylists to stand for long periods.

- Always give each client clean, freshly laundered towels.

- Never share combs, brushes, clips, and disposable caps between clients.

- Do not use tools or implements that fall on the floor that must be cleaned and disinfected with an Environmental Protection Agency (EPA) grade disinfectant solution.

- Client capes or coverings must never come in contact with bare skin. Use a towel or paper neck strip when draping a client.

- Pets are prohibited in the salon, except those animals that assist the visually impaired or physically challenged.

- Do not allow young children to run in the salon; they should be supervised by a parent or guardian to prevent injury.

- Open flames, gas burners, or lit candles are prohibited. When finishing the end of any synthetic braid extension, be sure to comply with your state rules and regulations regarding "open flame finish."

- Avoid cross-infection by not touching your face, hair, mouth, eyes, or arms when you service a client.

- Wear plastic gloves whenever possible. Gloves will protect the stylist's hands from dirt and debris when removing braids or weaves.

- Never reuse synthetic or human hair worn by another person.

- Wash hands with an antibacterial soap before and after every service. Liquid hand sanitizer or wipes should be available at every station for use by staff and clients. Make sure that both the back of hands and nails are thoroughly scrubbed.

- Never touch a client or coworker who has an open sore or cut. If you are cut, stop work immediately and follow the proper procedure for a blood spill.

- Keep the salon well lit and ventilated.

Your Professional Responsibility

As a salon professional, you have many responsibilities, but none is more important than protecting your clients' health and safety. Never take shortcuts for cleaning and disinfecting. You cannot afford to skip steps or save money when it comes to safety.

- It is your professional and legal responsibility to follow state and federal laws and rules.

- Keep your license current, and notify the licensing agency if you move or change your name.

- Check your state's Website weekly for any changes or updates to rules and regulations.

Myth: Afro Hair Doesn't Grow Long

The truth is that all hair grows. Regardless of the hair type, people's hair can grow on the average of 0.25 inch to 0.5 inch (0.6 cm to 1.3 cm) per month. Hair may appear not to grow, because it continually breaks from the lack of moisture, lack of natural oils, regular trims to remove brittle split ends, regular conditioning treatments, and a proper styling regimen. The key to all healthy textured hair is performing a regular conditioning treatment with moisture, protein, and essential oils that will create a complementary environment for the hair to flourish.

2-1 Proper Hand Washing

Hand washing is one of the most important procedures in your infection control efforts. Every state requires hands to be washed before performing any service.

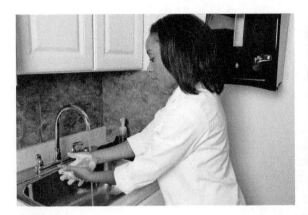

1 Turn on the warm water, wet your hands, and then pump soap from a pump container into the palm of your hand. Rub your hands together, all over and vigorously, until a lather forms. Continue for a minimum of 20 seconds.

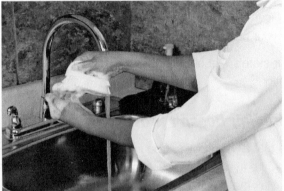

2 Choose a clean, disinfected nail brush. Wet the nail brush, pump soap on it, and brush your nails horizontally back and forth under the free edges. Change the direction of the brush to vertical and move the brush up and down along the nail folds of the fingernails. The process for brushing both hands should take about 60 seconds to finish. Rinse hands in running warm water.

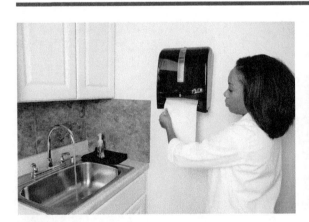

3 Use a clean cloth or paper towel, according to the salon policies, for drying your hands.

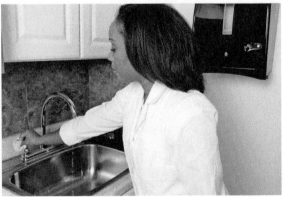

4 After drying your hands, turn off the water with the towel and dispose of the towel.[6]

Review Questions

1. Describe the basic principles and procedures for infection control.
2. Give some examples of state laws and rules regarding infection control.
3. Name the different types of bacteria and their classifications.
4. How are bloodborne pathogens transmitted?
5. Name the three types of decontamination practices, and list their differences.
6. What are Universal Precautions?

Chapter References

1. (2013). *Milady standard esthetics: Advanced* (2nd ed.). Clifton Park, NY: Milady, a part of Cengage Learning.
2. Ibid.
3. Ibid.
4. (2012). *Milady standard cosmetology.* Clifton Park, NY: Milady, a part of Cengage Learning.
5. Ibid.
6. Gerson, J. (2013). *Milady standard esthetics: Fundamentals* (11th ed.). Clifton Park, NY: Milady, a part of Cengage Learning.

CHAPTER 3

Basic Principles for Personal and Professional Success

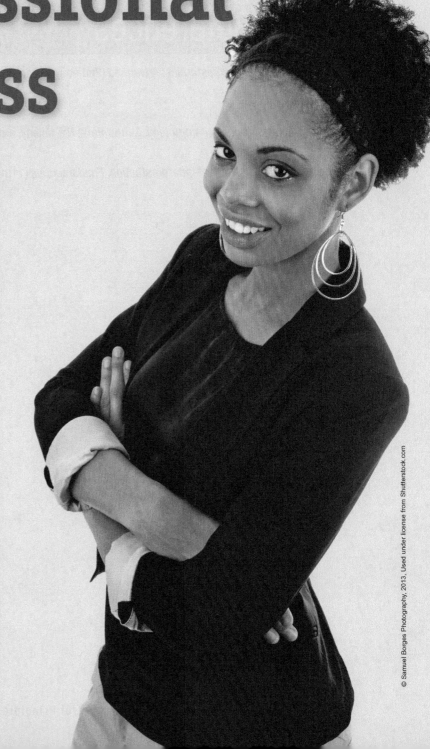

Chapter Outline

- Why Study Basic Principles for Professional and Personal Success?

- Life Skills

- Goal Setting

- Time Management

- Ethics

- Personality Development and Attitude

- Building Client Trust Through Touch

- Maintaining a Professional Attitude

- Preparing Clients for the Natural Hair Care Service

- Nurturing the Client's Total Well-Being

Learning Objectives

After completing this chapter, you should be able to:

☑ **LO1** List the principles that contribute to personal and professional life management skills.

☑ **LO2** Discuss the practical steps to success.

☑ **LO3** Explain how to set long-term and short-term goals.

☑ **LO4** Define ethics.

☑ **LO5** Discuss the most effective ways to manage time.

☑ **LO6** Define personality development and attitude.

☑ **LO7** Discuss how to build client trust.

☑ **LO8** Describe how to maintain a professional attitude.

☑ **LO9** Describe how to nurture the client's total well-being.

Key Terms

Page number indicates where in the chapter the term is used.

L ife has many challenges, and going to school to learn a new skill is just one of many that you will face as you walk this journey. Developing practical life and work skill is vital to your success. Life skills are difficult, and hard-and-fast rules that apply to more structured industries are sometimes absent in the salon. By its nature, the salon is a creative workplace where you are expected to exercise your artistic talent. The salon is also a highly social atmosphere that requires strong self-discipline and excellent people skills. Besides making a solid connection with each client, you must always stay focused on the task at hand. You must display competence, sensitivity, awareness, and enthusiasm every time you service the client. There are distinctive attributes in the relationship between the natural stylist and the client. In general, the beauty industry focuses primarily on efficiency and services that enhance the outer self. In the field of natural hair care, the stylist must be able to recognize the interrelationship between the client's hair, body, emotional, and physical environment in order to achieve the best results and have a satisfied customer. To the natural hair stylist, true beauty is the balance between the inner self and the outer self. Providing excellent service may encourage the client to begin her journey.

No matter how you feel personally, no matter how tired you may be or how many hours you have worked, you must always focus on the client and provide excellent service. Life skills are really the tools to manage, address, or handle any challenge or difficulty that you may encounter personally or in your career. A successful personal life and career are totally dependent on self-discipline, respect for others, good manners, and a positive attitude.

Why Study Basic Principles for Personal and Professional Success?

The natural stylist should study and have a thorough understanding of the basic principles for professional and personal success to have the best start to achieve all your life's goals. These fundamental rules of order are principles that will follow you throughout your life. The following principles are tools to succeed in the salon and in your life:

■ The practice of good life skills will lead to a more satisfying and productive career in the natural hair care industry.

■ The natural stylist works with a variety of personality types; having good life skills will help you to have positive and productive interactions with your clients.

■ Working well with work associates and management will require effective life skills.

■ Having good life management skills is a personal decision to have balance and wellness in your personal life as well as in relationships with others.

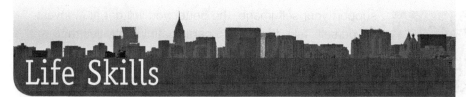

Life Skills

Having **life skills** is having the ability to manage your life successfully in order to resolve social issues. These abilities include anger management, money management, communication skills, conflict resolution, career management, and other essential life components that extend through your entire life.

life skills the tools needed to manage, address, or handle any challenge or difficulty that you may encounter personally or in your career.

The following attributes are just a few of the life skills you will need to be successful in life and in the salon:

- Have good self-awareness.

- Have good self-esteem.

- Genuinely care about servicing and helping others.

- Make and maintain good, healthy friendships.

- Have a good sense of humor when difficulties arise.

- Maintain a cooperative and positive attitude **(Figure 3–1)**.

- Have a strong work ethic and principles.

- Have a strong sense of responsibility.

- Successfully adapt to change and to challenging people.

- Create goals and complete them.

- Become more organized, so that you're not distracted or confused.

- Use your common sense, or sound practical judgment, when making decisions. ✔ **LO1**

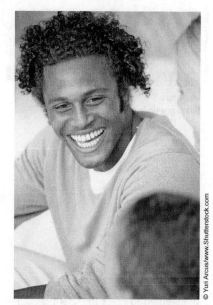

▲ Figure 3–1
Maintaining a positive attitude is integral to success.

The Road to Success

Though it is the most tangible form of success, money is not the only thing that matters in achieving your goals. In operating a profitable salon business, money is certainly a necessity, but defining success is a very personal experience. Some basic principles form the foundation to all personal and business success. The path to success can begin with the following principles:

- Build **self-esteem**. Self-esteem is based on inner strength, respect for yourself, and a trust in your ability to achieve your goals.

- **Visualize success**. To imagine or visualize is to create a mental picture of your dream salon or career. It begins with trusting in your ability to achieve your goals. It all begins with knowing that if you can conceive an idea, you can achieve your goals.

- Build on your strengths, not your weaknesses. Do the things that make you feel good, support your positive self-image, and let these things feed your soul. The more you do things that uplift and

self-esteem an inner strength and respect for yourself, and a trust in your ability to achieve your goals.

visualize success the practice of imagining or creating a mental picture of your dream salon, career, life, and so on.

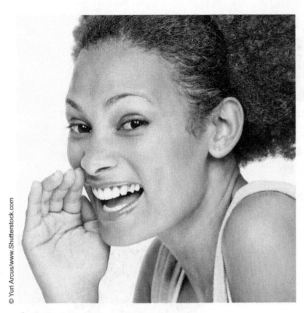

▲ Figure 3–2
Salon gossip is always bad news.

support your self-image, the better you will get at it. Invest in yourself: Take the time to participate in activities that replenish you and you are good at doing.

- Be kind to yourself. Overly self-critical thinking or negative thoughts will work against you, so don't beat yourself up with negative thoughts. Mistakes happen, and when they do, learn from them and correct them. Tell yourself you will do better next time.

- Practice new behaviors. Creating success is a skill. It takes time to learn, but you can develop your skill for success by practicing positive new behaviors. Positive new behaviors might include being on time, using better grammar, and standing tall and erect.

- Keep your personal life separate from your work. Talking about coworkers, associates, or management is counterproductive. It only harms the work environment; it does not help. Avoid all salon gossip **(Figure 3–2)**.

- Find balance. To be successful, a person needs a balance between work and personal time. Know when to put down the appointment book or comb to enjoy your friends, family, social entertainment, and activities.

- Good manners and respect for self and others are vehicles to success. Exercise good manners by using words like *please, thank you,* and *excuse me.* Displaying good manners and a respectful attitude are the greatest tools of influence in the salon. Practice **reflective listening** by listening to the client and repeating, in your own words, what you think the client has told you. This is the first step to creating a connection with the client.

- Stay productive. Three bad habits can keep you from maintaining peak performance: procrastination, perfectionism, and lack of a game plan. You will see an almost instant improvement in your productivity when you eliminate these behaviors.

  1. **Procrastination** is putting off until tomorrow what you can do today. This destructive habit is a characteristic of poor study and work habits (for example, "I'll study tomorrow instead of today"). Make this your motto: "Do the worst first." The project you most want to avoid doing is the one that you must do first. Get it out of the way, and then every task you do after that becomes easier.

  2. **Perfectionism** is an unhealthy compulsion to do things perfectly. Success is not defined as doing everything perfectly. In fact, someone who never makes a mistake may not be able to take risks necessary for growth and improvement. Taking calculated risks is a part of every successful career or business. The best definition of success is not giving up, even when things get really tough.

reflective listening the practice of listening to what the client is saying and repeating it in your own words.

procrastination the habit of delaying something that usually requires immediate attention.

perfectionism an unhealthy compulsion to do things perfectly.

3. Lacking a **game plan**. Having a game plan is the conscious act of planning your life instead of letting things just happen. Although the overall game or life plan is usually organized into large blocks of time (5 to 10 years), it is just as important to set daily, monthly, and yearly goals. Where do you want to be in your career five years from now? What do you have to do this week, this month, and this year to move closer to your goal? ☑ **LO2**

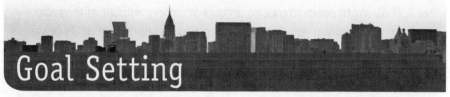

Goal Setting

Some people never have a fixed goal in mind. They go through life one day at a time without really deciding what they want, where they can find it, or how they are going to live their lives once they get it. They drift aimlessly from one activity to the next. Does this describe you? Or do you have direction, drive, desire, and a dream? What vision do you have for your future? Do you have a reasonable idea of how to attain your goals?

Goal setting is the identification of long- and short-term goals that help you decide what you want out of your life. When you know what you want, you can draw a circle around your destination and chart the best course to get you there. By mapping out your goals, you will see where you need to focus your attention and what you need to learn in order to fulfill your dreams **(Figure 3–3)**.

How Goal Setting Works

There are two types of goals: short term and long term. An example of a short-term goal is to get through a competency exam successfully. Another short-term goal would be graduating from school. Short-term goals are usually considered to be those you wish to accomplish in a year or less.

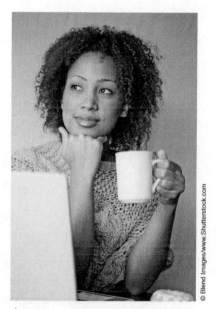

▲ Figure 3–3
Think about and map out your goals.

© Blend Images/www.Shutterstock.com

REAL-LIFE GOAL SETTING

Many salon managers help you set goals based on the salon's criteria. One common goal is for team members to sell retail products to a specific number or percentage of clients or in an amount equal to a percentage of billed services. For example, stylists might be required to retail at least 30 percent of gross.

Another common salon goal is that a technician should be booked a certain amount of the time and maintain a specific client retention rate. Usually, you cannot raise your prices unless you are booked 80 to 90 percent of the time and retain about 70 percent of your clients.

Goals that salons set are almost always tied to your income. In turn, goals that technicians will set for themselves are often based on what they want to earn. Salon managers will help you break down financial goals into attainable, daily goals. For example, if you want to gross $10,000 more a year, you need to earn an additional $27.39 per day. Of course, you don't work seven days a week. A more realistic number is based on working five days a week, 52 weeks out of the year. You need to gross $38.46 more per day, and fortunately there are many different ways to do it in the salon business. You can sell retail to half your clients; you can upsell braiding services and back-bar treatments; or you can get more clients.

Long-term goals are measured in larger sections of time—5 years, 10 years, or even longer. An example of a long-term goal is becoming a salon owner in 5 years.

Once you have organized your thinking around your goals, write them down in short-term and long-term columns, and divide each set of goals into workable segments. In this way, your goals will not seem out of sight or overwhelming. For example, one of your long-term goals should be to get your license to practice natural hair care and braiding. At first, getting this license might seem to require an overwhelming amount of time and effort. However, when you separate this goal into short-term goals (such as going to class on time, completing homework assignments, and mastering techniques), you see that each step on the way to the long-term goal can be accomplished without too much difficulty or stress.

The important thing to remember about goal setting is to have a plan and to reexamine it often to make sure that you are staying on track. Even people who have fame, fortune, and widespread respect continue to set goals for themselves. Although they may adjust their goals and action plans as they go along, successful people know that goals move them toward additional successes. ☑ **LO3**

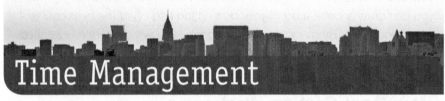

Time Management

One thing that all time management experts agree on is that each of us has an *inner organizer*. When we pay attention to our natural rhythms, we can learn how to manage our time efficiently, allowing us to reach our goals faster and with less frustration. Here are some of the most effective ways to manage time:

prioritize the process of ordering tasks on your to-do list from most important to least important.

- Learn to **prioritize** by ordering tasks on your to-do list from most important to least important.

- When designing your own time management system, make sure it will work for you. For example, if you are a person who needs a fair amount of flexibility, schedule in some blocks of unstructured time.

FOCUS ON

THE GOAL
Determine whether your goal-setting plan is an effective one by asking yourself these key questions:

- Are there specific skills I will need to learn in order to meet my goals?
- Is the information I need to reach my goals readily available?
- Am I willing to seek out a mentor or a coach to enhance my learning?
- What is the best method or approach that will allow me to accomplish my goals?
- Am I open to finding better ways of putting my plan into practice?

- Never take on more than you can handle. Learn to say no firmly but kindly, and mean it. You will find it easier to complete your tasks if you limit your activities and do not spread yourself too thin.

- Learn problem-solving techniques that will save you time and needless frustration.

- Give yourself some down time whenever you are frustrated, overwhelmed, worried, or feeling guilty. You lose valuable time and energy when you are in a negative state of mind. Unfortunately, in some situations—such as when you are in the classroom—you cannot get up and walk away. To handle these difficult times, try practicing the technique of deep breathing. Just fill your lungs as much as you can and then exhale slowly. After about 5 to 10 breaths, you will usually find that you have calmed down and your inner balance has been restored.

- Carry a notepad, an organizer, or your electronic notepad with you at all times. You never know when a good idea might strike or when you will need to add a task to your schedule. Write these things down before they slip your mind!

- Make daily, weekly, and monthly schedules that show exam times, study sessions, and any other regular commitments. Plan your leisure time around these commitments, rather than the other way around.

- Identify times during the day when you are typically energetic and times when you typically want or need to relax. Plan your schedule accordingly.

ACTivity

It is estimated that as much as four hours in the average person's day are spent checking e-mail, looking at Websites, and watching videos. The average teenager sends nearly 80 text messages a day! To find out if you are managing your time well, try this exercise:

- Write down the time in the morning when you first go online, check e-mail, or send a text message.
- Do what you normally do online, then note the time you finish these activities.
- Throughout the day, try to estimate (and add to your list) how much additional time you spend on these activities.
- Add up the total time at the end of your day.

Are you surprised? Time management experts recommend that you work for the first 45 minutes to an hour of the day, avoiding e-mailing, Web browsing, and texting during that time. Instead, use the time to plan your day, review reading materials for school, or do other work. This first hour of the day can be the best time to accomplish something concrete, because it is quiet and often free of interruptions. Starting your day by being productive helps you develop good time management skills for life.

- Reward yourself with a special treat or activity for work well done and time managed efficiently.

- Do not neglect physical activity. Remember that exercise and recreation stimulate clear thinking and efficient planning.

- Schedule at least one block of free time each day. This will be your hedge against events that come up unexpectedly, such as car trouble, babysitting problems, helping a friend in need, or any other unforeseen circumstance.

- Understand the value of to-do lists for the day and the week. These lists help you prioritize tasks and activities, a key element to organizing your time efficiently.

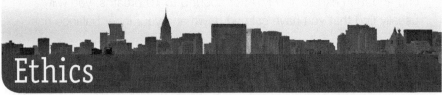

Ethics

Ethics are a set of standards, moral judgments, and compliances determined by the state board for the practice and licensing of natural hair care and braiding. There are standards of behavior that professional hair care specialists are expected to reflect. Ethics are not just rules and regulations, but informal expectations of a professional in the industry. Ethics are the morals, principles, or code of conduct that we live by. As a businessperson, the stylist must handle transactions with many different people effectively. Coworkers, managers, clients, repair people, and sales distributors are the kinds of people you can come in contact with daily. ✓ **LO4**

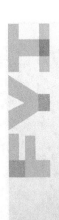

REAL-LIFE TIME MANAGEMENT
In the salon, the most important aspect of time management is staying on schedule with your bookings so that you can greet each client at the scheduled appointment time. This means completing the service during the time allotted. Some salons book haircuts on the hour; others book them in intervals of 45 minutes. Accomplished technicians do a cut in half an hour, but they usually schedule clients for longer so they can upsell more services if the opportunity presents itself.

Making sure that you arrive at the salon on time, starting your first client as soon as he or she arrives, and staying on schedule will take you a long way toward success as a natural stylist. The front desk and salon manager can be a tremendous help if you find yourself falling behind or if you have the opportunity to add on a service and need help fitting it into your day. With experience, you'll learn to accommodate late clients and add-on services like a pro (Figure 3–4). ✓ **LO5**

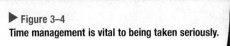

▶ Figure 3–4
Time management is vital to being taken seriously.

Code of Conduct

Ethical conduct will create honest, stress-free relationships with these people that will not only enhance your professional image, but help operate your business profitably. Ethical conduct improves your reputation in the community and builds a client's confidence in you, so much so that your clients begin to refer others to you. Personal referrals are the best form of promotion to keep your business successful.

The following is a basic code of conduct you should practice:

1. Be responsible for the energy that you bring into the salon. The service you offer is a reflection of you. Your work is an extension of yourself.

2. Give everyone the best quality you can physically offer. Be capable and competent.

3. Avoid making offers of services you cannot efficiently provide. If a client requests a style you cannot do, do not try to do it.

4. Be honest with all people. Your reputation depends on it.

5. Be courteous. You will meet people from different cultures and backgrounds. Respect their feelings, religious beliefs, and customs.

6. Comply with all state regulations. By following them, you are contributing to the health and welfare of your clients.

7. Maintain a safe environment not only for your clients, but your coworkers, too.

8. Sell products and services that the client needs or wants. Do not be overzealous in promoting a particular line of goods unless you truly believe in it.

9. Good credit is necessary if you want to borrow more money to open a business or buy a house. Good credit is built by paying your bills on time and by paying off balances in full.

Maintain Your Image

To improve and maintain a professional image, natural stylists should always look to upgrade their skills and education, and work on self-improvement. Whenever the opportunity presents itself, a technician should look at improving or keeping up with the following:

- Braiding and styling techniques

- Industry innovations

- Management skills and technology

- Self-image

- Communications skills

Here's a Tip!..........

Good Credit and Your Student Loan

You lose good credit by making late payments or defaulting on a loan, including your student loan. Repaying your student loan promptly is a good step toward building a good credit rating. Not paying your student loan on time will result in a poor credit rating. Here are some tips to help you when it comes to borrowing and repaying your student loans:

- Borrow only what you need for school and school-related expenses.

- Know what you are borrowing. Read all the information.

- Attend and pay attention to your entrance and exit loan counseling sessions.

- Pay your loan on time.

- Keep in touch with your loan servicer—they are there to help!

- Keep your paperwork organized.

- Know that you must repay your loan whether you drop out of school or graduate, and whether you find a job or not.

- Understand the consequences of defaulting on the loan:

  - The entire loan will become due and payable immediately

  - Garnishment of federal income tax refunds

  - Garnishment of wages

  - Ineligible to receive any additional federal student aid (including grants)

Personality Development and Attitude

Some occupations require less interaction with people than others. For example, computer programmers do not usually interact with all different sorts of people every day. Natural stylists, however, deal with people from all walks of life—every day, all day. It is useful, therefore, to have some sense of how different personality traits and attitudes can affect your success.

Refer regularly to the following characteristics of a healthy, positive attitude to ensure that they match your self-description.

- *Diplomacy.* Being assertive is a good thing because it helps people understand your position. However, it is a short step from assertive to aggressive or even bullying. Take your attitude temperature to see how well you practice the art of diplomacy. Diplomacy, also known as tact, is the ability to deliver truthful, even sometimes critical or difficult, messages in a kind way.

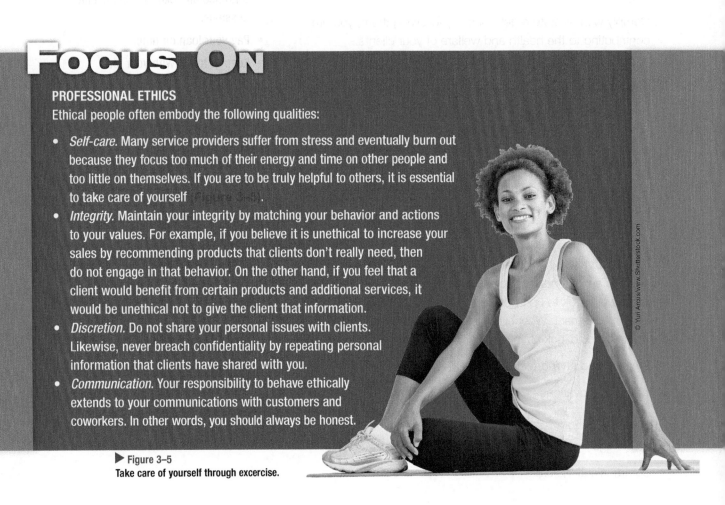

FOCUS ON

PROFESSIONAL ETHICS

Ethical people often embody the following qualities:

- *Self-care.* Many service providers suffer from stress and eventually burn out because they focus too much of their energy and time on other people and too little on themselves. If you are to be truly helpful to others, it is essential to take care of yourself **(Figure 3–5)**.
- *Integrity.* Maintain your integrity by matching your behavior and actions to your values. For example, if you believe it is unethical to increase your sales by recommending products that clients don't really need, then do not engage in that behavior. On the other hand, if you feel that a client would benefit from certain products and additional services, it would be unethical not to give the client that information.
- *Discretion.* Do not share your personal issues with clients. Likewise, never breach confidentiality by repeating personal information that clients have shared with you.
- *Communication.* Your responsibility to behave ethically extends to your communications with customers and coworkers. In other words, you should always be honest.

▶ Figure 3–5
Take care of yourself through excercise.

© Yuri Arcurs/www.Shutterstock.com

- *Pleasing tone of voice.* The tone of your voice is an inborn personality trait, but if your natural voice is harsh or if you tend to mumble, you can consciously improve by speaking more softly or more clearly. Also, if you have a positive attitude, this will shine through in a pleasant delivery, even if your tone of voice is not ideal (Figure 3–6). ☑ **LO6**

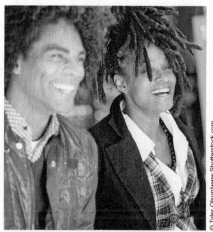

▲ Figure 3–6
Having a positive attitude can translate from your mood to your tone of voice.

Nurturing the Whole Person

A holistic approach to nurturing the client is one of the unique aspects of this rewarding industry. The natural stylist focuses on the client's physical, psychological, and emotional needs. The client deserves to have a unified self; to connect the inside self with the outside one. A holistic approach to natural hair services integrates these factors into a program designed for the client's complete well-being. This includes a healthy and balanced diet, vitamins and supplemental herbs, and regular exercise; it also includes dance, yoga, biking, playing sports, and living more consciously to replenish our bodies, our minds, and our earth. How we live in the world affects the world, our community, our homes, our families, our careers, and our bodies. An external stressor could be as simple as waiting in heavy morning traffic. Internal stressors could include anger, depression, anxiety, as well consuming processed foods with preservatives and sugary drinks. The stylist must be knowledgeable of some of the external and internal stresses that affect the client's total well-being. We will discuss how to integrate nutrition and healthy hair in Chapters 7 and 8. With this harmonized approach to natural hair care, the stylist views the client's beauty and health as being equally important. A natural stylist must never endanger the client's hair in order to create a fashionable style. The natural stylist's view is, "It is better to prevent than to cure." Avoiding harsh chemicals, abusive tools, and excessive styling and heat practices are preventative measures in keeping hair healthy (Figure 3–7).

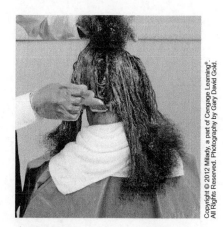

▲ Figure 3–7
Chemical relaxers can damage the hair.

Your Health

Healthy hair is the result of a healthy body and mind. The natural stylist is acutely aware that an attractive client is a healthy client (Figure 3–8). The whole person is equal to the sum of his or her parts and, as a result, a healthy client will have healthy hair. Our "inner" health is reflected in our hair. Good nutrition, exercise to maintain good circulation, and a peaceful or stress-free state of mind are the components to healthy hair. We do not live in a vacuum. Therefore, our environment affects our hair. Poor air and water quality, lack of vitamin D (from the sun), and stressful work or home environments are some of the external pressures that affect the hair and cause hair loss.

The Holistic Approach

With the holistic approach, the stylist is aware of these interrelated factors and is capable of educating clients, raising client consciousness, and reconnecting them with their natural hair. And so with the natural hair care salon, the stylist offers a quieter, relaxed, spa-like environment that includes soothing music, proper lighting, ample ventilation, and inspiring or invigorating colors.

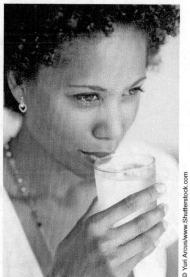

▲ Figure 3–8
Remember to drink water every day.

Building Client Trust Through Touch

Touch is a form of therapy and healing. Being touched and having the ability to touch is a vital human need. The natural hair care professional is basically licensed to touch. Touching another person and being touched is important to our emotional, physical, and total well-being. It is a part of communication. A simple touch makes us feel connected, reduces anxiety, creates bonds, and can improve our appearance. For professional natural hair stylists, their hands are "healing" tools that help build client trust. Shampooing, massaging, braiding, or locking should be calming, lulling, and gentle. The client should always be in a relaxed state. Some protective styles with extensions are more soothing than others. In cases where the braiding may be more stressful, you should inform the client before starting the service. The touch used in providing any natural or braiding service not only is a relaxing technique but also can be a stimulating technique. A soft but firm, deliberate touch is what will create the style. When braiding, the stylist executes the technique by using the fingertips—*not* the entire weight of the hand.

Within a period of one year, a stylist may service each client at least 6 to 12 times. During this service, a stylist is privy to many of the client's life-changing experiences, such as births, deaths, graduations, divorces, and weddings. This sharing and personal exchange leads to an extended-family–like environment within the salon. The trust that evolves over time creates a bond and a sense of security that positions the stylist as the client's confidant. ✓ **LO7**

The stylist's touch is also therapeutic and nurturing to the client. The repeated massaging and touch releases stress and begins to break down the client's inhibitions. The client becomes more open, spiritually and emotionally. The natural stylist's goal is to reassure and comfort the client so that he or she makes the right styling choices. The stylist must also realize that healthy hair is more than what is used topically on the head. Healthy hair is the result of a healthy body and mind. For example, in our hectic lives, stress can be a major factor in certain hair-loss problems. So in a natural hair care salon, it is imperative for the specialist to offer a quiet, relaxed, spa-like environment. Services that will begin to set the tone for the client–stylist relationship may be a relaxing shampoo/massage, followed by a soothing steam treatment **(Figure 3–9)**.

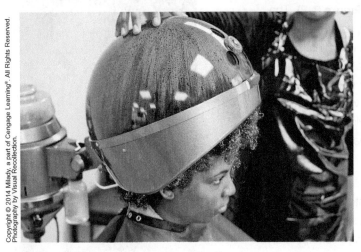

▲ Figure 3–9
The soothing touch.

Hair Doctors?

Some clients look to the stylist to motivate, nurture, and respond to their day-to-day life stories. At this special moment, a more personal bonding takes place between the client and stylist. The relationship between the natural hair stylist and the client can be compared with the relationship between a doctor and a patient. In that sense, natural hair care specialists become more than artists or hair designers. They become what those in the industry typically call "hair doctors."

The client–stylist intimate contact generally begins with these three procedures:

1. A relaxing, rhythmic shampoo that is also a stress-releasing scalp massage. It removes more than dirt and oil; it also removes the client's inhibitions, tension, and clarifies.

2. Conditioning treatments, ranging from stimulating and refreshing to slow and relaxing, create a soothing aromatic experience.

3. Herbal rinse or protein conditioning to fortify the hair.

While the stylist performs these three procedures, clients may begin to expose themselves, their flaws, and their concerns. As a client becomes more comfortable to the specialist, the stylist often begins to see a different side of that client's personality. This relationship intensifies as the client reveals his or her imperfections. The interaction builds to a level of total acceptance as the client experiences less fear and self-doubt. This acceptance also allows the client to feel safe and not judged. Acceptance, and a wonderful shampoo/conditioning experience, deepens the relationship between the stylist and the client; trust starts to flourish.

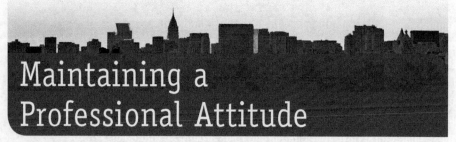

Maintaining a Professional Attitude

The key to a professional relationship with your clients is learning to develop effective communication skills and maintaining a level of professionalism without alienating the client.

Here are some of the various forms of communication:

- Attitude

- Tone of voice

- Body language

- Manner of dress

- Personal grooming

passive–underreact a personal communication style characterized by almost never taking responsibility for mistakes. These people let others make decisions for them, usually have a soft low voice, and have low self-esteem.

aggressive–overreact a personal communication style characterized by taking too much responsibility for others. This person gives unasked-for advice, makes decisions for other people, and criticizes others (constructive or otherwise). They may have a loud voice, be pushy and/or bossy, and always seem to know better than everyone else.

assertive–effective a personal communication style characterized by responding to situations in a positive and appropriate manner. This person is willing to listen, is open, has high self-esteem, shares observations and respects others' viewpoints, presents a good attitude, and stays balanced. They control their emotions and do not let emotions control them.

role playing to act out the attitudes, actions, and discourse of another in a mock situation in order to understand a differing point of view or social interaction.

Styles of Communication

People have three basic communication styles: passive, aggressive, and assertive.

1. **Passive–underreacts** to situations. People who use this style almost never take responsibility for mistakes; let others make decisions for them; usually have a soft, low voice; have low self-esteem.

2. **Aggressive–overreacts** to situations. A person using this communication style takes too much responsibility for others; gives unasked-for advice; makes decisions for other people; criticizes (constructive or otherwise); has a loud voice; is pushy and/or bossy; always knows better than everyone else.

3. **Assertive–effective** in a positive way. Someone using this style reacts to situations appropriately; is willing to listen; is open; has high self-esteem; shares observations and respects others' viewpoints; presents a good attitude; stays balanced; controls emotion, and does not let emotion control her.

By using effective communication techniques, the client and stylist become more comfortable in one another's presence. Good communication also helps the stylist to meet the client's expectations. Clients often view the stylist as a professional, simply because they think of a professional as one

ACTivity

ROLE PLAYING

Role playing is an activity that requires the students in the class to pretend or act out the characteristics of a personality type or communication style. To set up a game, choose three students to play the parts of a manager, a stylist, and a new client coming in for a consultation. Then, assign the three different communication types to each student/actor: The manager can pretend to have an assertive communication style, the stylist may display an aggressive communication style, and the client can display a desire for service, but pretend to be passive. Students can explore many different combinations of role playing with these characters. Have fun! Change the roles around so that each student has a different role to play, and each character displays a different communication skill. Discuss which communication styles work in the salon and which ones create a problem in providing service for the client. Have the students practice some of these techniques when role playing:

- Listen to what is being said—and what is not said.
- Learn to filter your words before speaking.
- Always try to mirror the client, matching verbal and nonverbal communication using positive body language.
- Give feedback, and answer questions and comments.
- Smile and use direct eye contact.
- Try to respond to the client's needs.

who earns his or her livelihood by performing specific skills and services. Therefore, at all times the stylist must project a proper image and positive attitude, be of good character, and adhere to simple moral codes of ethics. ✓ **LO8**

Preparing Clients for the Natural Hair Care Service

Keeping in mind that the special relationship between the client and stylist is holistic, the kinds of services a specialist provides are mostly therapeutic—not in a medical sense, but in a manner that gives the salon a soothing spa-type quality. The average client who walks into a natural hair salon generally has a history of chemically treated hair. The client is looking for someone to guide him or her through the *transition* of "going natural" or wearing "chemical-free" hairstyles. For clients who have suffered any amount of hair loss or scalp damage, the natural stylist or braider is particularly needed to restore, treat, and correct the abused hair. For clients who have little or no history of chemically treated hair, the specialist can offer preventive services to aid the client. Clients with natural, healthy hair are offered an array of sculpting and grooming services to maintain healthy hair.

In some cases, the stylist can work in conjunction with a dermatologist, or help clients with scalp disorders to treat and camouflage their hair loss. The natural stylist is available to coach clients in discovering themselves without the use of chemicals, to help them abandon the social confines of what is traditionally accepted as beautiful, and to redefine their natural aesthetic.

The following basic hair care services are particularly essential for the natural stylist:

- Help clients understand and appreciate the natural beauty that is inherently their own through historical photos and braid style books.

- Focus on the positive attributes of textured hair—its strength, luster, and ability to grow.

- Help clients to see their hair's potential by demonstrating the benefits and features of new products.

- Redefine how clients view their hair by teaching them to respect their hair in its natural state.

- Build clients' self-confidence by helping them to look good as well as feel good about their natural state.

- Demonstrate and explain the internal and external factors that directly affect healthy hair.

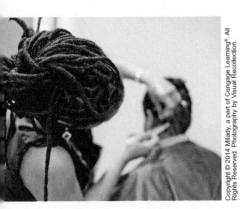

▲ Figure 3–10
Trust between the stylist and the client is extremely important.

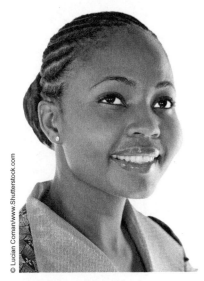

▲ Figure 3–11
This braided style is work appropriate.

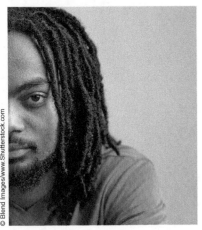

▲ Figure 3–12
Dreadlock style.

beauty wellness a holistic approach to natural hair services that views the client's beauty and health as being equally important.

Nurturing the Client's Total Well-Being

When the stylist has gained the client's trust, the client respects the stylist as a professional, and there is a clear understanding of what services are being provided **(Figure 3–10)**. The final step in the client–stylist relationship is learning how to nurture the client's total well-being. Perhaps in no other field of cosmetology today is this aspect of hair care so vital to the natural stylist and braid designer.

Protective styles, braids, and locs have been controversial in the workplace. Some salons provide counseling for clients determined to wear what is culturally aesthetic to them as well as for clients who have been the object of discrimination **(Figure 3–11)**. Intricate braiding styles and fashions can take 8 to 10 hours, sometimes days, to complete. They are generally not disposable hairdos that can be washed away or brushed out. With proper care, a braiding pattern can last up to three months. Clients must understand that they will be living with a particular hairstyle for long periods of time. Therefore, they must be committed to the hair design and have a positive self-image to carry it off through what can be called a "hair recovery/transitional phase." This transitional phase consists of the time and/or process in which the client's hair grows significantly in length and volume. This process can take several months or up to two years, depending on the damage level of the hair and the hair length the client wishes to obtain.

Referring Clients to Other Stylists

It is not unusual for a stylist to refer clients to another stylist simply because a client is too apprehensive and not quite ready for the total natural or braided look. The last thing a stylist wishes to do is spend hours on a braiding style and have the client reject it, demanding that all the braids be removed. Not only is it time-consuming for the stylist, but it could mean a loss of income for the business. Consultations, which are discussed in Chapter 4, are extremely important in determining a client's readiness—especially when the client wants the ultimate natural style: locks **(Figure 3–12)**.

Your clients are looking for someone to guide them through the transition to going natural. The principles of nurturing and supporting clients are not simple matters for most hair salons. Some clients have put their jobs in jeopardy simply because they chose to wear natural or African braid styles to work. At the start of the client–stylist relationship, a stylist must decide what level of support to offer the client. Another aspect of the client's well-being is helping him or her to understand the general physical connection to having healthy hair—**beauty wellness**. Because this is a process of re-education for many clients, the stylist may have to discuss, support, and inform the client about a nutrient-rich diet, supplements, herbs, botanicals, and oils or butters.

Be Observant of Your Client

When working with a client, a stylist can quickly identify early signs of stress and thinning hair. This problem is more readily observed when the hair is natural as opposed to being chemically treated. With chemically treated hair, such problems as hair loss, thinning, and breakage can be directly related to hair products, so these problems are not often seen as stress-related hair loss. Yet, helping clients learn to cope with stress may be another way for the stylist to support their total well-being. Once again, good communication skills will help determine the needs of each client.

To support the well-being of the client, the stylist must be prepared to do the following:

1. Coach the client through the hair recovery and/or transitional phase of natural hair care.

2. Dispel the myths and stigmas of naturally textured hair.

3. Educate the client about health and nutrition, suggest reading materials, and provide relevant information.

4. Refer new clients to other clients who are successfully wearing natural and African hairstyles.

5. Keep an open dialogue with the client to allow them to release and discuss their concerns.

6. Follow up with clients, helping them to see themselves as others see them.

Ethical conduct will create honest, stress-free relationships with those around you. Sharing and personal exchange leads to an extended-family-like environment within the salon. There are basically three styles of communication: passive, aggressive, and assertive. The natural stylist is available to coach clients in discovering themselves without the use of chemicals. The final step in the client–stylist relationship is learning how to nurture the client's total well-being. Help the client to understand the general physical connection to having healthy hair. ☑ **LO9**

Myth: Pressed Hair Is Natural and Can Return to Its Original Texture

Although thermally pressed hair is mechanically straightened with direct heat and not chemically, it is not virgin. Natural hair is unaltered virgin hair. Using excessive heat on textured hair can permanently damage the curl pattern or coil configuration. In some cases, after only one service with a hot comb or flat iron, the natural hair texture will never go back to its natural curl. There are better options to lengthening and elongating natural hair that will allow the tresses to return to their original texture without causing breakage or damage. Gentler controlled heat with professional blowdryers that are temperature-controlled and stretching the hair can offer straight options while keeping the hair healthy.

Review Questions

1. What are the three bad habits that can keep you from reaching and/or maintaining your peak performance?
2. List three ways a stylist can improve and maintain a professional self-image.
3. True or false: The stylist views the client's beauty and health as being equally important.
4. Define life skills. Why are life skills important to have as a natural stylist?
5. What are three basic styles of communication? Which style of communication is the most effective when dealing with clients and coworkers in a natural salon?
6. Why is reflective listening important?

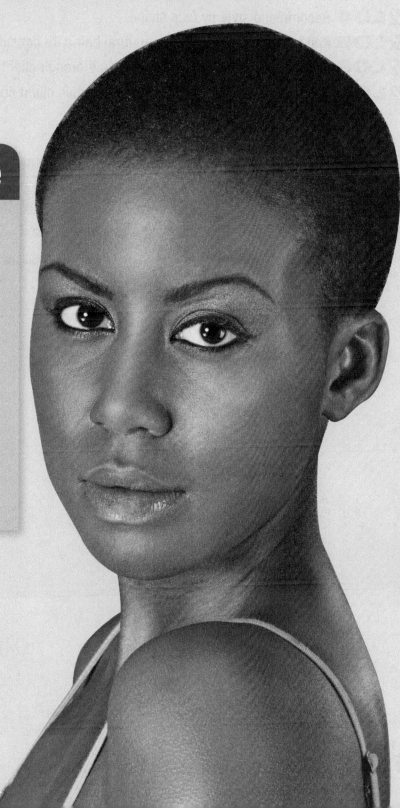

Chapter Outline

- Why Study the Professional Consultation?

- Communicating and Establishing the Client Journey

- The Natural Stylist: Determining Your Signature Look

- The Client's Journey

- Redefining the Client's Perception of Beauty

- Types of Facial Structures

- Consultation Basics

Learning Objectives

After completing this chapter, you should be able to:

☑ **LO1** Explain why communication is important to the natural stylist.

☑ **LO2** Address issues with clients due to insecurity about appearance.

☑ **LO3** Determine the importance of facial shape in the outcome of a style.

☑ **LO4** Recommend style by face shape.

☑ **LO5** Know the terms specific to a natural hair care consultation.

☑ **LO6** List the 17 questions necessary for a thorough client consultation.

☑ **LO7** Explain the steps necessary for an effective client consultation.

Key Terms

Page number indicates where in the chapter the term is used.

client consultation form
p. 84

effective communication
p. 77

reflective listening
p. 84

signature look
p. 78

The consultation between the new client and the natural stylist is the greatest opportunity for the stylist to determine precisely what a potential client's needs are and to ensure client satisfaction with the end result.

Why Study the Professional Consultation?

Natural stylists should study and have a thorough understanding of the professional consultation because:

- Performing a consultation will ensure that clients get what they want and need from their services.

- A thorough client consultation will help you avoid any unwanted reactions.

- Effective client consultations keep your clientele feeling great and can generate repeat customers.

Communicating and Establishing the Client Journey

Natural stylists are in the business of personal service. It is important to have effective professional communication skills that build trust, clarity, and lasting relationships. As natural hair care specialists, we are to provide counseling in specialized areas of natural hair care and styling. Although it is important to have technical and artistic skills, that is just the first stage of developing your career.

Mastering Communication

It is vital to master the art of communication and relationship building. Successful communication in the salon is important because:

- It is the foundation to all lasting relationships with employees, coworkers, and clients.

- **Effective communication**, or the successful sharing of information, will be necessary when handling interpersonal issues that require clarity and resolution.

- Professional communication guarantees that clients will receive great service and enjoy their salon experience, and it encourages continued patronage.

- Controlled, effective communication is vitally important when helping clients who are "going natural" or who are in "transition" to know all the possibilities that their hair texture can offer and when assisting them in taking their personal path of self-discovery. ☑ **LO1**

effective communication
the act of successfully sharing information between two people or a group of people so that the information is successfully and completely understood.

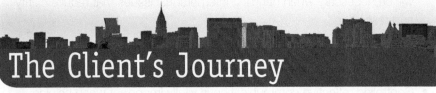

The Natural Stylist: Determining Your Signature Look

To serve your clients well, you must be truthful and honest with them. First, you must be clear about what your own **signature look** or service will be in the salon. You cannot be everything to everyone. What do you do best? What is your passion? Is it contemporary lock grooming and styling, or traditional hair sculpting like cornrows, or do you provide more comprehensive services for textured hair? It is important to know your niche or specialty. Your signature look is one of the reasons a client is in the salon—to receive your particular service, reflecting your personality and your signature touch.

Market Yourself and Be Honest with Your Client

This is the time to sell your service and yourself. Be warm and friendly, using direct eye contact to help the client feel at ease **(Figure 4–1)**.

No stylists in business for themselves would suggest turning clients away. Sometimes, though, it is in the stylist's best interest to be forthright and honest with potential clients and, if necessary, to refer their business to another salon that can offer a particular service. In the end, the stylist earns more respect, and the client—if he or she decides to receive a service—will be even more satisfied with the process. Trust is earned. Be honest and clear about your skill set, and give the client the opportunity to choose from the options you offer. Your open and candid conversation will create a feeling of trust, confidence, and respect. This is also a key step in developing a bonding relationship between the stylist and client.

The Ultimate Goal

Your ultimate goal is to make the client happy with herself and proud of her natural style. There is no time for guesswork during a consultation. The stylist must be very honest and sincere with the client, and carefully avoid insulting or belittling everyone who comes in for a consultation.

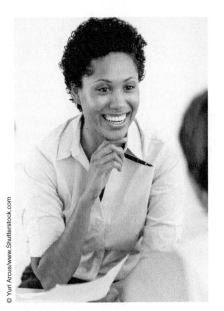

▲ Figure 4–1
Make direct eye contact with your clients.

The Client's Journey

The consultation offers you the opportunity to guide, nurture, and support the client as she develops the self-confidence and determination to redefine what real beauty is to her. It takes real courage to step outside the beauty box. With your assistance and expertise, the path to natural hair and wellness will be easier to walk.

Listen to Your Client and Learn Their Hair History

After the client has been seated, take time to ask the important questions and use the consultation as an opportunity to learn as much about the client's hair history as possible. Whether the client is in transition or has a full Afro, extensions or locks, it is a good time to explain the natural hair care experience you offer. You want it to be more than just a hair service. You want it to be a natural hair experience.

Create a Client Experience That Nurtures the Whole Self

You can differentiate your salon from other conventional salons by offering specialized hair services and by providing an intimate hair experience and environment that will replenish the entire being. Good examples of this experience are the "spa"-type hair salons. From the moment the client enters the salon, the soothing, aromatic environment reflects beauty and wellness. This is one way to differentiate your salon. Providing the client with filtered water or cool slices of fresh fruit are other opportunities to introduce the client to a natural hair salon experience **(Figure 4–2)**. The spa environment for a natural hair salon is the perfect setting for the client to remove those daily stressors, relax, and be nurtured.

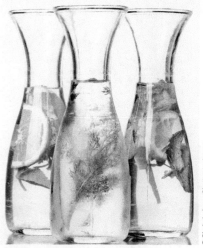

▲ Figure 4–2
Try infused water to create a relaxing experience for your client.

The Natural Stylist's Responsibility to the Client

Every client desires to receive a great service experience. However, the ultimate experience the client must have is with you. As a natural hair stylist, you have an obligation (1) to create a natural hair salon experience that will comfort, reassure, and encourage the client to have trust and confidence in your ability and skills; and (2) to provide the service and signature look that only you can offer.

Be excited and delighted about taking the new client on a journey that will motivate her on the path to self-love, acceptance, and care. This is a key step in developing a bonding relationship between the stylist and client. The relationship between the client and stylist begins the minute the client enters the salon.

Provide Your Client with Mental and Physical Comfort

Start the consultation service by making direct eye contact with your client and giving her a gentle, open greeting. Offer her a comfortable seat. In a consultation setting, the stylist is focused on the client's perceived needs and personal expectations. A positive, unconditional reception of the client can build trust and confidence almost at the first meeting. When speaking to and servicing your client, it is important to be "client-centered"; to consult and provide styling options that are centered around the client's needs and expectations. According to *The New Psy-Cosmetologist: Blending the Sciences of Psychology and Cosmetology*, unconditional positive regard communicates to clients that you accept them as they are without condition.[1] This client-centered approach frees clients to be more expressive about their self-image and initiates an emotional, almost spiritual, bond. Bonding with the client means developing a relationship, creating a connection personally and professionally during the first meeting.

Provide Adequate Time to Consult and Consider Special Consultation Needs

Time must be allotted for the consultation and the client. Consultation appointments must be made before the service. An adequate time for consultation can range from 10 to 15 minutes. However, more time may be needed for clients who are interested in getting the "big chop," those who would like protective styling with extensions or weaves, and those who suffer from scalp disorders or hair loss. Clients who suffer from hair loss or any scalp disorders may want to discuss it in privacy. Always offer the option of privacy to any client. By offering your clients the option of privacy, you help remove any inhibitions they may have. This will be the first step to building an ongoing relationship between you and your client.

Redefining the Client's Perception of Beauty

Facial features that are specifically characteristic of African structure do not have to be minimized unless the client is uncomfortable or considers the feature a problem. Typical African features such as high or large foreheads, wide and/or flat noses, big or full lips, and highly textured hair should not have to be minimized or covered up. Features like these distinguish this ethnic group, are beautiful, and should be celebrated. African features set this ethnic group apart from others, and they also make the people of this culture wonderfully unique. These features are attractive and should be acceptable within the African culture all over the world. The entire purpose of redefining what is beautiful is to allow all people to decide what they believe is beautiful and acceptable despite what they may have been conditioned to believe is "perfect." The natural stylist must be able to help the client "unlearn" these beliefs about perfection and embrace a more complimentary and realistic view of themselves.

The following techniques may assist the stylist when creating a finished look that will enhance unique features rather than simply camouflage them:

- Full or partial bangs, wisps, and fringes will minimize a large or wide forehead.

- Center parts, updos, and styles that move away from the face can minimize a flat or wide nose because they tend to make the face look longer.

- Keeping braid styles close to the face, or creating fullness around or behind the ears, can cover protruding or large ears. ☑ **LO2**

Types of Facial Structures

As a natural hair stylist, understanding facial types will enable you to create flattering styles that will enhance your client's best features. During the consultation, ask the client what they consider to be their best characteristics. Most people do not focus on the things they like about themselves; however, they can easily tell you what they consider to be flaws, imperfections, or negative facial characteristics.

It does not matter whether clients have decided that their forehead, nose, ears, lips, or eyes are unattractive. The important point is that the stylist can help clients choose natural and protective styles that flatter and affirm what they consider to be their positive features. As a professional stylist, it is your responsibility to assist clients to make the best decisions when choosing a hair style that nourishes their entire being and complements their facial structure.

The following paragraphs, containing general descriptions of facial types, will assist you in choosing a flattering natural hair or protective style for each client.

Oval Facial Type

Traditional textbooks refer to the oval facial structure as the ideal facial type due to its evenly contoured or proportional features. The distance from the forehead to the chin is usually equally spaced. Generally, the forehead is slightly wider than the chin. This client can wear most protective or natural styles. Special considerations must be made for features such as eye glasses, the size and shape of the nose, and the size and shape of the mouth **(Figure 4–3)**.

Round Facial Type

The round face is wide with a round or oval hairline. The chin is full and round. To create the illusion of thinness, add height to the style when completing the finished look. Updo styles add length to the face. Asymmetrical styles that show the ears can create a slenderizing look for this facial type. Weaved or braided styles with waves or full curls help to create balance and frame the face **(Figure 4–4)**.

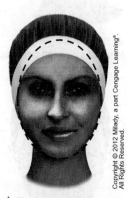

▲ Figure 4–3
Image of an oval face shape.

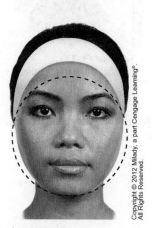

▲ Figure 4–4
Image of a round face shape.

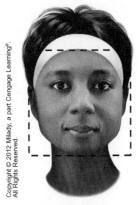

▲ Figure 4–5
Image of a square face shape.

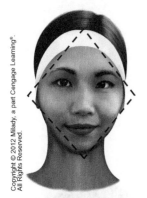

▲ Figure 4–6
Image of a diamond face shape.

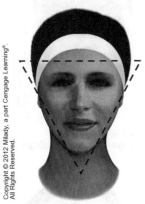

▲ Figure 4–7
Image of a heart face shape.

Square Facial Type

The square face is wide with a square jawline and an unusual or straight hairline. To create the illusion of length and soften facial lines, full styles that frame the face around the forehead, temples, and jawline are best. Wisps of hair or tapered fringe work best to soften any lines **(Figure 4–5)**.

Diamond Facial Type

The diamond-shaped face tends to be wide across the cheekbones. The forehead and chin are narrow. To minimize width across the cheekbones and help create an oval appearance, use styles that are full around the forehead or jawline. Full bangs or partial bangs will reduce the significance of a wide forehead. Keep the hair or braids close to the head along the cheekbones. Avoid updo styles and styles that move away from the cheeks or hairline **(Figure 4–6)**.

Heart-Shaped Facial Type

The heart-shaped face features a wide forehead and a very narrow chin. The goal is to minimize the width of the forehead by styling the finished look with partial bangs or wisps of hair or braids that frame the face. This style will help to add fullness around the chin **(Figure 4–7)**.

Pear-Shaped Facial Type

The pear-shaped face is recognized by its narrow forehead and wide chin or jaw. Soft fringes around the forehead will camouflage a small forehead without closing up the face. To give balance and fullness around the crown of the head, direct attention away from the narrow forehead. Styles that frame the cheekbones and are close or behind the ears can minimize the look of a wide jawline **(Figure 4–8)**.

Oblong Facial Type

The oblong face is usually very long and narrow and features small, hollow cheekbones. Creating full styles can make the face appear shorter or wider. The fullness must not be overpowering. Soft partial bangs or wisps of curls along the face can soften facial lines. The hair and/or braids should not be very long—keep braid styles at a medium length. Avoid middle parts, because they add length to a long, narrow face **(Figure 4–9)**. ☑ **LO3** ☑ **LO4**

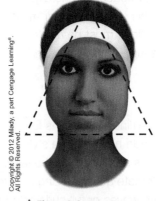

▲ Figure 4–8
Image of a pear face shape.

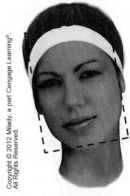

▲ Figure 4–9
Image of an oblong face shape.

Consultation Basics

Effective communication is the act of successfully sharing information between two people or a group of people so that the information is successfully and completely understood. Each client is different. Some clients know what they want in a new style when they come to the salon, and others have no idea of what hair effect they are trying to achieve. By using effective communication, the natural stylist can best understand the clients' needs and provide them with excellent service.

The following steps are a guide to conducting a thorough consultation:

Step 1. **Meet the client**—Greet all new clients pleasantly **(Figure 4–10)**. Be polite and friendly. Smile and introduce yourself, then give the client your name and status. Let the client know whether you are the receptionist, assistant stylist, stylist, or owner. Make sure you remember your client's name, because names are a good communication tool. Exhibit a professional and courteous attitude when speaking with a client to help develop an open exchange. Remember, clients come to you for your professional skills. You must be clear and direct. Convey interest and sincerity by maintaining direct eye contact. Look at your client while he or she is talking; it shows that you are an "active listener" and that you are dedicated to fulfilling that client's needs.

Step 2. **Seat the client**—Offer the client a seat before the consultation begins. She should be seated comfortably in front of a mirror. It is also appropriate at this time to physically examine the hair and scalp. Stand next to or behind the seated client while facing a mirror. In this position, you can maintain eye contact through the mirror image while you consult. Also, be aware of your body language, and do not appear to stare or gaze for long

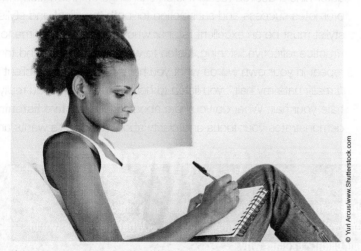

▲ Figure 4–10
A client waiting to have a consultation.

© Yuri Arcus/www.Shutterstock.com

client consultation form a questionnaire used to gather pertinent information about the client.

periods of time. That may make the client feel intruded upon or uncomfortable. Provide a **client consultation form**.

It is imperative for you to learn what the client's experience has been with chemicals and other processes. Let her talk about her hair history, experiences, and mishaps. Be a good listener, take mental notes, or use the client consultation form to record the client's hair history.

Step 3. **Review the client consultation form**—This card should request basic background information: the client's name, address, date of birth, hair and chemical history, and home care products being used. Also included in the information will be information about the client's hair care regime as well as any special disorders or scalp problems. The client consultation form will help the stylist to determine the condition of the hair. With the proper evaluation, the stylist can focus on correcting any styling problems that may occur.

Step 4. **Determine the client's ideal image and preferences by using "show and tell"**—While the client is seated, present magazines or pictures of different natural styles. Encourage her to flip through your style book, or ask her to present a mobile phone, tablet, or laptop to point out styles that are of interest to her. If you don't have your own style featured in a portfolio or on a social media page, start today. Every great style you have ever done can be featured and presented as your body of work. It shows the client your skill set and will start the dialogue about what the client is looking for in a hairstyle. Is the client in transition? What goal or effect is she trying to obtain with her hair? Is she interested in extensions as a protective style, or is her ultimate goal to obtain locks? After the client has filled out the card, it is time to review that information together and start a conversation about it.

Step 5. **Start a dialogue with your client**—As previously mentioned, the consultation is a dialogue, the verbal communication needed to determine a desired result. It is an exchange of information that promotes success and satisfaction for both the client and stylist. The stylist must be an excellent listener who gives the client time to talk. Practice reflective listening. Listen to what is being said and then repeat in your own words what you have heard. When a client says, "I really hate my hair," you listen to her and then say, "You really hate your hair. What do you hate about it?" **Reflective listening** demonstrates your focus and clarity about the client's wants and

reflective listening the practice of listening to what the client is saying and repeating it in your own words.

ACTivity

Bring to class pictures of models and celebrities from magazines. Look at them with classmates to analyze the facial shapes. Which styles were complimentary or uncomplimentary? What hairstyles would you suggest if the person pictured were your client? Explain why.

Trending natural hair terms to familiarize yourself with:

- *Big chop (BC)*—cutting off all the relaxed or chemically treated hair.
- *Co Wash*—to use conditioner to shampoo hair.
- *Cones*—silicones; not water soluble.
- *DT or DC*—deep treatment or deep conditioner applied over an extended period of time or period of time with dry heat or moist steam heat.
- *Dusting*—a very fine trim; can range from 0.25 inch (0.6 cm) or less, meaning as little hair as possible, so it resembles dust on the floor.
- *No Poo*—no shampooing, use conditioner to shampoo (see co wash).
- *Plopping*—quick-dry method for curly hair using paper towel or T-shirt.
- *SLS*—sodium laurel sulfate; surfactant, cleansing agent, and detergent that can be irritating, toxic, and drying to hair and scalp.
- *TNC*—twist and curl, double-strand twist, and rod or flex set.
- *TWA*—teeny weeny Afro.
- *Wash n Go*—a co wash following a leave-in conditioner, and texture enhancer; hand style, air dry, or diffuse.
- *Twist-out*—double-strand twist set that is dried, opened, and styled.
- *Hair Typing System*—general classification of hair textures for social media communication and product selection. Hair typing or classification is often with a numerical hierarchy, from 1-4 or 1-8. This system describes natural hair textures based on the wave/curl/coil patterns, elasticity, porosity and density.
- *CBL*—hair length reference, meaning "collarbone length."
- *PJ*—product junkies, a person who continually buys hair products, looking for a magic potion that will enhance hair texture.

needs **(Figure 4–11)**. Asking the right questions is crucial to the communication process. It is important to know your clients, how they are managing their hair at home, and the language used on social networking blogs and natural Websites. ☑ **LO5**

Consultation Questions

When providing your client with a thorough client consultation, it is necessary to ask effective, open-ended questions. This will allow the natural stylist to gather as much information as possible. The following list provides examples of questions you will want to ask your client:

1. Do you generally go to a professional for hair services?

2. What is your hair care maintenance and daily styling routine?

3. How often do you shampoo?

4. What products are you currently using?

5. What detangling tools are you currently using?

6. Are you using any heat applications: flat irons, hot combs, blowdryers?

7. Density: Do you consider your hair very thick, thick, medium thick, thin, or fine?

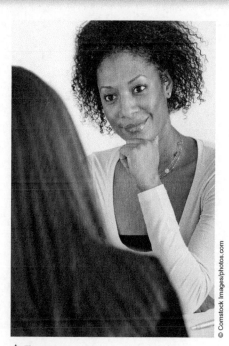

▲ Figure 4–11
Listen to what your client's wants and needs are.

© Comstock Images/photos.com

8. Hairline: Is your hairline healthy, thinning, or bald?

9. Length: How would you describe your hair length: short, medium, or long?

10. Scalp condition: How would you describe your scalp: dry, itchy, flaky, normal, oily, or tender?

11. Hair condition: How would you best describe the health of your hair: normal/healthy, dry/dehydrated, damaged/heat distressed, weak/breaking, dull/brittle, or limp/lacks volume?

12. How would you describe your natural hair texture: wavy, loose curls, tight curls, coily, highly textured, or wiry?

13. How often do you have your hair trimmed? When did you receive your last trim?

14. Transitioning: How long have you been growing out the relaxer? Do you want to transition over the long term (6 to 12 months) or short term (6 months or less), or would you consider totally cutting the remainder of the relaxed hair? What are your hair goals? What vision do you have for your hair and for your lifestyle? What particular style do you have in mind? What are your styling abilities?

15. Cutting relaxer or "the big chop": Are you prepared to see yourself with short hair? Are you prepared to manage your short hair? Do you have the support you need from family and friends to take this adventure? What options are you looking for in a style (business, evening, or casual look)? What silhouettes or shapes are you looking for in your new cut?

16. Protective styling: Have you ever considered wearing twists and/or braids with or without extensions, weaves, or wigs? Will protective styling affect how others perceive you at work or at home? What fibers or textures are you interested in using? Are you allergic to any fibers?

17. Lifestyle: Are you a student, professional working woman, artist, or stay-at-home mom? How often do you go to the gym, swim, or spend any time engaged in outdoor activities? Are you looking for a "statement style"—a style that reflects your personal style? Or, do you want a style that is easy care without much styling preparation? ☑ **LO6**

Step 6. **Select the materials to be used for the style**—When discussing a particular protective style, inform your client that it may require using human hair or synthetic hair extensions. Various braiding styles require particular materials. The pros and cons of the materials cost factor must be discussed in detail with the client. Find out what kind of experiences, both negative and positive, the client has had. Regardless of the problems the customer has had with a stylist in the past, remind her that you will avoid similar mistakes. For example, if the client had problems with synthetic hair extensions, recommend styles that feature other extension materials, like human hair fiber. Avoid putting the client through the same experience—trial and error is too costly in this business.

Step 7. **Analyze the hair and scalp** (Note: Protective gloves are optional.)—The objective is to examine the texture of the potential client. Different hair textures react differently to the same service. It is important to find a style that enhances the distinct features of the client's hair type. Conduct the hair analysis by separating the hair at the scalp and then looking for the different curl/coil patterns in the head. Pay close attention to areas where the hair is thinner, damaged, or broken. (And be sure to note these trouble spots on the profile card.) If the client suffers from a particular scalp disorder or is balding, make a notation and ask if she is under any medical supervision or taking any medications. Some medications will change the condition and texture of the hair. Always remain sensitive to the client's discomfort when discussing such problems. Chapter 5 provides a further discussion of hair characteristic and qualities.

Step 8. **Look for scalp abrasions**—Examine the scalp for cuts or sores. Be careful not to irritate or scratch the affected area. Avoid touching open sores. If open sores are apparent, recommend that the client see a dermatologist or a medical doctor. Again, remain sensitive to the possible discomfort of the client.

Step 9. **Examine the hairline**—With a soft brush, take a 1-inch (2.5 cm) hair section and brush it forward into the face to examine the hairline to see if it is receding or balding. If the hairline is damaged, certain natural and protective extension styles will be very difficult to execute. Avoid styles that place direct tension on the hairline or involve parting along the hairline.

Step 10. **Ask about the client's history with using hair chemicals and extreme heat**—Even though you are a natural hair care specialist, it is imperative that you learn what the client's experience has

Did you know?

Extreme heat with flat irons and straightening combs are chemically free services, but over a period of time, direct heat will break down the disulfide bonds of the cortex in the hair shaft and reduce or diminish texture. A warm flat iron or hot comb once a year may not break down the cuticle; however, under no circumstances should direct extreme heat (400 degrees F) from a pressing comb or flat iron be applied to hair that is in transition or chemically relaxed. The hair will lose all of its elasticity and break. In some cases with extreme heat application, the hair will smell scorched; the hair cuticle will stay intact but will be slightly burned. Remember: Direct heat diminishes texture.

FOCUS ON

YOUR COMMUNICATION SKILLS

If you feel uncertain about how to communicate with salon owners, managers, and clients from a different generation, watch and listen to your peers. Visit colleagues in various professional settings. Stop by a high-end clothing store and listen to the salesperson. Ask questions at these businesses yourself, and listen closely to the responses. Find someone whose communication skills you admire, and emulate that style. Practice using *yes, no, please, thank you,* and *excuse me* in daily conversation. (Avoid using *yeah, nope,* and *thanks.*) Use a dictionary to increase your vocabulary. You can even record yourself (audio or video) and assess your own communication style. The more confident you become when communicating with people from different walks of life and people with different types of jobs, the better.

been with chemical and extreme heat from flat irons. The client who is "going natural" will often use a flat iron on the hair to create that smooth look and avoid using chemicals. At first glance, it appears that heat straightening can be an option for those in transition. However, even though using heat services on the hair is chemical free, using direct heat on the hair eventually will reduce, and in many cases, destroy the natural curl or coil pattern of the hair. ✓ **LO7**

Most clients looking for extension and weave styles view them as a way to repair or protect the hair damaged by chemicals. All extension styles can cause a minimal amount of stress on the hair. If the hair has been weakened by past chemical or heat treatments, the stylist must avoid creating certain extension styles that will add more stress to the hair. Wait until the client's hair is strong and healthy enough to withstand any braid extension technique. Chemical treatments have various effects on hair color, elasticity, and texture. They often leave the protective cuticle layer of the hair fragile and damaged. The client's history of using hair chemicals will also affect the stylist's choice of shampoos and conditioners to use in repairing and smoothing down the protective cuticle layer.

The consultation is the opportunity to determine what a client needs and to avoid dissatisfaction **(Figure 4–12)**. It is important for the stylist to help clients choose styles that flatter their positive features. Everyone is beautiful in their own right. As natural stylists, it is our duty to avoid creating clones of what mainstream or pop culture considers beautiful, and to personalize every service and help clients to see their own beauty. If, after the service, your client expresses concerns about the style or says there is too much tension on the hairline, then it is obvious that you did not listen properly during the consultation. If the client is displeased in any way, you must take the responsibility for poor communication. On the other hand, if a client remains unclear during a consultation, trust your instincts and ask the client to defer to your judgment—after all, that is why customers come to you.

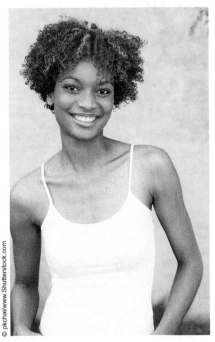

© pkchai/www.Shutterstock.com

▲ Figure 4–12
A good consultation will lead to a satisfied client.

Myth: *Textured Natural Hair Is Dry, Dull, and Brittle*

Yes, all untreated textured hair can feel dry, dull, and brittle. Textured hair does not reflect light or shine in the same manner as straight hair. Curly/coily hair absorbs light, giving it a dull brittle finish. To reduce this dull finish, textured hair requires products with moisturizing humectants to keep hair moist, supple, give it elasticity, and add luster and shine. Proper products such as essential oil treatments, styling creams, or nonalcoholic gels are the key to keeping textured hair moist, shiny, and pliable. Do the research—read ingredients and dedicate some time to finding out what works for all the specific hair types. In general, the key to reducing breakage to dull brittle hair is to address the needs of the hair by using products that offer nurturing ingredients that moisturize, hydrate, and help the hair to retain moisture.

Note: Textured hair and natural hair are interchangeable in the book.

Review Questions

1. Name the reasons that communication is important to the natural stylist.
2. Explain how a client's face shape can influence the outcome of a style.
3. What style would you recommend for a pear-shaped face?
4. Name some ways that a natural stylist can handle client insecurity about facial features and physical appearance.
5. Name the 17 questions essential to a thorough client consultation.
6. List the 10 steps to a successful client consultation.

Chapter Reference

1. Scoleri, Donald W. and Dr. Lewis Losoncy. *Salon Today Publication,* Reading, PA (1988).

Hair Types, Structure, and Textural Differences

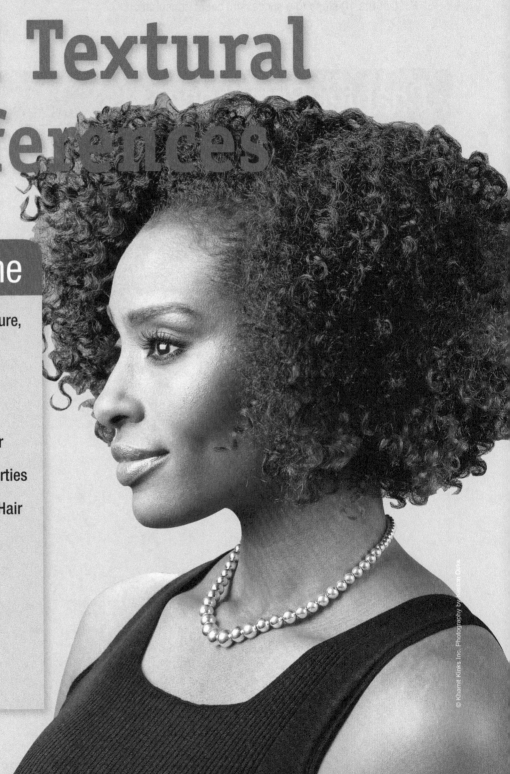

© Khamit Kinks Inc. Photography by Nelson Deka

Learning Objectives

After completing this chapter, you should be able to:

☑ **LO1** Name and describe the structures of the hair root.

☑ **LO2** List and describe the layers of the hair shaft.

☑ **LO3** Discuss the qualities and characteristics of the varying hair textures.

☑ **LO4** List the different factors to consider during hair analysis.

☑ **LO5** Describe the three growth phases of hair.

Key Terms

Page number indicates where in the chapter the term is used.

amino acids p. 97	**diameter of the hair** p. 103	**hair texture** p. 98	**peptides** p. 97
anagen phase p. 94	**disulfide bonds** p. 98	**hair type** p. 98	**salt bonds** p. 97
arrector pili muscle p. 94	**emollients** p. 96	**humectants** p. 96	**sebaceous glands** p. 94
catagen phase p. 94	**hair bulb** p. 94	**hydrogen bonds** p. 97	**sebum** p. 94
COHNS elements p. 97	**hair elasticity** p. 105	**hydrophilic** p. 104	**telogen phase** p. 94
cortex p. 96	**hair follicle** p. 93	**hydrophobic** p. 104	**terminal hair** p. 93
curl configuration p. 99	**hair porosity** p. 104	**keratinization** p. 97	**vellus hair** p. 93
cuticle p. 95	**hair root** p. 92	**keratinized protein** p. 97	
dermal papilla p. 94	**hair shaft** p. 92	**medulla** p. 96	

The primary function of hair is to insulate the body from the heat and the cold and to protect the head from injury and physical trauma. The secondary purpose of hair is for adornment. It has been said that our hair is our "crowning glory." The crown represents the regal beauty and power of the tresses. The word *glory* symbolizes a source of pride, self-care, and esteem. Natural hair is truly significant in lives because it shapes self-perception and redefines cultural aesthetics.

Natural hair has structural properties that can be shaped, molded, colored, stretched, and sculpted to beautify and reflect a person's most distinctive features. The basic structural composition of the hair fiber determines its physical properties. Volume, texture, shine or sheen, tensile strength, moisture absorption, and the ability to stretch and grow are all determined by the structural components of hair. As natural stylists, our most common interests are in hair growth, hair typing, hair care, and styling.

Why Study Hair Types, Structure, and Textural Differences?

You should have a thorough understanding of structural properties of the hair, scalp, and textural differences because:

- Services to natural hair are better performed when there is a clear understanding of the structural properties, growth process, color, and textural form of hair.

- Identifying hair textures is a vital part of being able to offer the appropriate products and services to your client.

- Spotting an unhealthy scalp that could be harboring a communicable disease or even be causing permanent hair loss aids your client in caring for and restoring the client's hair and scalp to a healthy balance.

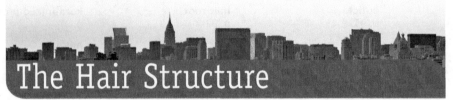

The Hair Structure

Hair is considered an appendage of the skin. Hair is defined as a slender, threadlike outgrowth of the epidermis of the skin and scalp **(Figure 5–1)**.

A mature strand of hair is divided into two parts: the root and the shaft.

1. **Hair root**—hair structure beneath the skin surface; it is the structure from which the hair grows. Hair doesn't grow from its outer structure, the shaft, but from its inner rooted stem.

2. **Hair shaft**—hair structure, also known as the stem, that extends above the skin surface. This is the portion that we see and manipulate; however, it is biologically inactive.

hair root hair structure beneath the skin surface; it is the structure from which the hair grows.

hair shaft hair structure, also known as the stem, that extends above the skin.

Structure of Hair Root

The basic hair structure contains the follicle, bulb, papilla, arrector pili muscle, and sebaceous glands **(Figure 5–2)**.

Hair Follicle

The **hair follicle** is the deep, angular, pocket-like depression in the scalp. Every single strand of hair is enclosed in its own follicle. It has been observed that in some cases, more than one hair can grow from a single follicle. We are born with about 100,000 to 150,000 follicles on our heads. Except for the lips, the palms of the hands, and the soles of the feet, people have over 500,000 hair follicles throughout the entire body. Some hair follicles contain **vellus hair**—short, fine "baby" hair; other follicles contain **terminal hair**—the coarser, longer hair found throughout the body. As we age and the skin shrinks, we can lose varying numbers of follicles. The follicle may vary in size, shape, and thickness depending on the genetic phenotype of the hair. The follicle acts as a "mold" for the creation of the hair shaft. Hair types fall into three very general divisions: Asian, European, and African. When we refer to one's hair type, we refer to hair in its most basic characteristics or in its general attributes. When we discuss hair texture, we are referring to the hair's specific physical structure and visual characteristics that encompass a full range of properties from straight to tight coily/wiry. Each of these general hair types exhibits its own distinct follicle shape, and each one of these hair types is created through the follicle. The round follicle generally creates straight hair and is usually seen in Asian hair types. The oval, curved, or round follicle generally creates wavy to straight hair and can be seen in European hair types. African hair types can vary from wavy/curly to coily/wiry, as well as combinations of varying degrees of highly textured hair, in which the follicle can vary from almost flat/elliptical to flat/spiraled.

One reason for the dry, fragile quality of the African hair type is that the tightly coiled hair makes it difficult for the natural oils or sebum to be distributed along the entire hair shaft. Other dermatologists suggest that the basic nature of its curved or spiraled follicle creates a lack of moisture, thus making the African hair shaft brittle and dry. The tighter the coil configuration, the more difficult it is for the hair to retain moisture; therefore, the hair will loose its natural elasticity, become more fragile, and break. Often the client will complain about how "hard" her hair may feel. She may apply a basic moisturizer or oil and still feel as if her hair were dry. In many cases, her hair may be dehydrated; however, often it is the natural texture or curl pattern she is feeling.

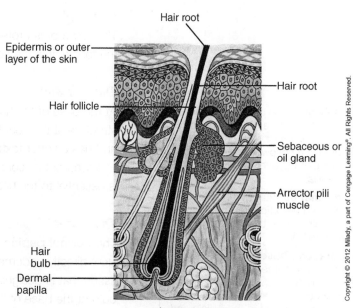

▲ Figure 5–1
Structures of the hair.

hair follicle a deep, angular, pocket-like depression in the scalp; contains the hair root.

vellus hair short, fine, white and downy hair, usually without a medulla. Vellus hair is found on any area of the body except the palms of hands and soles of feet.

terminal hair pigmented hair found on the scalp, arms, legs, nose, and ears. This hair is coarser than vellus hair, although it varies in texture, color, and length.

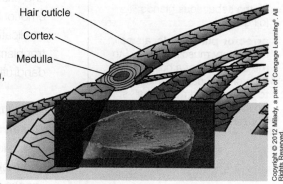

▲ Figure 5–2
Cross-section of the hair cuticle.

Hair Root

The hair root is protected in the dermis of the skin and is cocooned within the follicle. It is the actual stem beneath the skin.

The Hair Bulb

At the base of the hair root is the **hair bulb**. It is an enlarged, thick, round structure at the very bottom of the hair root. The bulb is whiter in color and has a softer texture than the hair shaft. The base of the bulb is a hollowed-out or concave ball that fits over and covers the papilla. The bulb is essential to the health and growth of the hair shaft.

The Dermal Papilla

The **dermal papilla** is made up of cells from the dermis (inner layer of the skin) directly underneath the hair follicle. It is the cone-shaped connective tissue that is designated to enclose the base or bulb of the hair follicle bulb at the base of the hair follicle. The dermal papilla is responsible for supplying the hair with oxygen-rich blood, nerves, and keratin protein cells that nourish the hair, and stimulate growth and regeneration. Through the papilla, the foods we eat provide nourishment to the hair bulb. The papilla plays a huge role in determining the hair's growth cycle and renewal process. It directly determines how and when the hair grows through the inter-fiber relationship with growth cycles: the **anagen phase**, the **catagen phase**, and the **telogen phase**. A healthy papilla will generate hair cells in the bulb and produce new hair growth. Here is where the hair can most benefit from good nutrition, chemically free products, scalp massage to increase the blood circulation, and stimulating herbal and botanical treatments. Increased blood flow feeds the dermal papilla. A well-fed and nutrition-enriched papilla will help to keep it active. The papilla is active during the anagen phase, separated during the catagen phase, and totally inactive during the telogen phase of the hair growth cycle.

Sebaceous Glands

Sebaceous glands are sac-like structures that provide the follicle with natural oils. They are the hair's natural conditioners. The oil glands secrete a substance called **sebum**, which adds luster and pliability to the hair and scalp. The production of sebum is directly associated with nutrition, emotional stress, and blood flow, as well as the impact of drugs and medication on the endocrine glands. Sebaceous glands frequently become troublemakers by overproducing and bringing on a common form of oily dandruff.

Arrector Pili Muscle

The **arrector pili muscle** is a small, involuntary muscle attached to the underside of a hair follicle. Fear or cold causes this muscle to contract and makes hair stand up straight, giving the skin the appearance of "goose bumps." Eyelash and eyebrow hair does not have arrector pili muscles. ✔ **LO1**

---

hair bulb the almost transparent, round structure at the very bottom of the hair root. The base of the bulb is a hollowed-out or concave ball that fits over and covers the papilla.

dermal papilla small cone-shaped elevations at the end of hair bulb at the base of the hair follicle.

anagen phase the period of hair development when the bulb is moving up through the follicle. During this phase, new cells are being produced in the follicle and new hair is produced. This phase can last up to seven years.

catagen phase the transition or resting stage of hair development. During this phase, after years of growing, the hair cells stop reproducing. The hair begins to lose moisture and separates from the papilla. It is the signal of the end of the growth phase. This phase lasts from one to two weeks.

telogen phase during this phase of hair development, the bulb is totally separate from the root; new hair cells divide and multiply, creating a new shaft. New hair sprouts to the surface of the scalp, pushing out the old strands, or remains until the original hair returns to the next phase (anagen). This stage begins the new cycle, and it lasts two to four months.

sebaceous glands the sac-like structures that provide the follicle with natural oils.

sebum the substance secreted by the sebaceous glands (oil glands).

arrector pili muscle a small, involuntary muscle attached to the underside of a hair follicle. Fear or cold causes this muscle to contract and makes hair stand up straight, giving the skin the appearance of "goose bumps."

As natural hair stylists, we nourish the hair from the outside. We must recognize and help the client to embrace the idea that the keys to healthy hair are a healthy body and mind. Healthy hair starts from the inside out. The body cannot produce healthy hair without good nutrition, physical fitness, and minimal life stressors **(Figure 5–3)**. Be very aware that what happens to the hair root and follicles—which are connected to the blood vessels, oil glands, and nerve supplies—is extremely important to the health and condition of the hair shaft.

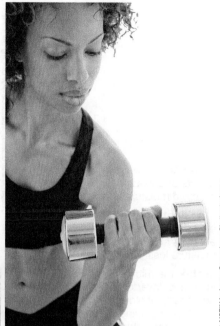

▲ Figure 5–3
Physical fitness promotes healthy hair.

Hair Shaft Structure

Understanding hair structure is vital because it is the foundation on which hair care and styling is built. Knowing its structure helps us to better determine how hair interacts with hair care products, chemicals, and the environment. The human hair shaft is also known as the stem. It extends above the epidermis layer of the scalp. The shaft is made up of dead protein cells. They are biologically inactive before they reach the surface of the scalp. Advertising and marketing claims of protein-filled products that "repair" the hair shaft are not accurate. We cannot revive dead hair or skin cells. The hair shaft is most brittle when dry. It will easily break and is most susceptible to heat and mechanical manipulation. Applying moisturizing products will coat the shaft, fill in the raised top layer, and prevent breakage. Most hair products we use topically to shampoo, condition, or treat the hair are only temporary fixes until the next service is applied. Most of the nourishing products that we use can only reinforce and assist in keeping clients' hair healthy, manageable, and protected from the environment, chemical processing, and physical abuses **(Figure 5–4)**.

Parts of the Hair Shaft

The hair shaft consists of three parts:

• Cuticle: outer layer **(Figure 5–5)**

• Cortex: middle layer **(Figure 5–6)**

• Medulla: inner layer

The **cuticle** on the hair shaft is made up of dead protein, called keratin, as well as amino acids such as cystine. The cuticle is the first line of defense for the cortex. It is the outermost layer, the surface of the shaft, protects and seals the hair. The cuticle consists of flattened keratin cells arranged like shingles on a roof. The scale-like cells overlap and lie close together, forming a tight, flat sheath around the shaft. When the cuticle is intact, the hair stays healthy. The hair is healthy when the cuticle layers are in good

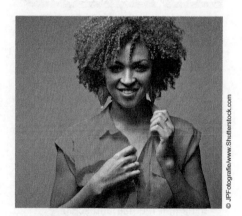

▲ Figure 5–4
Nourishing products make hair manageable.

cuticle the outer layer of the hair shaft; it is made up of dead protein cells (keratin) as well as amino acids such as cystine and is arranged in overlapping scales, like shingles on a roof.

humectants water-binding agents or substances that promote moisture retention.

emollients oily or fatty ingredients that coat the hair, aid in its elasticity, and prevent moisture loss.

cortex the thickest and innermost layer of the shaft composed of elongated cells. This layer contains melanin and is also responsible for the hair's elasticity.

medulla the innermost core of the shaft, consisting of sponge-like, baggy cells. In very thin, light-colored hair, it may be hollow or not exist at all. For the most part, the medulla does not require any hair care services.

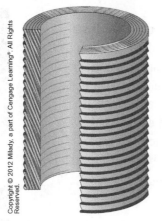

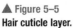

▲ Figure 5–5
Hair cuticle layer.

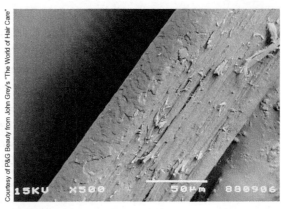

▲ Figure 5–6
Hair shaft with part of the hair cuticle stripped off, exposing the cortex.

Did you know?

Have you heard the expression "You are what you eat"? Although a healthy diet does not always guarantee healthy hair and scalp, it is mainly true that what you eat will affect your hair and scalp. The body can produce 11 of the 20 amino acids that make up hair, but your daily diet must include the remaining nine essential amino acids that the hair and scalp need. This is why crash dieting and anorexia can cause hair loss, lackluster hair, and unhealthy scalp conditions. Proteins in meat, fish, eggs, and dairy products are good sources of these amino acids, as are food combinations such as peanut butter and bread, rice and beans, and beans and corn.

condition, the scales are flat, and the cuticle surface is porous. The hair shaft appears to have a smooth surface that reflects the light or shines.

Unfortunately, African hair textures do not reflect light. Instead they absorb light, giving the cuticle a dull finish. For textured hair to have sheen or reflect light, an oil-based product must be applied. When the cuticle is aged or "weathered" through chemical processing, styling processes, sun exposure, or heat damage, the cuticle edges begin to lift and separate from the shaft. Though the cuticle has from 7 to 10 layers, once the cuticle lifts, it chips away from the hair shaft; the cortex and medulla are then exposed. This weakens the shaft and leads to breakage. The cuticle is very porous and softens when wet. Keeping the cuticle layers intact and tight is the best barrier against breakage. When hair is wet, it is flexible and can stretch about 25 to 50 percent past its original length. To avoid breakage, moisture is the key to keeping the cuticle smooth so that it doesn't lift up and stays intact. Keeping the cuticle well hydrated with moisturizing products is paramount to having healthy hair. Some examples used to keep hair well hydrated include moisturizers, humectants, emollients, sealants, and protection with protein-based products. In general, moisturizing products are mixtures of **humectants** or hydrators, which are water-binding agents or substances that promote moisture retention. Most moisturizing products are a combination of humectants and **emollients**, which are the oily or fatty ingredients that coat the hair, aid in its elasticity, and prevent moisture loss.

The **cortex** is the thickest part of the hair shaft. It takes almost 90 percent of the weight of the shaft. It is filled with keratin and protein cells that originate in the matrix. These cortical cells travel lengthwise, become elongated, and contain melanin pigmentation. Melanin is the element that gives hair its color. Within the cortical cells are long protein filaments called microfibrils. Microfibrils give hair its length. These fibers determine the strength, resilience, and moisture content of the hair.

The **medulla** is the innermost core of the shaft. In thick, coarse hair, it is made up of porous, sponge-like, baggy cells. In very thin, light-colored hair, the medulla may be hollow or not exist at all. ☑ **LO2**

Chemical Composition of Hair

Hair is composed of living protein cells within the hair follicle. These fibrous protein cells, which originate in the dermal papilla, travel up the follicle, where they are still living cells. As the cells move up, harden, and mature through a process called **keratinization**, the cells lose their nuclei and die. As the hair shaft emerges and grows through the dermis, the cells are no longer alive; the result is known as **keratinized protein**. This protein makes up 90 percent of the hair fiber. This protein is made up of **amino acids**, which consist of the five main elements that create the hair fiber—carbon, oxygen, hydrogen, nitrogen, and sulfur, also known as the **COHNS elements (Table 5–1)**.

Amino acids are linked together like beads on a necklace. **Peptides** are the links that bond the amino acids together **(Figure 5–7)**. Long chains of amino acids linked with peptides are known as polypeptides. These polypeptides form a coiled chain called a helix.

The polypeptides are cross-linked by side bonds. These bonds hold the keratin fibers in place and give hair its strength, elasticity, and molding ability. These side bonds can be one of three types: hydrogen bonds, salt bonds, and disulfide bonds **(Table 5–2)**.

Hydrogen bonds are easily broken by water or heat. They account for one-third of the hair shaft's resilience and fiber strength. The hydrogen bonds are weak and change easily when hair is shampooed or wet. The hydrogen bond loses its shape when wet and reforms when heat applied to dry the hair. That is why hair is so fragile when wet—because the hydrogen bonds can be easily manipulated or broken.

Salt bonds are more temporary and are easily broken or weakened by strange alkaline or acidic products. They account for one-third of the hair shaft's strength.

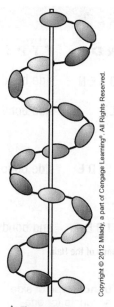

▲ Figure 5–7
Polypeptide chains intertwine in a spiral shape called a helix.

keratinization the process of cells moving upward inside the follicle, maturing and hardening as the cells lose their nuclei and perish.

keratinized protein mature keratin cells in the hair shaft that have grown away from their roots and have lost their nuclei are considered to be made of dead protein.

amino acids, units that are joined together end to end, by strong, chemical peptide bonds to form the polypeptide chains that comprise proteins.

COHNS elements the major elements that make up human hair, carbon, oxygen, hydrogen, nitrogen, and sulfur.

peptides a chain of amino acids that are bonded together to make keratin protein for hair, nails, and body.

hydrogen bonds a type of side bond that accounts for one-third of the hair shaft's resilience and fiber strength. Hydrogen bonds are weak and change easily when hair is shampooed or wet.

salt bond a type of side bond that is temporary and is easily weakened by strong alkaline or acidic solutions.

THE COHNS ELEMENTS	
ELEMENTS	**PERCENTAGE IN NORMAL HAIR**
CARBON	51%
OXYGEN	21%
HYDROGEN	6%
NITROGEN	17%
SULFUR	5%

Table 5–1 The COHNS Elements.

BONDS OF THE HAIR

BOND	TYPE	STRENGTH	BROKEN BY	REFORMED BY
HYDROGEN	side bond	weak, physical	water or heat	drying or cooling
SALT	side bond	weak, physical	changes in pH	normalizing pH
DISULFIDE	side bond	strong, chemical	1. thio perms and thio relaxers 2. hydroxide relaxers 3. extreme heat	1. oxidation with neutralizer 2. converted to lanthionine bonds
PEPTIDE	end bond	strong, chemical	chemical depilatories	not reformed; hair dissolves

Table 5–2 Bonds of the Hair.

disulfide bonds type of side bond that accounts for one-third of the hair's resilience and strength; disulfide bonds join the sulfur atoms in the amino acids to create cystine. These bonds are broken only by a chemical solution, thus attesting to their strength.

hair type the most basic form and general characteristic of the hair fiber.

hair texture the measurement and curl configuration of a hair fiber.

Disulfide bonds are side bonds that join the sulfur atoms in the amino acids to create cystine. There are fewer disulfide bonds than hydrogen or salt bonds, but they are much stronger and do not break down or change due to water or heat. The disulfide bonds are strong and always want to return to their natural shape. The disulfide bonds can be broken down by permanents and chemical relaxers. These bonds are reformed with a new, modified shape (straight or wavy) by neutralizing or stopping the reforming process.

Hair Types and Texture Properties

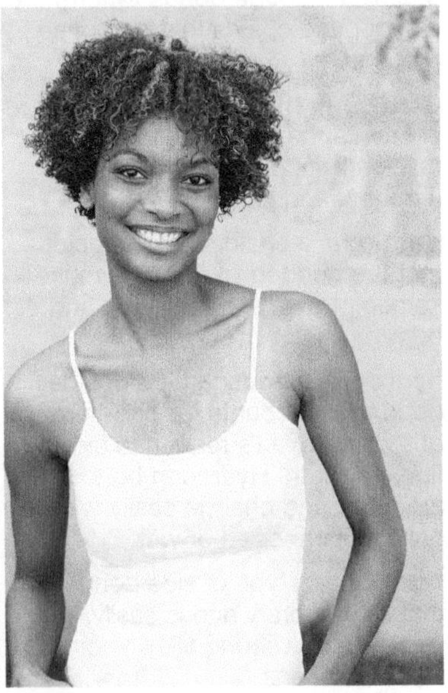

When clients come in for a consultation or service, the very first thing you will note is their hair type and texture. In general terms, **hair type** is the most basic descriptor of the hair fiber (**Figure 5–8**). It is an easy term to use when describing the most general characteristics of the hair, because it is the most basic hair category when discussing hair differences or textures (**Table 5–3**). When speaking of hair types based on race, these references in general have overtones of bias, are vague, and are unreliable in helping the stylist to determine the true texture of the hair.

Hair texture is the curl configuration or coil pattern of the hair. As we know, our family lineage determines our hair type or texture; however, there are many exceptions. Generally speaking, Asians and Native Americans have extremely straight hair; Caucasians mainly have straight hair, but it can range from wavy to curly to tightly curled. Often, clients who are biracial or multiracial have hair patterns that can range from very straight to wavy to tight and coily. African hair types have great texture range as well. African hair types can range in texture from soft waves to tight curls and from strong coils to wiry tresses.[1]

© pkchai/www.Shutterstock.com

▲ Figure 5–8
Identifying hair type is one of the most important parts of the consultation.

HAIR TYPES AND CROSS SECTION

1. Straight hair is usually round.

2. Wavy hair is oval to round.

3. Curly hair is almost flat.

4. Coily hair is flat and spiral in shape.

Table 5–3 Hair Types and Cross Sections.

What determines the differences in hair types? Some scientists say that when the follicle is straight, the hair will grow straight. When the follicle is genetically programmed to grow slightly bent or curved, the hair shaft will curl or coil. Another theory to explain how natural hair coil patterns grow is based on the shape of the cross section of the hair shaft. When the cross section of the hair is round, the hair will be straight. When the cross section is oval to slightly round, the hair will be wavy to curly. When the cross section is very flat or spiral in shape, the hair will be coily or in tight ringlets.

The hair texture is the most specific and detailed descriptor. When talking about hair texture, we are referring to the **curl configuration** and its different characteristics: the straight, wavy, curly, coily, kinky, or wiry shape of the hair shaft. A successful natural hair stylist must have a full understanding of hair and appreciate all hair types and the varying textures from people all over the world. As a professional stylist, it is important to know that all hair is "good" no matter the type or texture. Good hair is healthy hair. Bad hair can no longer be determined by whether it is straight, wavy, or coily; straight hair has always been the preferred hair type in the modern aesthetic. Today, however, we can acknowledge that bad hair is simply unhealthy, damaged, or "weathered" hair.

curl configuration the natural external form of a hair fiber; refers to the straight, wavy, curly, coily, kinky, or wiry shape of the hair shaft.

There is no longer a need for a listing or hierarchy of hair textures. Categorizing or classifying hair textures by numbers or letters, or within consumers'/laymen's social networks is just another divisive way to diminish the African hair texture. Consumer "hair typing" is all product based. Product manufacturers are finding opportunities in the movement toward appreciation and celebration of natural hair. Thanks to the newfound options from social media such as Websites, hair blogs, and YouTube, we have great resources that make the exchange of information incredibly fast and efficient. However, not all the information from these sources is accurate or beneficial. Professional hair typing should not be based on the generalized system of numbers and letters used by consumers or social media. Be a professional; do your own strand testing. Use your professional skills as a natural stylist to determine the specific texture. Refer to the texture guide that follows in this text; look at the hair to determine curl configuration. Run your fingers down the shaft to feel the curl pattern; or gently spray water on a small section

Study the reference guide and then conduct your own strand test. This will give you practice in providing a strand test. It's not difficult to do. To get good at something, you must do it repeatedly. Tell four or five different friends that you would like to test their hair strands. Have each friend give you a strand of hair. Place each strand on a light-colored sheet or cloth. With each strand, place the thumb and forefinger on the fiber and slowly go down the shaft. Is the hair smooth or bumpy? Is the strand thicker than the others? When stretched out, is it fine, thick, corkscrewed, brittle, or soft? Take notes and compare strands.

of hair, note any shrinkage, and gently pull strands back and forth to observe porosity, elasticity, and the size of the curl pattern. Most people have more than one texture, so take samples from three different parts of the head—the nape, crown, and front—to determine the differences in textures your client may have. Professionals and nonprofessionals alike have flooded the network with information that in most cases is informative and entertaining, but it is not always useful for your professional needs. Regardless of their race, anyone can have straight, wavy, curly, or coily hair.

Reference Guide for Natural Hair Textures

The reference guide in this section is just that—a set of guidelines to use when studying hair types and textures. It provides general description of hair textures, shapes, or configurations as well as of the hair qualities or properties that make a particular texture uniquely beautiful. Why is it so important to understand this guide? It will help you to give your clients better service. With an understanding of hair types, hair qualities, and textures, you will be better prepared to offer any service you can provide. You will conduct more complete consultations, see the needs of the hair, and address those needs to enhance, nurture, and embellish the client's texture. Use this guide to help you choose the correct hair treatments, styling procedures, and finishing techniques **(Table 5–4)**.

REFERENCE GUIDE FOR NATURAL HAIR TEXTURES

TEXTURED HAIR	CURL FORM/ CONFIGURATION	HAIR PROPERTIES
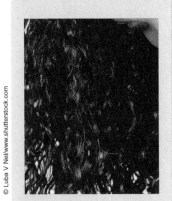 ▲ Soft waves.	SOFT WAVES	• Soft, medium wave pattern • Diameter fine to coarse • Density average • Volume limited • Moderate elasticity • Easy movement • Requires low-pH products to close cuticle and retain moisture • May need wave enhancer to reduce frizz • Reflects light/shines

© Luba V Nel/www.shutterstock.com

Table 5–4 Reference Guide for Natural Hair Textures. (*continued*)

REFERENCE GUIDE FOR NATURAL HAIR TEXTURES

TEXTURED HAIR	CURL FORM/ CONFIGURATION	HAIR PROPERTIES
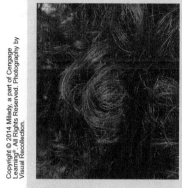
▲ Wavy hair.

| **WAVY** | • Small wave pattern
• Diameter fine to coarse
• Density slightly above average
• Volume moderate
• Moderate to excessive frizzing
• Good elasticity
• Gentle movement
• Requires regular moisture/hydration regime
• Will frizz and tangle
• Will need wave enhancers to reduce frizz
• Reflects light/low shine
• Requires low-pH products to close cuticle and retain moisture |
|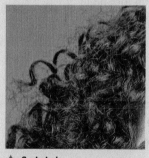
▲ Curly hair.

| **CURLY** | • Large to medium ringlets, spirals, or loops
• Diameter fine to coarse
• High volume
• Density above average
• High elasticity
• Moderate to excessive frizzing and tangles
• Requires low-pH products to close cuticle and retain moisture
• Requires regular moisture/hydration regime
• Reflects a little light/sheen |
|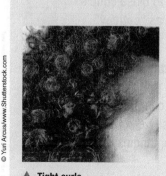
▲ Tight curls.

| **TIGHT CURLS** | • Medium to small ringlets, spirals, or corkscrews
• Diameter fine to medium
• Easily tangles; frizz and knots at ends
• Some elasticity
• High volume, shrinkage
• Very dense
• Can feel dry to the touch
• Requires daily moisture/hydration
• Requires low-pH products to close cuticle and retain moisture
• Does not reflect light; use oil for sheen |

Table 5–4 *(continued)*

REFERENCE GUIDE FOR NATURAL HAIR TEXTURES

TEXTURED HAIR	CURL FORM/ CONFIGURATION	HAIR PROPERTIES
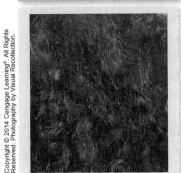 ▲ Coily hair.	COILY	• Small, spiral-shaped curls; small ringlets • Diameter fine to coarse • High volume, shrinkage • Dense • Fragile; tangles and breaks easily • Requires low-pH products to close cuticle and retain moisture • Requires additional hydration and moisture, oil for sheen
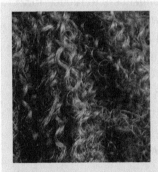 ▲ Tight coils.	TIGHT COILS	• Very small, tight, spiral curls or corkscrews • Volume and density can range • Lots of shrinkage • Fragile, tangles at the ends, breaks easily • Needs repeated moisture/hydration applications and oil for sheen • Often referred to as "spongy"
▲ Kinky hair.	KINKY	• Very small, tight curls or coils • Lots of shrinkage when wet • Diameter fine to coarse • Very dense • Very fragile, tangles very easily, frizz • Requires daily moisture/hydration; oil often for sheen • Requires low pH to close cuticle • Often referred to as "cottony"
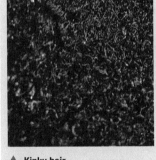 ▲ Wiry hair.	WIRY	• Feels coarse or rough to the touch • May have zigzag pattern • Diameter fine to coarse • Volume and density can range • Extremely fragile, tangles very easily, frizz • Low porosity • Requires low-pH products to close cuticle • Requires intensive moisture regime; oil often for sheen • Protein to minimize breakage ✓ **LO3**

Table 5–4 (*continued*)

Hair Analysis and Qualities

To provide creative natural services, the stylist must analyze the client's hair texture and scalp condition. During the hair analysis, you must use all your senses—hearing, touch, smell, and sight—to observe, prepare, and provide excellent hair services. When you are conducting a hair analysis for naturally textured hair, the most important factors to consider are the curl configuration and pattern as well as the hair shaft diameter, porosity, and elasticity.

Hair Properties for Hair Typing

The finished style depends on whether the hair is straight, wavy, curly, coily, kinky, or wiry. It is important to be familiar with the different curl or coil patterns to better provide the hair with what it needs to be healthy, supple, and resilient. As you can see in the Reference Guide to Natural Hair Textures, different hair types have different needs and require an array of care regimens, including moisturizing and nurturing options to keep the hair in peak condition.

As we know, a client can have more than one hair texture, so the natural stylist must make careful note of each different texture and address the needs of each one. Fully understanding the needs of the varying curl configurations will allow you to select the correct cleansing, conditioning, and finishing products that will best address the needs of varying hair types. Clients with multiple textures require a full range of conditioning and styling options. Varying textures require different styling products. The soft, fine hair around the hairline may require a waxy gel, but the hair at the nape and sides require a water-based gel with lots of hold. You may also have to create a conditioning "cocktail" that will address the different needs of each texture. When learning the range of hair types and textures, remember that the natural hair care industry does not have a "one size fits all" policy. For us, it's all about fulfilling the needs of the individual, creating and maintaining the unique qualities of the hair texture and the person **(Figure 5–9)**.

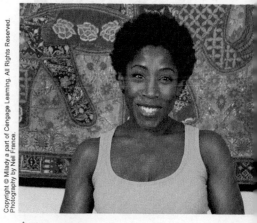

▲ Figure 5–9
Each client requires special attention.

Diameter of the Hair

The **diameter of the hair** refers to the size of the individual strands and the degree of coarseness, thickness, fineness, or thinness. It is another aspect of determining hair texture. The true test of whether a hair strand is thick or thin is measured by its diameter. Human hair diameter ranges from very fine (about 15 microns) to very thick (about 170 microns). The average diameter is between 60 and 110 micron (1 micron = 1/1000 millimeter). Like the curl configuration, the hair strand diameter may vary in different areas of the head. Coarse hair has the largest diameter, is stronger, and often requires more processing time when using chemicals. Coarse hair can be associated with any curl pattern. Tightly coiled to wiry hair is often classified as coarse; however, these textures may have varying degrees

diameter of the hair the size of the hair shaft and the individual strands. It determines the texture and degree of coarseness, thickness, fineness, or thinness.

hair porosity the hair's ability to absorb water, moisture, or chemicals through the cuticle into the cortex.

hydrophobic describes moisture-resistant hair with low porosity.

hydrophilic describes hair that is overly porous (high porosity), releasing needed moisture when dry and absorbing excessive amounts of water, moisture, and chemicals when wet.

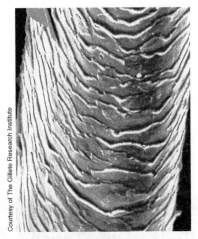

▲ Figure 5–10
Low porosity (resistant hair).

of diameters. In actuality, these hair types may feel coarse because of their natural curves, spirals, and corkscrews. Hair that is medium in diameter is most common and generally easy to manage. Fine hair is smaller in diameter, can be very fragile, breaks easily, and can easily be overprocessed.

Hair Porosity

Hair porosity refers to the hair's ability to absorb water, moisture, or chemicals through the cuticle into the cortex. The cuticle layer covers and protects the hair shaft like shingles of a roof. Moisture is diffused in and released out through the cuticle layer. All hair types have some level of porosity. The degree of porosity is directly related to the condition of the cuticle layer. Healthy hair usually has low porosity **(Figure 5–10)**; the cuticle layers lie flat and tight, so that very little moisture is allowed into or out of the shaft. Low porosity occurs when the hair is resistant and absorbs the least amount of moisture. This moisture-resistant hair is referred to as **hydrophobic**. Hair with high porosity is considered overly porous, releasing needed moisture when dry and absorbing excessive amounts of water, moisture, and chemicals when wet. Hair with high porosity is also known as **hydrophilic**.

Hair with average porosity is considered normal **(Figure 5–11)**. This hair type usually absorbs water, moisture, and chemicals as expected, based on its texture—that is, the hair condition, diameter, and curl pattern. Different degrees of porosity can be found in all hair types and textures. In general, naturally coarse, coily hair will have low porosity or be more resistant to moisture absorption, leaving the hair feeling dry and brittle. In some cases, fine, kinky hair may have high porosity or be overly porous, thus allowing moisture to easily escape or becoming chemically overprocessed because the cuticles have degenerated.

Hair with high porosity is known to absorb moisture or solution very quickly due to overprocessing. This overprocessed hair is damaged, dry, and fragile, and breaks very easily **(Figure 5–12)**. Hair damage has occurred,

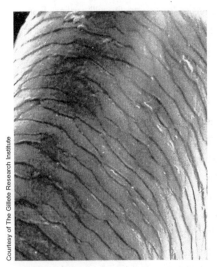

▲ Figure 5–11
Average porosity (normal hair).

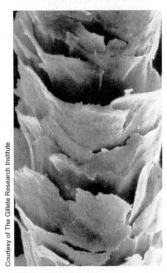

▲ Figure 5–12
High porosity (overly porous).

and hair loss may begin. Hair with low porosity requires more alkaline solutions to lift the cuticle and permit uniform saturation. Products with less alkaline or low pH can prevent further damage.

Texture

When speaking of texture, we first need to address the curl/coil pattern or lack of a curl configuration. The second element is determining the thickness of the hair strand. The diameter of the strand (coarse, medium, or fine) will also determine the porosity. Thick, coarse hair is generally more resistant; fine hair may often be extremely porous, absorbing moisture very easily. Tightly curled, coily, and kinky hair textures are generally dry with open cuticles that make the hair very porous. The diameter of the strand does play a role in porosity; however, when it comes to these very porous textures, the coarseness or fineness just increases the vulnerability of the hair strand.

Elasticity

Hair elasticity refers to the hair's ability to stretch and return to its original size and shape without breaking. Normal elasticity is springy and lustrous in appearance. Good elasticity is evident because the side bonds that hold keratin fibers are in place and strong. Dry hair can stretch about one-fifth of its length. Wet hair can stretch up to 50 percent of its original length. When combing wet, coily hair, you may find that the hair can stretch up to twice its unencumbered length. Blowdrying will also elongate the coil. Avoid extreme heat. Using a hood dryer on loose twists can elongate the hair. The elasticity is often surprising to the client. ☑ **LO4**

hair elasticity the hair's ability to stretch and return to its original size and shape without breaking.

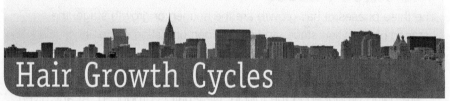

Hair Growth Cycles

Is hair alive? The answer is both yes and no. The hair that extends beyond the scalp and covers our head has no blood or nerve endings and therefore feels no pain when cut. On the other hand, from a metaphysical and holistic viewpoint, all hair is believed to hold a life force. It is part of our integrated system of being. Hair responds to all of life's elements: the sun, water, wind, and temperature. Hair also reacts to the internal elements of the body: stress, emotional and physical shock, diet, drugs, and chemicals.

The portions of the hair that are totally alive—the papilla, bulb, root, and follicle—are under the scalp. The human body has two main hair types: vellus hair and terminal hair.

Vellus Hair

Vellus hair is short, fine, and has a downy feel. This type of hair is commonly found on infants and young children until puberty, giving

Did you know?

In the African tradition, some tribes believe that the hair is a spiritual transmitter.

it the nickname of "baby hair." On adults, vellus hair can be seen throughout the body, as well as on seemingly hair-free places like the forehead, eyelids, earlobes, and bald scalps. There is no vellus hair on the soles of the feet or palms of the hands. Vellus hair is colorless. Women normally have 55 percent more vellus hair than men do. This fine, short hair keeps the body cool by helping it to effectively evaporate perspiration.

Terminal Hair

Terminal hair is long, mature hair found on the scalp, legs, arms, backs, and bodies of both men and women. Except for gray hair, terminal hair is coarser and darker than vellus hair. All hair follicles can produce either vellus or terminal hair; this ability is determined by age, genetics, sex, and hormones.

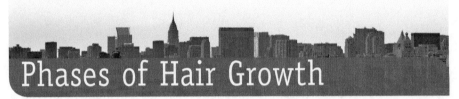

Phases of Hair Growth

Hair is completely renewable! It is the only body structure that can regenerate itself if the follicle is not damaged or scared. The regeneration of hair is known as a growth cycle. The cycle has three phases that are repeated throughout each person's lifetime. The three phases are the anagen or growth stage, the catagen or transition stage, and the telogen or the resting stage.

The Three Phases

The three phases of hair growth are the anagen or growth stage, the catagen or transition stage, and the telogen or resting stage.

1. **Anagen: The growth phase**—the period of development when the bulb is moving up through the follicle. During this phase, new cells are being produced in the follicle. New hair is produced. At any given time, 70 to 90 percent of hair is in this phase of growth. This phase can last up to seven years, but in some cases has lasted up to 10 years. The longer the anagen phase, the longer the hair will grow. The average growth of healthy hair is approximately ¼ inch (0.6 cm) to ½ inch (1.3 cm) a month. The secret to having long, healthy hair is to promote the long duration of the anagen phase. Most women's scalp hair grows faster than that of men. Scalp hair generally grows fuller and faster between the ages of 15 and 30, but slows down after the age of 50.

2. **Catagen: The transition phase**—the transition or resting stage. After years of growing, the hair cells stop reproducing. The hair begins to lose moisture and separates from the papilla. It is the signal of the end of the growth phase. During this phase, the follicle shrinks and separates from the papilla. The hair bulb and the root shrink. About 1 to 2 percent of

the hair is at this phase at any one time. This happens while another new hair begins to grow at the root. This phase lasts from one to two weeks.

3. **Telogen: The resting phase**—the bulb is totally separate from the root. New hair cells divide and multiply, creating a new shaft. New hair sprouts to the surface of the scalp, pushing out the old strands or remains until the original hair returns to the next anagen phase. This begins the new cycle. This stage lasts two to four months **(Figure 5–13)**.

The beauty of the entire process of hair growth is that each hair strand is at a different stage at a particular time. At any given time, a strand is growing, resting, or shedding. All the hair we see in the brush or comb is usually the hair that has been shed naturally. Fifty to 100 hairs per day can be in the shedding stage.[2] ✓ **LO5**

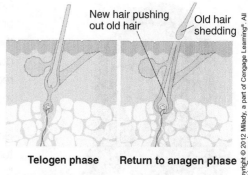

New hair pushing out old hair

Old hair shedding

Telogen phase   Return to anagen phase

▲ Figure 5–13
Cycles of hair growth.

Structural Differences of Textural Hair

With textured hair, the follicle is curved or spiral in shape. The hair shaft conforms to the shape of the follicle, so the follicle determines the coil configuration. This structure is consistent throughout all major racial groups. The physical attributes of the shape and the amount of curl or coil are thought to be related to the cross-links in the cortex, which is genetically programmed during the molding of the hair shaft.

There are different degrees of waves, curls, and coils. The coil can be small, medium, or large in its curved configuration. A small coil, for example, is tight in its winding pattern and may vary in other physical characteristics (such as being fine or coarse to the touch). The smaller the coil pattern, the greater the possibility of tangling (meshing for locks) and breakage during grooming.

A medium coil or curl can also vary in its corkscrew pattern. This texture is easier to groom, and it tends to break less when combed. The meshing/locking process takes slightly longer. The longer coil or curl still requires proper grooming. The degrees and patterns of coils are almost endless. These are just general descriptions of textured hair. The professional loctician addresses the specific needs of those clients who are interested in locking. Locticians are experts on the subject of texture and the techniques necessary to get the varying hair textures to lock. Cultivating locks is truly a hands-on art form. Cultivated locks are natural or chemically free hair, groomed in a systematic way to be symmetrical, circular, or manipulated into a style. By studying the cultivation of locks, we can gather more information about the varying coil and curl patterns.

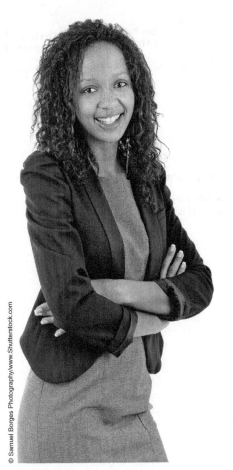

© Samuel Borges Photography/www.Shutterstock.com

▲ Figure 5–14
Example of a woman with different textures throughout her hair.

Coil patterns can differ on the same head. One client may display three or more textures throughout her head **(Figure 5–14)**. When labeling the client texture, it is very normal to see several textures with different qualities on one head. Generally, the texture of hair along the occipital region is tighter in its coil configuration; in some cases it may be dryer, more brittle, and easier to break. The hair in this area tends to lock first during the locking process (see Chapter 10, "Natural Hair and Braid-Sculpting Techniques"). You will notice the difference in texture along the temples or sides of the head around the ear. This area may display a "softer" texture with medium to fine curls or coils. The hair is less brittle, and the coil pattern may vary from very tight or loose to a medium to large corkscrew pattern. The hair in this area generally locks next in the process. The front and crown regions have the greatest variety of textures, ranging from fine, wiry waves to coarse, curly clusters or medium, grainy coils. The texture at the top of the head is often the last to lock.

During the braiding service, hair in the frontal area must be noted for its different or varying textures. Applying too much extension fiber can lead to breakage and permanent hair loss (see Chapter 6, "Hair and Scalp Diseases and Disorders").

CAUTION

Extremely porous hair stretches more than hair with poor porosity, such as overprocessed hair or hair damaged by chemical color services. It tends to stretch like a rubber band and then break.

Myth: *You Should Shampoo Natural Hair Every Day*

Cleansing daily with shampoos that contain sodium lauryl sulfate, an abrasive detergent that produces creamy foam or suds, can strip the cuticle and leave hair dry and brittle. Instead, choose gentle shampoos made of natural botanicals and oils that cleanse and nourish the hair. Natural shampoos have gentle ingredients that leave the hair soft, moist, and pliable. Cleansing the hair and scalp once per week or every two weeks for locs and braided styles with a sulfate-free cleansing shampoo is adequate for all types and textures. Clients often prefer to co-wash between weekly or biweekly shampoos and salon visits. Less is more when it comes to botanical concentrated hair care products.

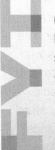

Coily or spiral textured hair grows in a similar pattern; however, because it has a corkscrew pattern, it appears to grow more slowly. The flattened shaft gets thinner at every turn of the coil's bend. As the shaft bends, the flattened strand becomes weaker and more fragile. At this point, when stress through combing or brushing takes place, the shaft often breaks.

Review Questions

1. Why is it imperative for natural hair stylists to understand hair typing and hair texture?
2. What follicle shapes produce coily and curly hair fibers?
3. What are the three growth phases of hair, and how long does each one last?
4. According to the text, is hair physically alive? Define keratinization.
5. Name two parts of the hair structure. What part of the structure does the natural stylist manipulate?
6. Where is the dermal papilla located, and what is its function?

Chapter References

1. (2012). *Milady standard cosmetology*. Clifton Park, NY: Milady, a part of Cengage Learning.
2. (2012). *Milady standard cosmetology*. Clifton Park, NY: Milady, a part of Cengage Learning.

CHAPTER 6

Hair and Scalp Diseases and Disorders

Chapter Outline

- Why Study Hair and Scalp Diseases and Disorders?

- Hair Loss and Your Client

- Hair Disorders and Treatments

- Scalp Disorders and Treatments

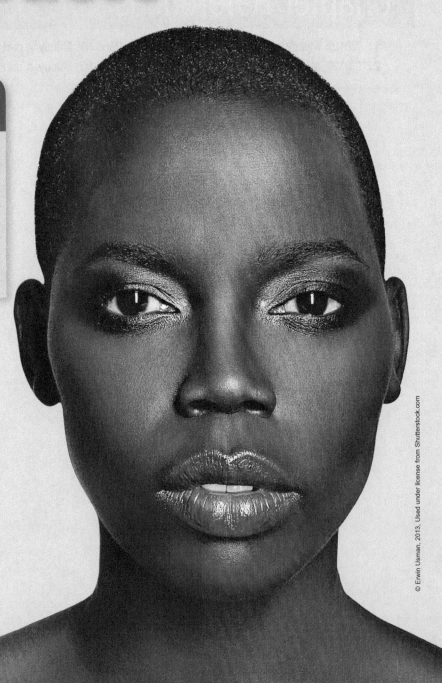

Learning Objectives

After completing this chapter, you should be able to:

☑ **LO1** Discuss the types of hair loss and their causes.

☑ **LO2** Describe the treatment procedures for hair loss.

☑ **LO3** Name and describe the varying hair disorders and treatments.

Key Terms

Page number indicates where in the chapter the term is used.

acne keloidalis
p. 129

alkaline
p. 117

alopecia
p. 122

alopecia areata
p. 124

alopecia totalis
p. 124

alopecia universalis
p. 124

ammonium thioglycolate (no-lye)
p.115

androgenetic alopecia
p. 124

calcium hydroxide (no-lye)
p. 115

canities (congenital and acquired)
p. 115

cradle cap
p. 120

dermatologist
p. 112

diffuse alopecia
p. 124

epidermis
p. 119

fragilitas crinium
p. 116

guanidine hydroxide relaxer
p. 117

hypertrichosis
p. 116

inflammatory response
p. 124

keloidal tissue
p. 129

keratin treatments
p. 115

lithium hydroxide relaxer
p. 117

lye/sodium hydroxide
p. 115

malassezia
p. 119

miniaturization
p. 124

monilethrix
p. 116

no-lye perm
p. 117

papilla
p. 115

parietal front
p. 124

pediculosis capitis
p. 130

perifolliculitis keloidalis occipital (PFKO)
p. 129

pityriasis
p. 119

postpartum alopecia
p. 124

potential hydrogen (pH)
p. 115

psoriasis dermatitis
p. 112

relaxer base
p. 117

ringed hair
p. 116

seborrheic dermatitis
p. 121

sodium hydroxide relaxer (lye perm)
p. 117

sub-occipital
p. 118

thioglycolate perm
p. 118

tinea
p. 130

traction alopecia
p. 114

trichoptilosis
p. 116

trichorrhexis nodosa
p. 116

psoriasis dermatitis skin disease characterized by red patches covered with silver-white scales; usually found on the scalp, elbows, knees, chest, and lower back.

dermatologist physician who specializes in diseases and disorders of the skin, hair, and nails.

Everyone wants to have healthy, beautiful hair. A client's personal goal to obtain attractive, healthy hair can be greatly diminished by the weakened condition or traumatized state of the scalp. Some diseases of the scalp are infectious, others may be an allergic reaction to chemicals, and still others are an autoimmune response; all of them cause problems. Each disease or disorder has its own specific symptoms or conditions. Others, such as seborrheic dermatitis and **psoriasis dermatitis**, may have similar inflammatory conditions. Although these two scalp disorders manifest similar topical conditions, seborrheic dermatitis is the most common and can be helped in the salon with the application of non-fatty skin and scalp products designed for sensitive skin. Psoriasis dermatitis in general requires a visit with a dermatologist or physician to eliminate the skin disorder. The natural stylist should have on hand a list of dermatologists who are experienced in treating people of color with multi-textured hair and skin disorders. The relationship between the **dermatologist** and the natural stylist should be complementary and interactive. For a natural hair stylist, the focus is on hygiene, wellness, beauty, and care; on the other hand, the dermatologist's primary goal is to analyze, treat, prevent, and cure. Both professions address and fulfill the inherent need we have to be attractive, healthy, culturally aware, and socially accepted.

Why Study Hair and Scalp Diseases and Disorders?

Natural stylists should study and have a thorough understanding of the history of natural hair care and braiding and the career opportunities available because:

- You need to know how and why the hair grows and falls out in order to differentiate between normal and abnormal hair loss.

- To protect you and your client, you need to be able to identify certain scalp disorders that could be harboring communicable diseases.

- Knowing what creates natural texture is a part of offering the appropriate service for the client with the most effective treatment and hair enhancement camouflage.

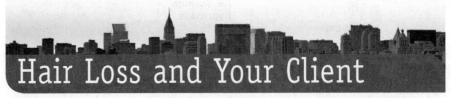

Hair Loss and Your Client

The emotional impact of hair loss is very real for men and women. Although it has been noted that hair loss occurs more often in men than in women, both are affected by the agonizing and intense feelings of shame, embarrassment, social anxiety or discomfort, and lack of attractiveness. When hair loss occurs, the client's self-image is impaired. For both men and women, losing hair, or even addressing the issues of a hair or scalp disorder, can be problematic and stressful. Some things an individual might experience with hair loss are

- lack of assertiveness.

- personality changes; they may become less personable or likable.

- looking much older, by five years or more.

Clients with hair loss may come to you first before going to a physician. As a natural stylist, you will be the first authority to address their emotional, aesthetic, and hair health needs. It is vital for you to recognize the disease or disorder so that you can cosmetically treat the problem.

The natural stylist's role is to educate the client on proper products, services, and techniques that will diminish the problem. If the affected area of hair loss is a recent problem for the client (occurring in the last 3 to 12 months), the natural stylist may be able to determine whether the hair loss is the result of chemical, physical, mechanical, or emotional effects in order to appropriately refer their client. The longer the scalp injury or disorder persists, the more permanent the hair loss. Some clients cover up painfully extensive hair loss and scalp disorders by camouflaging the condition with poorly made wigs, tight weaves, and heavy extensions, all of which can intensify the problem. The natural stylist must assist the client by offering support in self-care and a maintenance regimen that addresses or diminishes the problem **(Figure 6–1)**.

Causes of Hair Loss

During the hair growth cycle, people can lose an average of 50 to 100 hairs a day during the telogen/shedding phase. When a client's hair begins to thin, break, or fall out, or when male-pattern baldness becomes apparent, the body is often sending a signal that something is wrong **(Figure 6–2)**. Hair loss can be introduced or can result in the following ways:

- Hereditary, male or female-pattern baldness due to inherited genes

- Aging

- Emotional stress

- Sudden weight loss

- Poor nutrition

- Hormonal changes (pregnancy, menopause)

- Medications/drugs

- Surgery

- Endocrine disorders, thyroid problems

- Viral diseases, cancers, lupus

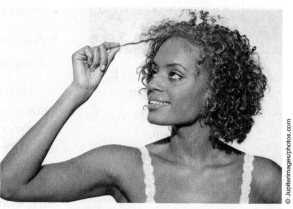

▲ Figure 6–1
Assisting clients in understanding their hair will help them improve their self-care.

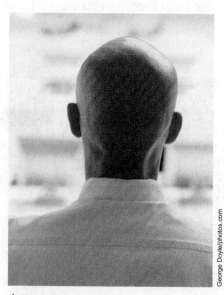

▲ Figure 6–2
Young man with completely bald head.

traction alopecia hair loss that occurs due to traction placed on hair. Traction alopecia is commonly seen with braids, ponytails, and other hairstyles that create traction on the scalp.

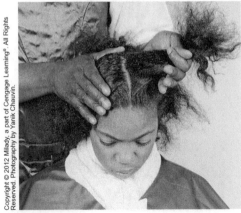

▲ Figure 6–3
Scalp analysis.

- Infection due to improper sterilization
- Autoimmune disease
- Excessive heat and chemical hair treatments

The internal factors that may cause hair loss usually require professional medical attention for proper diagnosis. Generally, a dermatologist will recommend a prescription shampoo, a topical scalp treatment, and/or a steroid injection provided during an office visit. Often the client will bring his prescribed hair treatment and request that you use it instead of the salon products. As with all products, read the labels and instructions before using it on the client. ☑ **LO1**

Caring for Your Client

If the medical condition can be arrested, often the hair will return when the body heals. Clients who are living with autoimmune diseases such as cancer, lupus, HIV, diabetes, and many other long-term degenerative diseases are very sensitive both physically and emotionally. The natural stylist must be supportive and patient and listen to each client's special styling needs. Often natural twists, soft braided/weave styles, or wigs can be created to camouflage as well as diminish the hair-loss problem. Take special note of any tenderness, scalp abrasions, or lesions when servicing clients with degenerative diseases to avoid causing infection **(Figure 6–3)**.

Your clients who have hair loss must avoid wearing heavy, thick braid extensions or feeling extreme tension from cornrows or weaves. These techniques will only accelerate the problem, because the weight of extensions will weaken already fragile hair strands. Placing large amounts of hair extensions on small amounts of thin, fragile hair creates stress on the hair shaft and can only cause further damage; it can be painful and will eventually lead to **traction alopecia** (discussed later in this chapter). In most cases, advise your clients not to use larger braid extension services (such as Casamas braids, corkscrews, or knots) during a transitional period of hair growth. You will avoid applying stress on damaged hair or the scalp as new, sparse hair returns. Using the "feed-in" method of cornrowing would best suit and protect hair in this transitional period.

For better results, offer non-extension braid services. Treat these clients with nurturing hair and scalp treatments, scalp massages, and a supportive, positive outlook. Your attitude and disposition will help clients relax and eventually build trust in your ability to nurture and groom their hair. Another alternative for major hair loss is to offer the client a stylish, contemporary wig. This approach will allow you to continue hair treatments without causing styling stress on the affected areas of the scalp. Styling and cutting a wig is a regular service you may offer clients with special needs.

Hair growth does not occur overnight. Inform your client that whatever caused the hair loss problem took months or years to develop. It will take much more time to stop the problem and for the client's hair to return. The longer the client has the hair-loss problem, the longer it will take for the scalp to recover from the trauma. If the scalp is badly scarred or chemically burned, or if the hair's **papilla** (the bulb of a hair strand) is totally destroyed, permanent hair loss will occur. Never create false hope. Be realistic with clients. Offer all possibilities to your client: the natural cut, Afro and twists with or without soft extensions, or soft, braided styles that will encourage hair growth and enhance the client's appearance.

The Chemical Effect

Since the late 1950s, women with curly and coily textured hair have been chemically straightening their hair. Its social and cultural rewards have been the major factor in its mainstream popularity. Removing and diminishing texture was the ultimate goal of every young black woman around the world. Every visual image on television, movies, and videos as well as in books, social settings, and the work environment has reinforced the concept that black women need to have thermal heat straightening or chemically straightened hair. Applying a sodium hydroxide relaxer (lye) on tight curly or coily (highly textured) hair may at first glance seem to make the hair more manageable and shiny; however, the harsh, corrosive chemicals negatively affect the hair and scalp. In many cases, a client can suffer from severe skin abrasion, burning, and inflammation from the improper use of chemical products and poor technical skills. Unfortunately, when clients receive a relaxer service, the burning and scalp discomfort have become the norm. Clients believe the longer the chemical stays on and/or burns the scalp, the straighter the hair becomes. On social media, you can find hundreds of blogs on the topic of what to do for scalp burns associated with the product. Standard chemical treatments, whether they use **lye/sodium hydroxide**, **no-lye/calcium hydroxide**, or **no-lye (ammonium thioglycolate)**, or **keratin treatments** with **pH (potential hydrogen)**, are harsh on the sponge-like scalp. The skin absorbs the chemicals. Repeated exposure to caustic chemicals will lead to hair loss and scalp damage.

papilla the small root area at the base of hair, which receives the nutrients needed for hair growth.

lye/sodium hydroxide sodium hydroxide, commonly known as lye, is a very strong alkali used in chemical hair relaxers, callous softeners, and hair depilatories.

calcium hydroxide (Ca(OH)$_2$ no-lye) a non pre-formulated straightener, and inorganic compound with the chemical formula combining a cream containing calcium hydroxide (slaked lime) with an "activating solution" of guanidine carbonate.

ammonium thioglycolate (HSCH$_2$CO$_2$NH$_4$; no-lye) a chemical compound also known as perm salt. Being the salt of a weak acid and weak base, ammonium thioglycolate exists in solution as an equilibrium mixture of the salt itself.

keratin treatments straightening systems that are keratin based. Keratin fills in gaps in the hair cuticle that are cracked, dry, or damaged. Some treatments contain varying levels of formaldehyde; when applied to the hair with keratin protein and sealed in with the heat of a flat iron, it straightens the hair. Because formaldehyde is a known carcinogen, many companies formulate natural progressive treatments with an organic compound made from L-cystine.

potential hydrogen (pH) represents the quantity of hydrogen ions.

canities (congenital and acquired) technical term for gray hair; results from the loss of the hair's natural melanin pigment.

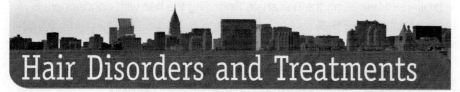

Hair Disorders and Treatments

Gray hair or **canities** is the technical term for graying hair. Its immediate cause is the loss of natural pigment or melanin in the hair. There are two types:

1. **Congenital canities** exists at or before birth. It occurs in albinos (people whose hair and bodies lack melanin) and occasionally in persons with normal hair. A patchy type of congenital hair graying may develop either slowly or rapidly, depending on the cause of the condition.

2. **Acquired canities** is due to the aging process or may occur prematurely in early adult life. Hair graying can be observed as early as age 13 in curly/coily hair types. The decrease or loss of melanin has been correlated to the hair growth cycle. As we age, during the

ringed hair a variety of canities characterized by alternating bands of gray and pigmented hair throughout the length of the hair strand.

hypertrichosis (hirsuties) condition of abnormal growth of hair, characterized by the growth of terminal hair in areas of the body that normally grow only velllus hair.

trichoptilosis technical term for split ends.

trichorrhexis nodosa technical term for the condition known as knotted hair; it is characterized by brittleness and the formation of nodular swellings along the hair shaft.

monilethrix technical term for a condition known as beaded hair.

fragilitas crinium technical term for brittle hair.

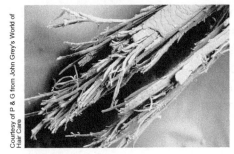

▲ Figure 6–4
Trichoptilosis.

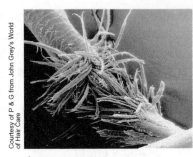

▲ Figure 6–5
Trichorrhexis nodosa.

telogen phase, the follicle and bulb shrink, reducing the process of hair pigmentation or melanin. Heredity, prolonged illness, and diet may also affect the hair pigmentation process.

Ringed hair is another variety of canities. It is characterized by alternate bands of gray and dark pigmented hair, a condition also known as salt and pepper.

Hypertrichosis, or hirsuties, refers to superfluous hair, an abnormal development of terminal hair on areas of the body normally bearing only downy vellus hair. Women with this disorder commonly have light mustaches, beards, or extreme facial hair. This condition is treated by tweezing hair or removing it with depilatories, electrolysis, waxing, or shaving.

Trichoptilosis is the technical term for split hair ends. Split ends are treated by applying conditioning hair oils to the hair to soften and lubricate the dry ends. Split ends are permanently removed by cutting **(Figure 6–4)**.

Trichorrhexis nodosa, or knotted hair, is a dry, brittle condition that includes formation of nodular swellings along the hair shaft. The hair breaks easily, and there is a brush-like spreading out of the fibers of the broken-off hair along the hair shaft. Softening the hair with conditioners is beneficial **(Figure 6–5)**.

Monilethrix is the technical term for beaded hair. The hair breaks between the beads or nodes. Scalp and hair treatments may improve the hair condition.

Fragilitas crinium is the technical term for brittle hair or split ends. The hairs may split at any part of their length. Conditioning hair treatments may be recommended. Cutting above the split hair is required to reduce further damage.

Chemical Damage

As a natural stylist, you are not legally allowed to apply chemical altering services. However, it is your responsibility to understand how chemical services work on textured hair **(Figure 6–6)**.

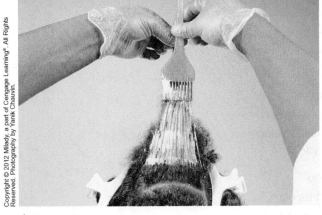

▲ Figure 6–6
Applying relaxer.

The external factors that can traumatize the scalp and cause hair loss usually stem from improper chemical relaxing and perm applications. Most women of the African diaspora and other women of color have straightened their textured hair with chemical relaxers—it is the most popular form of styling. About 90 percent of African American women have relaxed their hair at one time or another.

There are two basic types of chemical straighteners. One type of relaxer is sodium hydroxide or a lye perm the other types are **guanidine hydroxide** and **lithium hydroxide relaxers** or "no lye" perms. Due to the instability of the guanidine hydroxide relaxers, an "activator" or calcium hydroxide is added to the base to protect the new growth of textured hair. **No-lye perms**, as they are commercially called, dominate the retail market. Relaxer home kits can be bought at any neighborhood beauty supply store. They are the most popular relaxer kits for home use because they claim to be mild, safe, and gentle relaxers. These claims are misleading.

Sodium hydroxide relaxers (lye perms) have a high pH (potential hydrogen—the degree of acid mantle in the hair and scalp). The optimum neutral pH level for hair is 7. The lower the number on the pH scale, the more *acidic* the content. A pH higher than 7 indicates the **alkaline** level. The highest level on the pH scale is 14. Sodium hydroxide relaxers are the most caustic and reactive because of their high pH levels, which range from about 12 to 14 on the pH scale and are potentially dangerous to the hair and scalp. When this type of chemical touches the scalp, forehead, ear, or neck, burning irritation may occur. Before applying this type of relaxer, a pre-application of petroleum is required to protect the skin and scalp.

This type of highly alkaline relaxer, or **relaxer base**, requires the stylist to use an emollient such as petroleum, since manufacturers anticipate irritation to the scalp. The other type of relaxers, referred to as no-base relaxers, may be composed of guanidine hydroxide (no-lye). They are marketed as not requiring the use of a protective petroleum base. Although chemical burning is less frequent with a no-base, no-lye relaxer, some burning still may occur and a protective petroleum base should be applied to the hairline and scalp.

Despite manufacturers' claims, sodium hydroxide relaxers are irritants to the skin, scalp, eyes, and lungs; they are also environmental toxins. According to the Occupational Safety and Health Administration (OSHA), repeated use over a long period of time can promote temporary or permanent hair loss. Relaxers containing a concentrated solution with pH levels equal to 13.5 will cause the hair to dissolve and result in irreversible baldness and scalp burns. A burning sensation on the scalp, combined with a sore throat, nausea, vomiting, and shortness of breath, may be linked to certain cancers.

The most frequently noted side effect from using chemical relaxers is hair breakage. Anyone who has had a relaxer applied to their hair has experienced some type of breakage. Hair breakage is most common

Did you know?

Sodium hydroxide solutions are found in many different caustic products:

- Aids in the making of soap, detergents, and disinfectants
- Glass making
- Textile processing, metal processing, and degreasing
- Aluminum processing
- Adhesive preparation
- Paint remover
- Cellophane
- Rayon

guanidine hydroxide (GH) relaxer products using GH are known as no-lye relaxers; although they are technically not no-lye, the active ingredient is the hydroxide ion. GH contains two components that must be mixed immediately before using.

lithium hydroxide relaxer (LiOH; no-mix or no-lye) this substance is technically not lye, but the chemistry is identical. There is very little difference in performance of lithium hydroxide and lye. It is not widely used today.

no-lye perm/ammonium thioglycolate a chemical compound with the salt of a weak acid and weak base; ammonium thioglycolate exists in solution as an equilibrium mixture of the salt itself. Ammonium thioglycolate, also known as perm salt, is used to create permanent waves or curls.

sodium hydroxide relaxer (lye perm; NaOH) a strongly alkaline white deliquescent compound with a high pH. It is the most caustic and reactive because of its high pH levels, which range from about 12 to 14 on the pH scale, making it potentially dangerous to the hair and scalp. When this type of chemical touches the scalp, forehead, ear, or neck, burning irritation may occur. Before applying this type of relaxer, a pre-application of petroleum is required to protect the skin and scalp. It is also used in many industrial processes such as the manufacturing of soap and paper.

alkaline a solution that has a pH above 7.0 (neutral).

relaxer base a protective cream that is applied to the entire scalp before application of the relaxer.

sub-occipital the area underneath or below the occipital bone.

thioglycolate perm/no-lye perm a chemical compound with the salt of a weak acid and weak base; ammonium thioglycolate exists in solution as an equilibrium mixture of the salt itself. Ammonium thioglycolate, also known as perm salt, is used to create permanent waves or curls.

at the **sub-occipital** nape of the neck, where the chemical is often first applied and remains on the hair for the longest time. The frontal and temporal hairlines are secondary locations of damage because of long exposure to the chemical and overlapping processes during touch-up services.

For most women, touch-up services are applied much too often for chemically treated hair—usually every 3 to 4 weeks. This is not enough time to allow new natural hair to grow. Touch-ups are recommended every 6 to 8 weeks and even 10 weeks. The noted dermatologist Dr. Wesley Wilborn of Atlanta, Georgia, believes that frequent retouches are harmful. He says, "The relaxer invariably will overlap onto previously treated hair, causing resultant, irreparable damage to the hair shaft and subsequent breakage."[1]

In addition, Dr. Wilborn explains that:

> A depilatory effect may occur from the improper use of a chemical relaxer. The hair literally "melts away" when the cosmetologist chooses the incorrect relaxer strength or leaves the product on too long. The cosmetologist must be aware that all chemicals cause some kind of side effect and that it is their responsibility to minimize the occurrence, when using these products.

Here are some factors that affect the degree of breakage from relaxers:

- Strength of relaxer
- Application time
- Effective removal (neutralizing shampoo)
- Hair texture, phenotype
- Desired finished look

Many of the no-base relaxers are marketed for home use. Consumers buy the home kit to apply the relaxer themselves. Inevitably, the consumer will overlap or overprocess the hair. Most people will overlap hair in sections of the head that cannot be easily reached, such as the nape and crown. Although no-base relaxers are milder to the scalp, when used improperly, the chemicals can create breakage and scalp damage. Relaxer home kits are generally more drying, since they are formulated with calcium hydroxide. "Kiddie perms" are another popular chemical service offered as a home kit. Beautiful young girls with shiny, bone-straight hair are displayed on the boxes. The advertising is aimed toward vulnerable youths who want to look like the girls on the box. These advertisements might give the false impression that young children look more acceptable with straight hair.

In the 1970s and 1980s, "Jheri curls" and "California curls" or **thioglycolate perms/no-lye perms** were extremely popular. These chemical services offered African American men and women other styling options. First, the natural texture was removed or chemically straightened. Then the hair was rolled and saturated with an oxidizing agent or neutralizer to reshape the wave patterns, creating a loose curl. This two-step procedure lost its popularity after consumers reported severe scalp damage and breakage. The active ingredient, ammonium thioglycolate, was strong and depleted moisture from the hair. To maintain the curly style, the client was required to frequently replenish moisture with emollients that sealed in moisture and kept the hair wet and sticky. Clients often covered their heads with plastic bags and shower caps to retain the moisture. Hair breakage occurred during the straightening process if the hair was not kept hydrated. The same factors that affect breakage for relaxers hold true for curl or wave systems. Relaxed hair is stronger when dry, but curly, wavy, and coily (kinky) hair is more expansive and stronger when moist or wet.

Many clients reported that their hair was healthier and grew faster when they had a curly perm. However, it appears that the chemical service did not promote hair growth; rather, it was the moisturizing gels, sprays, and lotions that kept the hair wet and moist that aided in protecting the hair. Although the popularity of the curl perms has declined, the use of synthetic moisturizing agents has not. Moisture is the key to healthy and natural textured hair.

In this section, you have learned that many clients with a history of using chemicals on their hair wrestle with hair breakage and scalp damage. The natural hair care specialist must be emotionally supportive and patient and must listen to clients' special styling needs. You should offer all the possibilities to your clients, including natural or braided styles that will encourage hair growth. The factors that cause hair loss usually stem from improper chemical relaxing and perm applications. The lower the number on the pH scale, the more acidic the content. Although no-base relaxers are milder to the scalp when used improperly, the chemicals can create breakage and scalp damage.

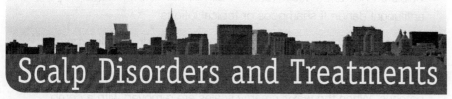

Scalp Disorders and Treatments

As a natural stylist, having a thorough understanding of scalp disorders and treatments will protect you and your client. A skilled and knowledgeable natural stylist will be able to identify certain scalp disorders that could be harboring communicable diseases.

Dandruff

The outermost layer of the scalp, the **epidermis**, continually sheds and replaces dead skin cells. A natural shedding of these small skin cells is a normal human occurrence and should not be confused with dandruff. Normal shedding is a light, powdery form of skin cells that disappear when the hair is washed or brushed. Dandruff, medically known as **pityriasis**, is the accumulation of large, visible clumps of scales on the scalp. It is characterized by the overproduction of skin cells. This excessive production is introduced to the scalp by the overgrowth of a fungal yeast, known as **malassezia**, that is a natural resident of the body. This fungus is normal to all human skin types, sexes, and races. However, when the fungal yeast grows out of control, the

epidermis the protective, nonvascular outer layer of the skin.

pityriasis a common skin problem that causes a rash. Although it can occur at any age, it is seen most often in people between the ages of 10 and 35.

malassezia naturally occurring fungus that is present on all human skin, but is responsible for dandruff when it grows out of control.

symptoms of dandruff occur. This scaly, painless scalp disorder occurs in about 45 percent of the human population. It is an aesthetic or cosmetic issue. Some individuals are also more susceptible to the irritating effects of malassezia. Factors such as stress, age, hormones, and poor hygiene can cause the fungus to multiply and dandruff symptoms to worsen.

Dandruff is usually accompanied by an itching sensation without skin inflammation or redness. Scales are often found on the shoulders, hair, scalp, neck, forehead, eyebrows, and sometimes breasts. When found on an infant's scalp, dandruff is called **cradle cap**. The infant usually grows out of this condition within a year. This excessive shedding of the cells may become worse in the cold, dry winter months. Simple and effective treatments are available to eradicate or control dandruff. Shampoos containing active antifungal base agents are very popular. Most clients prefer dandruff shampoos over topical creams. Dandruff shampoos conveniently address both the cleansing of the hair and removal of flakes while leaving an active coat on the scalp that reduces itching and scaling until the next shampoo. Many of the retail dandruff shampoos can be harsh on the hair. Natural stylists should advise their clients to use these shampoos for a limited time to avoid exposure to strong chemicals on the hair. Clients can also apply a secondary moisturizing shampoo to address the harshness and dryness to the hair.

cradle cap an oily, yellow scaling or crusting on a baby's scalp. It is common in babies and is easily treated. Cradle cap is not a part of any illness and does not imply that a baby is not being well cared for.

Types of Dandruff

There are two types of dandruff:

1. *Pityriasis capitis simplex* is considered the classic dandruff. This is the dry type associated with flaking, scattered scales, and itching. It is visible on hair and shoulders. It is easily removed with frequent use of antifungal dandruff shampoos or topical lotions.

2. *Pityriasis steroids* is considered more severe dandruff. This type of dandruff has large greasy or waxy scales that are combined with sebum, thus causing the scales to stick to the scalp in white creamy patches. When the waxy, creamy scales are removed with a comb, bleeding or oozing sebum may result. This severe dandruff may be accompanied by redness or inflammation. The client will experience more discomfort, and medical treatment is required. This type of dandruff is also very similar to seborrhea dermatitis.

Dandruff can be caused by the following internal factors:

- Poor circulation or metabolism

- Hormonal imbalance

- Poor nutrition

- Lack of water

- Stress and tension

- Glandular problems

- Biochemical changes to the scalp

The following external factors induce dandruff:

- Lack of proper cleansing
- Infrequent shampooing
- Topical medication ointments
- Oils or creams that irritate the scalp
- Increased activity of bacteria or fungi
- Poor scalp stimulation
- High pH in water
- High pH shampoos

Dandruff Treatments

Commercial dandruff shampoos all claim to treat dandruff problems. These shampoos are usually made with tar solutions that cosmetically and temporarily address the problem. The flaking generally reappears within 2 to 3 days, so frequent shampooing is required to control or minimize the problem. Daily shampooing is very drying and stressful to the hair as well as impractical for African Americans with highly textured hair types. Therefore, the stylist must look for products that offer longer, more effective results or that enhance commercial shampoos by adding natural extracts to aid the problem.

Shampoos, conditioners, hot-oil treatments, or ointments that contain the following substances have been noted to be effective as anti-dandruff products:

1. Selenium is effective in a shampoo that contains sulfur; it can be found in amino acids (cystine, cystini) and herbs (coltsfoot, horsetail, rosemary, sage) or plant oils (evening primrose, jojoba, eucalyptus, tea tree oil, or peppermint). See the herbal chart In Chapter 8.

2. Sulfur is found in the keratin fibers of protein in the hair and scalp. A deficiency of sulfur can weaken or impair the mucous membranes of the sebaceous gland (sebum), which can lead to dandruff, seborrhea, and hair loss.

3. Horsetail, coltsfoot, nettle, rosemary, and sage are botanicals rich in sulfur and amino acids. Vitamin B complex (panthenol and inositol) increases blood circulation and provides nutrients that are absorbed into the scalp to diminish seborrhea (excessively oily scalp).

4. Garlic or garlic extracts have anti-inflammatory properties and are used for their antifungal and antiseptic properties. They have a strong odor.

5. Apple cider vinegar as a pre-shampoo treatment cools and neutralizes the acidic base of the hair and scalp.

6. Tea tree oil is a very strong antiseptic and antifungal ingredient.

Seborrheic Dermatitis

Seborrheic dermatitis (SD) is a skin condition caused by an inflammation of the sebaceous glands. This condition is a form of eczema that can involve the

Did you know?

Dandruff is usually accompanied by an itching sensation and a scattering of scales. Since daily shampooing is very drying and stressful for African American hair types, weekly or biweekly medicated shampoo or cleansing is recommended.

seborrheic dermatitis a skin condition caused by an inflammation of the sebaceous glands. It is often characterized by redness, dry or oily scaling, crusting, and/or itchiness.

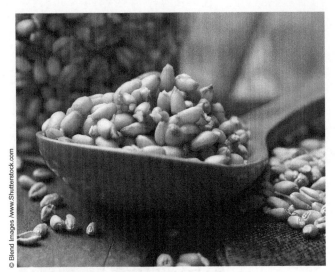

▲ Figure 6–7
Contributer to seborrheic dermatitis: wheat germ.

scalp, eyebrows, and chest—any area rich in sebaceous glands. Affected areas are characterized by greasy yellow scales. In dark skin types, areas may be drier and result in hypopigmented or hyperpigmented plaques. Left untreated, these plaques can spread to the entire face, neck, and upper torso.[2] Mild flares of seborrheic dermatitis are sometimes treated with cortisone creams. Severe cases should be referred to a dermatologist, who will often prescribe topical antifungal medications.

Seborrhea can also be an inflammatory reaction to some commonly used hair products. It may be induced by the following:

- Lanolin oil

- Soybean oil

- Wheat germ oil **(Figure 6–7)**

- Castor oil/peanut oil

The problem will lessen by simply avoiding certain hair products containing those ingredients. The following natural antiseptics can help benefit the client with seborrheic dermatitis:

- Aloe vera

- Chamomile

- Rosemary/sage

- Almond oil

- Lavender

Seborrheic dermatitis looks like wet dandruff. This greasy dandruff or excessive flaking consists of white, creamy, yeast-like film or patches that coat the scalp. However, unlike dandruff, this condition causes little flaking. The scalp is inflamed, itchy, and red. The oily discharge of sebum and skin scales adheres to the scalp. Although the scalp may be oily, in highly textured hair types the hair still may be dry. Therefore, daily shampooing is not recommended. A natural hair care specialist should suggest that the client use a pre-shampoo treatment consisting of essential oils, tea tree oil, peppermint oil, or rosemary mint oil, which are natural toxin removers that rid the scalp of yeast and fungus. Also suggest that the client shampoo her hair once a week with a medicated shampoo recommended by her physician or dermatologist. Be sure to tell the client to follow the prescribed or manufacturer's instructions for cleansing. Avoid heavy oils when treating this type of dermatitis, because they clog the pores.

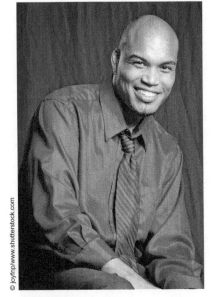

▲ Figure 6–8
Male-pattern baldness.

alopecia abnormal hair loss. |

Alopecia

Alopecia is the general term for a variety of problems, such as abnormal hair loss, balding, or reduced hair density **(Figure 6–8)**. It is an autoimmune disorder that mistakenly attacks the hair follicle during the anagen or telogen growth phase. There are several different types of alopecia, depending upon their location on the head, how they evolve on the scalp, and their underlying cause. In this section, we will discuss the seven most common hair-loss disorders: alopecia totalis, alopecia universalis, androgenetic alopecia, alopecia areata, diffuse alopecia, postpartum alopecia, and traction alopecia. These excessive hair-loss disorders should not be confused with normal hair shedding.

We all lose hair daily. The natural hair growth cycle involves continuous replenishing of new hair throughout our lifetime. As the old hair is shed during the telogen phase, it is replaced by another strand in the next new anagen phase, thus continuous new hair growth. Each follicle has its own individual time to regenerate and be replenished by new hair. The average life cycle of a hair strand is estimated at four to six years. A varying amount of hair is shed daily; anywhere from 50 to 150 hair strands are generally in the telogen, or shedding, phase. At any one time, 85 percent of our hair is normally in the anagen, or growing, phase. Ten to 20 percent of our hair is resting or in the weakened catagen phase. Telogen (shedding) hair continues for about 10 to 15 percent of this two- to five-month period. Both the anagen and telogen phases can be shortened, accelerated, or destroyed by alopecia and by a variety of contributing factors:

- Gender—men more frequently experience greater hair loss than women do.

- Age—young children have fine hair that easily can be removed by pulling or traction, without pain.

- Hair type—all hair types are vulnerable.

- Nutrition—acute deficiencies in protein, iron, zinc, sulfur, and essential/fatty acids affect hair growth.

- Heredity—those with a personal or family history of hair loss are prone to alopecia.

- Physical health—surgical operations, sudden or extreme weight loss, anemia, and hormonal changes (especially thyroid or postpartum shedding) can affect hair growth.

- Emotional health—hair growth cycles can be affected by extreme psychological depression/anxiety, stress, or trauma.

- Drugs or chemical ingestion—growth cycles can be affected by some medications (i.e., general anesthesia, antidepressants, steroids), exposure to some pesticides, arsenic poisoning, some over-the-counter drugs (i.e., products that contain boric acid: eye drops, gynecological topical solutions, and spermicides, just to name a few).

These extreme hair-loss disorders are accelerated when external or internal trauma takes place. These traumas can trigger the body's immune system to "defend" itself. When the body or the spirit has been traumatized, alopecia of some form may occur, signaling to the stylist that special services should be rendered. Hair loss due to psychological or emotional stress will reverse itself naturally once the stress is

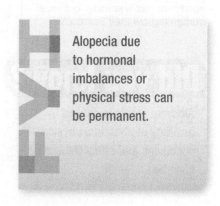

FYI

Alopecia due to hormonal imbalances or physical stress can be permanent.

alopecia totalis total loss of scalp hair.

alopecia universalis complete loss of body hair.

androgenetic alopecia (alopecia androgenetic) hair loss characterized by miniaturization of terminal hair that is converted to vellus hair; in men, this disorder is known as male pattern baldness.

miniaturization a condition of the hair follicle when long, thick, and pigmented (terminal) hair strands are replaced by short, thin, and unpigmented hair.

parietal front (parietal ridge) the widest area of the head, usually starting at the temples and ending at the bottom of the crown.

alopecia areata autoimmune disorder that causes the affected hair follicles to be mistakenly attacked by a person's own immune system; usually begins with one or more small, round, smooth bald patches on the scalp.

inflammatory response occurs when the body identifies an area of the scalp as the enemy and wants to destroy the hair follicle.

diffuse alopecia appears in both women and men; however, women are much more affected than men. Diffuse hair loss can occur at any age and is characterized by thinning of the entire scalp, followed by thinning of the hair (the hair loses its density). Diffuse hair loss is temporary; hair grows back as long as the hair follicle remains active.

postpartum alopecia (telogen effluvium) a classic short-term disorder that often happens to women soon after giving birth. The sudden change in hormone levels at birth is such a shock to the hair follicles that they shut down for a while. There may be some significant hair shedding, but most women regrow their hair quickly.

Did you know?

Alopecia areata is caused by a variety of abnormal physical conditions that affect the scalp condition or health.

addressed, alleviated, or managed. However, other more chronic alopecia disorders due to imbalances, diet deficiencies, autoimmune disorders, or other physical stressors can manifest permanent or long-term hair loss.

Types of Alopecia

Some of the most common types of alopecia are as follows:

- **Alopecia totalis**—starts with small, round patches of hair loss and progresses until there is total scalp hair loss.

- **Alopecia universalis**—all body hair is lost.

- **Androgenetic alopecia**—also known as male-pattern baldness; can occur in both men and women. This disorder can start as early as age 13 in young men and after puberty in women. It generally develops slowly over 15 to 30 years and increases with age in both sexes. Androgenetic alopecia affects 20 percent of men by age 20, and 50 percent by age 50. For women, the presence of this disorder is lower, but signs of reduced hair density can be seen as early as age 30. Usually between the ages of 50 and 60, and with hormonal changes after menopause, women will see their hair lose density and eventually experience the unavoidable androgenetic alopecia or male-pattern baldness. This disorder is characterized by a slow decrease in hair density along with reduced hair size. The terminal hair (long, thick strands with pigment) is replaced by intermediate hair. This hair is later replaced by vellus hair (short, thin, unpigmented hair), a condition called **miniaturization** of the hair follicle. In women, this disorder is usually seen at the crown of the head and at the temples. In men, this disorder is generally located at the **parietal front** and progresses to a horseshoe-shaped outline at the crown of the head to the occipital area.

- **Alopecia areata**—People with this type of alopecia experience the sudden or sometimes unrecognized falling out of hair in patches or spots. These smooth oval or round bald patches can vary in size from ⅛ inch to 4 inches (0.3 cm to 10 cm) in diameter. The affected areas are usually lighter in color (often pale) due to the poor blood supply to the area. Alopecia areata is an autoimmune dysfunction in which certain cells create an **inflammatory response** to the hair follicle that triggers the telogen or catagen phase hair growth cycle in a particular area of the scalp. The body identifies that area of the scalp as the enemy and wants to destroy the hair follicle. In most cases, the destruction or weakening of the hair follicle is temporary. The inflammatory response usually will decrease. The affected area generally grows back and can take up to a year or more for full recovery. **Diffuse alopecia**, or alopecia areata incognita, is a rare form of alopecia areata. It affects primarily young females, and the hair loss on the head is radical and sudden.

- **Postpartum alopecia** is temporary hair loss experienced at the end of a pregnancy. For some women, pregnancy seems to disrupt the normal growth cycle of hair. Very little normal hair loss occurs during pregnancy, but then sudden and excessive shedding takes place from three to nine months after delivery. Although this experience is usually very traumatic for the new mother, the growth cycle generally returns to normal within a year after the baby is delivered.

Traction Alopecia

Traction alopecia is the most common balding disorder among young women and girls with highly textured hair. Many suffer with this problem in early adolescence. Traction baldness occurs when the hair is pulled too tight. The hair is literally pulled out of the follicle, taking out the hair root and the bulb. Destroying the hair shaft may cause white bumps and pus, or scaling may occur around the affected area. If the tight pulling continues over a long period of time, permanent scarring or balding will develop **(Figure 6–9)**.

It takes about one to three years for the bald spot to develop. If the client continues to style or groom her hair the same way, day after day, without altering the tension, traction alopecia can begin very rapidly—sometimes within weeks. Hair loss is often apparent in the frontal and temporal regions of the head. The nape of the neck can also be affected by traction alopecia, depending on the hair texture and how the hair is styled.

Traction alopecia is directly related to improper grooming techniques and hairstyling practices. The main culprits in this disorder include tight braids and ponytails, but sponge rollers are the worst offenders.

Braids and Traction Alopecia

Initially, all braids create a small amount of tension on the hair **(Figure 6–10)**. However, when a braider properly starts the braid style, cornrows, or extensions—there should be no pain, discomfort, or irritation to the scalp. The braid stylist must always remember that the basic concept of servicing the client is to nurture and groom. The braid stylist should be aware of the following guidelines for braiding services:

• Improper tension—This can occur when starting the braid. Too often braiders start the braid very tightly when applying an extension to the

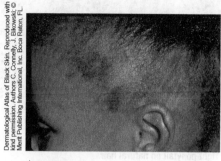

▲ Figure 6–9
"Severe" traction alopecia with tight braids.

Did you know?

When you have a client with traction alopecia, it is your responsibility to reeducate the client.

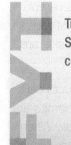

Traction baldness occurs when the hair is pulled too tightly. Some women ignore the warning signs of hair loss by continuing to wear damaging hairstyles.

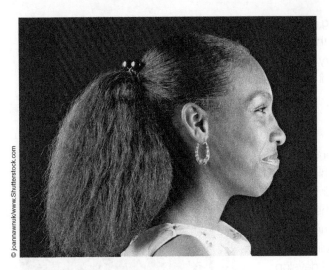

▲ Figure 6–10
Tight ponytail on natural hair.

hairline (frontal and temporal regions). Braiders often try to gather the fine or broken strands of hair while keeping the extension taut.

- Excessive amount of hair extension—Applying too much additional hair extension material disproportionate to the number of strands in the sectioned hair can cause excessive tension on the natural hair. The hair extension materials become too heavy for small amounts of natural hair, particularly when the hair begins to grow out from the base. When hair grows away from the base, the large, heavy braid extension is attached to only three or four strands of natural hair, causing tension.

- Braids worn too long—Six to eight weeks is the average length of time for an extended braid style. If worn longer, hair breakage may occur. As the natural hair grows, the extension grows away from the base and then starts to pull and stress the scalp area. Extension hair can also rub and erode the exposed area, leading to balding and breakage.

- Braided styles and hair pulled back—Braided and locked styles that are constantly pulled away from the face contribute to the tension. Single braids or cornrows that stress the hairline should be worn down occasionally, to relieve tension on the scalp. Braids that are styled upward all the time are also detrimental to the scalp. They should not be worn for more than 2 months. Try to style the braids so that they can be loosened at night or worn down to relieve the stress on the scalp.

- Pustules—Pustules are small white pimples that seep pus. They are a direct result of tension from excessive pulling and cause lack of circulation. If scratched or irritated, the pustules may become infected. This condition may require medical attention.

- Tight ponytails—Young girls and very busy working women find it easier to simply get a rubber band or some elastic band and pull the hair back into a ponytail. It appears to be neat, quick, and easy; however, it is also very damaging to the hair and scalp if the ponytail is constantly worn too tight.

- Tension on ponytails—The pulling tension from ponytails affects the scalp. Slick, sleek updos are very popular and contribute to this problem. When putting in a ponytail or updo, don't pull excessively or cause too much tension in the style. The braid stylist will know if the hair is too tight. The stylist will notice that the client's eyes and skin are pulled taut into an almond shape and look distorted.

- Hair accessories associated with ponytail styles—These products can be problematic, too. Rubber bands, elastic clips, bows, and clamps are all attractive and easy to use, but they are damaging to the hair. When in doubt, avoid all rubber bands or elastic ties. Some elastic ties are covered in cotton and are more appropriate when not doubled around the braid. Also, remember to instruct the client to remove the ponytail at the end of the day if it is not sewn on. This will relieve the scalp of any tension.

- Sponge rollers—Sponge rollers are the worst hair-setting tool on the market for textured hair, because they pull on individual strands and cause tension and breakage. The most commonly affected areas are the frontal and temporal regions. However, depending on the style and hair texture, the occipital area or nape can be badly damaged as well. The real problem with sponge rollers is that they do not "give" when the hair is wound around the pink sponge. Sponge rollers will create an excellent tight curl, but they also create tension and stress on affected areas. Once the hair is unwrapped, hair is always found stuck on the sponge, even when endpapers are used to protect the hair strands. Sponge rollers are made from a soft, synthetic material that helps the wearer sleep easier when wearing sponge rollers at night. However, when the client sleeps, the roller is rubbing and eroding the hairline. If the wearer does not pay close attention, a bald spot will begin to appear. If ignored, the hair loss can be permanent.

Clients with Traction Alopecia

There are five steps you should take when dealing with a client's alopecia:

1. Learn the client's history and styling practices, and note them on the profile card during the consultation.

2. Point out all the affected areas, and make a note of them.

3. Try to determine whether the damage appears to be permanent, and insist that the client stop any abusive behavior to the hair.

4. Suggest camouflage styling techniques to help the client feel and look better.

Once tension is removed and nurturing treatments are applied, new hair may come back. However, its growth will be intermittent.

How to Service Clients Who Have Alopecia

External treatments to stimulate blood flow and rejuvenate hair growth vary from person to person. Slow, therapeutic scalp and head massages are recommended to increase blood flow and create a nurturing environment, which helps relax the client. Massages with aromatic oils and herbs are helpful and create calmness through the olfactory system (smell). Aromatherapy with essential oils has been recorded since the 12th dynasty in Egypt to heal and nurture the body. Some stimulating oils are as follows:

- Peppermint
- Rosehip seed

Did you know?

Pam Ferrell, the author of *Where Beauty Touches Me*, noted that it was very common to see young girls and women with hairlines as far back as 2 inches (5 cm) as witnessed on one of her many trips to West Africa. She attributes this condition to abusive practices that are taught from one generation to another.[3] The same holds true for styling or curling the hair with sponge rollers. Our peers and mothers used them, so many of us continue to use them.

- Lavender

- Eucalyptus

- Rosemary

- Black seed

- Clover

- Tea tree

Clients with alopecia areata can be aided by using the following eleven steps:

1. Preheat oil needed for the hair treatment.

2. Shampoo once to remove surface debris from hair or braid.

3. Place warm oil on scalp in small amounts, section by section.

4. Massage the scalp slowly and rhythmically, kneading, stroking and rolling, and squeezing gently. Avoid disturbing braid extensions or tangling hair. Focus on the scalp.

5. Once the oil is distributed evenly, place a cotton strip around the client's entire head to keep oil from dripping into her eyes.

6. Place a damp towel or plastic cap on the head to retain moisture.

7. When using a hair steamer or heating cap, apply heat for 20 minutes. A conditioning rinse may also be applied to the hair.

8. Apply mild conditioning or medicated shampoo for the second cleansing.

9. Rinse oil from hair; towel dry.

10. Lightly spray hair or braids with a finishing rinse or comprehensive lotion to coat the hair for manageability.

11. Groom; blowdry with low, warm air for braided style.

Medical Hair Loss Treatments

As a natural stylist, you need to familiarize yourself with the medical treatments available for certain forms of hair loss. Of all treatments that are said to counter hair loss, only two products—minoxidil and finasteride—that have been proven to stimulate hair growth and are approved by the Food and Drug Administration (FDA) for sale in the United States.

Minoxidil is a topical (applied to the surface of the body) medication that is put on the scalp twice a day and has been proven to stimulate hair growth. It is sold over the counter (OTC) as a nonprescription drug. Minoxidil is available for both men and women and comes in two different strengths: 2 percent regular-strength solution and 5 percent extra-strength solution. It is not known to have any serious negative side effects. The most well-known minoxidil product on the market is Rogaine®.

Finasteride is an oral prescription medication for men only. Although finasteride is more effective and convenient than minoxidil, possible side effects include weight gain and loss of sexual function. Women may not use this treatment, and pregnant women or those who might become pregnant are cautioned to avoid even touching finasteride tablets because of the strong potential for birth defects.

In addition to the treatments just described, several surgical options are available to treat alopecia. A hair transplant is the most common permanent hair replacement technique. This process consists of removing small sections of hair, including the follicle, papilla, and hair bulb, from an area where there is a lot of hair (usually in the back) and transplanting them into the bald area. These sections grow normally in the new location. Only licensed surgeons may perform this procedure, and several surgeries are usually necessary to achieve the desired results. The cost of each surgery can range from $8,000 to over $20,000.

Hair stylists can offer a number of nonmedical options to counter hair loss. Some salons specialize in nonsurgical hair replacement systems such as wigs, toupees, hair weavings, and hair extensions. With proper training, you can learn to fit, color, cut, and style wigs and toupees. Hair weavings and hair extensions allow you to enhance a client's natural hair and create a look that boosts self-esteem. ☑ **LO2**

Folliculitis Keloidalis

The scalp disorder folliculitis keloidalis is common among young African American men. It is also known as **acne keloidalis** or **perifolliculitis keloidalis occipital (PFKO)** and commonly referred to as "razor bumps." This disorder is the chronic inflammation, irritation, and infection of the hair follicle. The infection leads to scarring or lesions usually found in the occipital region of the head or the back of the neck. The scarring usually occurs in areas where a razor or an electric trimmer is used to enhance the hairline.

In the early stage of this scalp disorder, soft papules (pimples) rise, harden with time, and eventually form **keloidal tissue (Figure 6–11)**. The skin has been traumatized by the repeated use of the uncleaned razor or clipper, thereby creating an infection of the follicle.

Currently, this disorder is increasing due to close-cut styles like fades, caesars, and bald cuts, which require using razors and liners to repeatedly touch the skin to remove coily and curly hair. More women are experiencing this disorder because short new cuts for women are increasing in popularity.

Two hereditary factors contribute to this severe keloidal scarring:

1. Coily/curly hair—The tight coil (highly textured) or conformation of the follicle determines the hair shape. Consequently, the curl shaft, when cut close, pierces and reenters the skin, forming pimples or papules.

acne keloidalis a destructive, scarring folliculitis that occurs almost exclusively on the occipital scalp of people of African descent, primarily men.

perifolliculitis keloidalis occipital (PFKO) a common scalp disorder among young African American men; it is often referred to as razor bumps. PFKO is the chronic inflammation, irritation, and infection of the hair follicle. It leads to scarring or lesions usually found in the occipital region of the head or back of the neck.

keloidal tissue a thick scar resulting from excessive growth of fibrous tissue.

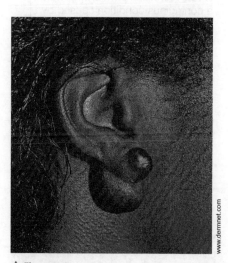
www.dermnet.com

▲ Figure 6–11
Keloidal tissue on ear.

Here's a **Tip**..........

Men and women prone to keloidal scarring should avoid fades or bald cuts and allow the hair to grow a little fuller and away from the scalp before having the hair cut with a razor.

2. African Americans are genetically prone to keloids. When the skin tries to heal itself after the razor cut, instead of creating a scab, the skin cells produce inflamed tissues. The soft papules dry and harden and then leave raised skin tissue or keloids.

Clients can avoid this keloidal scarring challenge by avoiding close haircuts or clean lines with an electric trimmer on the neck. Those prone to scarring should avoid fades or bald cuts. These clients should always allow their hair to grow a little fuller and away from the scalp. Wearing hair twisted or in locked styles is a great alternative.

If the infection is active, the natural stylist must recommend that the client see a dermatologist. A typical and/or systemic antibiotic is usually required to aid the healing process.

Remember—always clean and disinfect tools before every service. Infection of the follicle can be avoided if all razors, clippers, and and trimmers are cleaned and disinfected before and after every cutting service.

Vegetable Parasitic Infections

Tinea is the medical term for ringworm, which is caused by vegetable parasites. All forms of ringworm are contagious and can be transmitted from one person to another. The disease is commonly carried by scales or hairs containing fungi. Bathtubs, swimming pools, and uncleaned articles can also be sources of transmission.

Ringworm starts with a small, reddened patch of little blisters. Several such patches may be present. Any ringworm condition should be referred to a physician.

Tinea capitis, or ringworm of the scalp, is characterized by red papules, or spots, at the opening of the hair follicles **(Figure 6–12)**. The patches spread and the hair becomes brittle and lifeless. It breaks off, leaving a stump, or falls from the enlarged open follicles.

Tinea favosa, also known as favus or honeycomb ringworm, is characterized by dry, sulfur-yellow, cuplike crusts on the scalp, called scutula, which have a peculiar odor. Scars from favus are bald patches that may be pink or white and shiny. It is very contagious and should be referred to a physician.

Ringworm can be minimized by keeping tools and the work area sanitized with antifungal solutions or detergents.

Animal Parasitic Infections

Scabies "itch" is a highly contagious, animal parasitic skin disease caused by the itch mite. Vesicles and pustules can form from the irritation of the parasites or from scratching the affected areas.

Pediculosis capitis is a contagious condition caused by the head louse (animal parasite) infesting the hair of the scalp. As the parasites feed on the scalp, itching occurs and the resultant scratching can cause an infection. The head louse is transmitted from one person to another by contact with

tinea technical term for ring worm, a contagious condition caused by fungal infection and not a parasite, characterized by itching, scales and sometimes painful lesions.

pediculosis capitis, infestation of the hair and scalp with head lice.

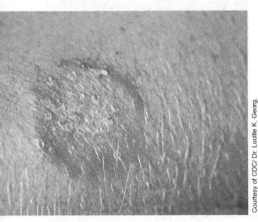

Courtesy of CDC/ Dr. Lucille K. Georg.

▲ Figure 6–12
Ringworm.

infested hats, combs, brushes, or other personal articles. To kill head lice, advise the client to apply larkspur tincture or other similar medication to the entire head before bedtime. The next morning, the client should shampoo with germicidal soap. Treatment should be repeated as necessary. Never treat a head lice condition in the salon or school. Advise the client to use caution when applying shampoos, creams, and lotions that contain *insecticides* (e.g., linden or larkspur solution). Pregnant women as well as infants should avoid all insecticide solutions. ☑ **LO3**

Myth: Heavy Grease and Pomades Help Natural Hair Grow

Ingredients made from petroleum, mineral oil, and lanolin are typically included in the category of heavy "grease" and pomade products, and they should be avoided. Some clients have an emotional attachment to the thick feel and fragrance of a heavy lacquered look. Educate the client on lighter herbal and botanically based products that add nutrients and fortify the hair instead of just coating the hair shaft and clogging the pores of the scalp.

Review Questions

1. List and describe the three stages of hair growth.
2. Why is it important for the natural stylist to understand the different types of hair disorders and hair loss?
3. Describe the difference between congenital canities and acquired canities.
4. Describe the two types of dandruff.
5. List the internal factors that cause dandruff.
6. What are the common treatments used for dandruff?
7. How many strands of hair are shed daily?
8. List the seven types of alopecia described in this chapter.
9. What types of styles are commonly seen with traction alopecia?
10. Which scalp disorder results in scarring that usually occurs in areas where a razor or an electric liner is used to enhance the hairline?
11. What is the medical term for ringworm, which is caused by vegetable parasites?
12. List and describe two types of animal parasitic infections.

Chapter References

1. Wilborn, W. S. (1994). Disorders of hair growth in African Americans. In E. A. Olsen (Ed.), *Disorders of hair growth: Diagnosis and treatment* (p. 395). New York McGraw-Hill.
2. Pierce, A. (2013). *Milady's aesthetician series: Treating diverse pigmentation*. Clifton Park, NY: Milady, a part of Cengage Learning.
3. Ferrell, P. (1993). *Where beauty touches me: Natural hair care & beauty book*. Washington, DC: Cornrows & Co.

Basic Anatomy, Physiology, and Nutrition

Chapter Outline

- Why Study Basic Anatomy, Physiology, and Nutrition?

- Anatomy, Physiology, and You

- Eleven Main Body Systems and Their Functions

- Nourishment from Within to Produce Healthy Hair

- Nutrition and Maintaining Healthy Hair

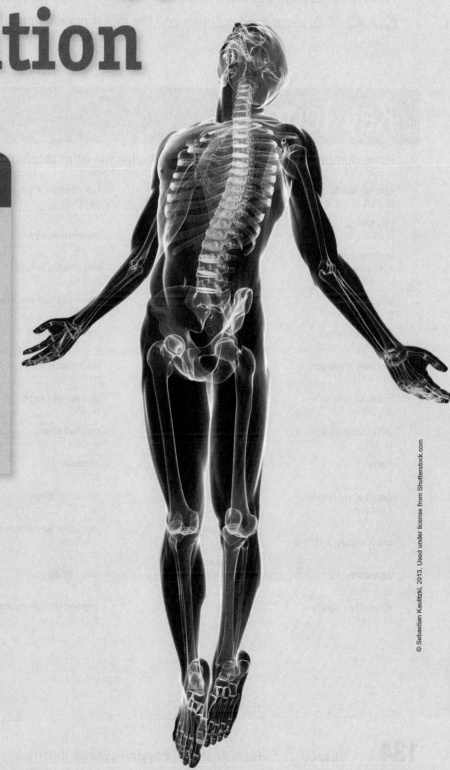

Learning Objectives

After completing this chapter, you should be able to:

☑ **LO1** Define and explain the importance of anatomy and physiology and how it relates to the profession of natural hair care and braiding.

☑ **LO2** Name 9 body organs and the 11 body systems.

☑ **LO3** Explain the basic functions of the 11 body systems.

☑ **LO4** Discuss good nutrition and the role it plays in maintaining healthy hair.

Key Terms

Page number indicates where in the chapter the term is used.

amino acids
p. 150

anatomy
p. 135

autonomic nervous system
p. 140

blood
p. 141

body systems
p. 136

carbon dioxide
p. 141

cardiac muscle
p. 139

cell enzymes
p. 150

cells
p. 136

central nervous system
p. 140

circulatory system
p. 141

cranium
p. 138

digestive system
p. 144

endocrine glands
p. 142

endocrine system
p. 142

epicranial aponeurosis
p. 139

epicranius
p. 139

ethmoid bone
p. 138

excretory system
p. 143

exocrine glands
p. 142

facial skeleton
p. 138

frontal bone
p. 138

frontalis
p. 139

hormones
p. 143

integumentary system
p. 136

lungs
p. 143

lymphatic/immune system
p. 142

muscular system
p. 138

nervous system
p. 140

nonstriated muscles
p. 138

nutriceuticals
p. 145

nutricosmetics
p. 145

occipital bone
p. 138

occipitalis
p. 139

organs
p. 136

parietal bones
p. 138

peripheral nervous system
p. 140

physiology
p. 135

reproductive system
p. 143

respiration
p. 143

respiratory system
p. 143

retinoic acid
p. 151

skeletal system
p. 137

skin
p. 136

skull
p. 138

sphenoid bone
p. 138

spinal cord
p. 141

striated muscles
p. 138

temporal bones
p. 138

tissue
p. 136

United States Department of Agriculture (USDA)
p. 149

A basic scientific understanding of the structure and functions of the human body will help the natural hair stylist to provide clients with the appropriate service. It is important to understand how the various body systems work as an integrated whole toward wellness.

A healthy, functioning body will produce healthy hair. Hair is a part of the whole. Although as a natural hair care specialist, you may never use the names of the bones, muscles, or nerves in the salon, a general understanding of how they work will increase your proficiency when performing many of the natural hair care services and braided styles. A general understanding of anatomy and physiology will enable you to recognize the differences between what is and is not considered a normal body function and whether a specific treatment is appropriate.

Why Study Basic Anatomy, Physiology, and Nutrition?

Natural stylists should study and have a thorough understanding of anatomy and physiology because:

- Understanding how the human body functions as a whole is a key component in understanding how a client's hair may react to various treatments.

- Understanding the bone and muscle structure of the body will help you properly provide services, apply products to the scalp, and perform manipulations of the face.

- Understanding nutrition is important for overall health and wellness, including the hair and scalp.

Anatomy, Physiology, and You

While you should have an overall knowledge of human anatomy, the work of the natural stylist is primarily limited to the skin, muscles, nerves, circulatory system, and bones of the head. Understanding the anatomy of these areas will help you develop techniques that can be used during scalp massage and as part of a ritual at the shampoo station. In addition, knowing the bones of the skull and facial structure is important in designing flattering hairstyles that gracefully drape the head. ✓ **LO1**

Anatomy is the study of the human body structures that can be seen with the naked eye and how the body parts are organized; it is the science of the structure of organisms or of their parts.

Physiology is the study of the functions and activities performed by the body's structures. The ending -*ology* means "study of."

anatomy study of the human body structure that can be seen with the naked eye and how the body parts are organized; the science of the structure of organisms or of their parts.

physiology the study of the functions and activities performed by the body's structures.

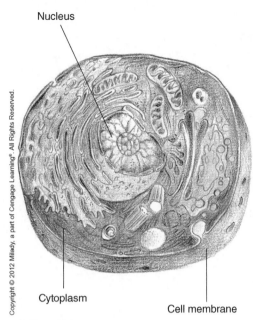

Nucleus

Cytoplasm

Cell membrane

▲ Figure 7–1
Basic structure of the cell.

cells basic units of all living things from bacteria to plants to animals, including human beings.

tissue collection of similar cells that perform a particular function.

organs structures composed of specialized tissues designed to perform specific functions in plants and animals.

body systems (systems) groups of body organs acting together to perform one or more functions.

integumentary system body system that protects the body from environmental elements, such as germs, chemicals, water, and sun exposure. This system includes accessory organs such as oil glands, sweat glands, sensory receptors, hair, and nails.

skin major organ that is the external protective coating that covers the body.

Cells

Cells are the basic units of all living things, from bacteria to plants to animals, including human beings. Without cells, life does not exist. As a basic functional unit, the cell is responsible for carrying on all life processes. There are trillions of cells in the human body, and they vary widely in size, shape, and purpose **(Figure 7–1)**.

Tissues

Tissue is a collection of similar cells that perform a particular function. Each kind of tissue has a specific function and can be recognized by its characteristic appearance. Body tissues are composed of large amounts of water, along with various other substances. There are four types of tissue in the body:

- **Connective tissue** is fibrous tissue that binds together, protects, and supports the various parts of the body. Examples of connective tissue are bone, cartilage, ligaments, tendons, blood, lymph, and *adipose tissue*, a technical term for fat. Adipose tissue gives smoothness and contour to the body.

- **Epithelial tissue** is a protective covering on body surfaces, such as skin, mucous membranes, tissue inside the mouth, the lining of the heart, the digestive and respiratory organs, and the glands.

- **Muscle tissue** contracts and moves various parts of the body.

- **Nerve tissue** carries messages to and from the brain and controls and coordinates all bodily functions. Nerve tissue is composed of special cells known as neurons that make up the nerves, brain, and spinal cord.

Organs and Body Systems

Organs are structures composed of specialized tissues designed to perform specific functions in plants and animals **(Table 7–1)**. **Body systems**, also known as *systems*, are groups of body organs acting together to perform one or more functions.

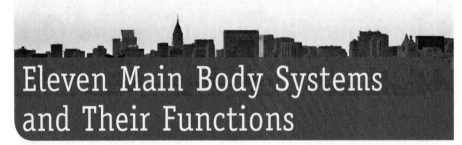

Eleven Main Body Systems and Their Functions

The groups of organs that work together for the common well-being of the human body are called systems. The body is composed of 11 systems that sustain the skin, bones, muscles, nerves, blood supply, lungs, waste elimination, stomach, and reproduction.

Integumentary System: Skin

The word *integument* means "natural covering." The skin is the natural covering and serves to protect the body. The **skin** protects the body

MAJOR BODY ORGANS AND THEIR FUNCTIONS

ORGAN	FUNCTION
BRAIN	Controls the body.
EYES	Control the body's vision.
HEART	Circulates the blood.
KIDNEYS	Excrete water and waste products.
LUNGS	Supply oxygen to the blood.
LIVER	Removes waste created by digestion.
SKIN	Covers the body and is the external protective coating.
STOMACH	Digests food along with the intestines.
INTESTINES	Digest food along with the stomach.

Table 7–1 Nine Major Body Organs and Their Functions.

from environmental elements such as germs, chemicals, water, and sun exposure. Included in this system are accessory organs such as oil glands, sweat glands, sensory receptors, hair, and nails. As the blood circulates through the skin, the blood and lymph contribute essential materials for growth, nourishment, and repair of the skin, hair, and nails. Networks of arteries and lymphatic vessels that send their smaller branches to hair papillae, hair follicles, and skin glands are found in the subcutaneous tissues.

Skeletal System: Bones

Bone structure provides the physical foundation of the body. It is composed of 206 bones of different sizes and shapes that are connected by movable and immovable joints. It shapes and supports the body and protects various internal structures and organs. It also serves to attach muscles and joints that act as levers to produce body movement.

Except for the tissue that forms the major part of the teeth, bone is the hardest tissue in the body. It is composed of connective tissue consisting of about one-third organic matter, such as cells and blood, and two-thirds minerals, mainly calcium carbonate and calcium phosphate.

The primary functions of the skeletal system are as follows:

- Give shape and support to the body.

- Protect various internal structures and organs.

- Serve as attachments for muscles and act as levers to produce body movement.

skeletal system body system that forms the physical foundation of the body. It is composed of 206 bones of different sizes and shapes that are connected by movable and immovable joints. It shapes and supports the body and protects various internal structures and organs. It also serves to attach muscles and joints, which act as levers to produce body movement.

skull The skull is the skeleton of the head and is divided into two parts:

- Cranium—an oval, bony case that protects the brain.
- Facial skeleton—the framework of the face that is composed of 14 bones.

cranium an oval, bony case that protects the brain.

facial skeleton the framework of the face that is composed of 14 bones.

occipital bone hindmost bone of the skull, below the parietal bones; forms the back of the skull above the nape.

parietal bones bones that form the sides and top of the cranium. There are two parietal bones.

frontal bone bone that forms the forehead.

temporal bones bones that form the sides of the head in the ear region. There are two temporal bones.

ethmoid bone light, spongy bone between the eye sockets; forms part of the nasal cavities.

sphenoid bone bone that joins all the bones of the cranium together.

muscular system muscles are fibrous tissues. This body system shapes and supports the skeletal system. Its function is to produce all movements of the body. It consists of more than 500 muscles, large and small, and comprises about 50 percent of the body's weight.

striated muscles also known as skeletal muscles. Muscles that are attached to the bones and are voluntary, consciously controlled.

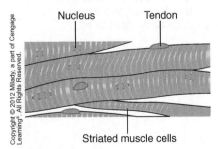

Nucleus   Tendon

Striated muscle cells

▲ Figure 7–2
Striated muscle cells.

- Help produce both white and red blood cells (one of the functions of bone marrow).
- Store most of the body's calcium supply, as well as phosphorus, magnesium, and sodium.

A **joint** is the connection between two or more bones of the skeleton. There are two types of joints: movable, such as elbows, knees, and hips; and immovable, such as the joints found in the pelvis and skull, which allow little or no movement.

Bones of the Skull

The **skull** is the skeleton of the head and is divided into two parts:

- **Cranium**—an oval, bony case that protects the brain.
- **Facial skeleton**—the framework of the face that is composed of 14 bones.

Bones of the Cranium

The following are the cranium's eight bones:

1. **Occipital bone**—hindmost bone of the skull, below the parietal bones; forms the back of the skull above the nape.

2. **Parietal bones**—bones that form the sides and top of the cranium. There are two parietal bones.

3. **Frontal bone**—bone that forms the forehead.

4. **Temporal bones**—bones that form the sides of the head in the ear region. There are two temporal bones.

5. **Ethmoid bone**—light, spongy bone between the eye sockets; forms part of the nasal cavities.

6. **Sphenoid bone**—bone that joins all the bones of the cranium together.

Muscular System: Muscles

The **muscular system** shapes and supports the skeletal system. Its function is to produce all movements of the body. It consists of more than 500 muscles, large and small, and comprises about 50 percent of the body's weight. Muscles are fibrous tissues. The natural hair care specialist should be concerned with the voluntary muscles of the head, face, neck, arms, and hands. Massage stimulates these voluntary muscles the most to help increase blood flow and relax muscles, which is the main concern of the natural hair care specialist.

There are three types of muscle tissue:

- **Striated muscles** also known as **skeletal muscles**—muscles that are attached to the bones and are voluntary, or consciously controlled. Striated muscles assist in maintaining the body's posture and protecting some internal organs **(Figure 7–2)**.

- **Nonstriated muscles**, also known as **smooth muscles**—muscles that are involuntary and function automatically, without conscious will. These

Copyright © 2012 Milady, a part of Cengage Learning®. All Rights Reserved.

muscles are found in the internal organs of the body, such as the digestive or respiratory systems **(Figure 7–3)**.

- **Cardiac muscle**—involuntary muscle that forms the heart. This type of muscle is not found in any other part of the body **(Figure 7–4)**.

A muscle has three parts:

- **Origin**—the part of the muscle that does not move and is attached closest to the skeleton.

- **Belly**—the middle part of the muscle.

- **Insertion**—the part of the muscle that moves and is farthest from the skeleton.

Pressure in massage is usually directed from the insertion to the origin of a muscle.

Muscles of the Scalp

The four muscles of the scalp are the following:

- **Epicranius**, also known as **occipitofrontalis** (ahk-SIP-ih-toh frun-TAY-lus)—a broad muscle that covers the top of the skull and consists of the occipitalis and frontalis.

- **Occipitalis**—the back (posterior) portion of the epicranius; the muscle that draws the scalp backward.

- **Frontalis**—the front (anterior) portion of the epicranius; the muscle of the scalp that raises the eyebrows, draws the scalp forward, and causes wrinkles across the forehead.

- **Epicranial aponeurosis**—the tendon that connects the occipitalis and frontalis muscles **(Figure 7–5)**.

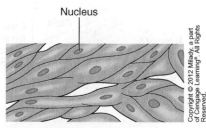

▲ Figure 7–3
Nonstriated muscle cells.

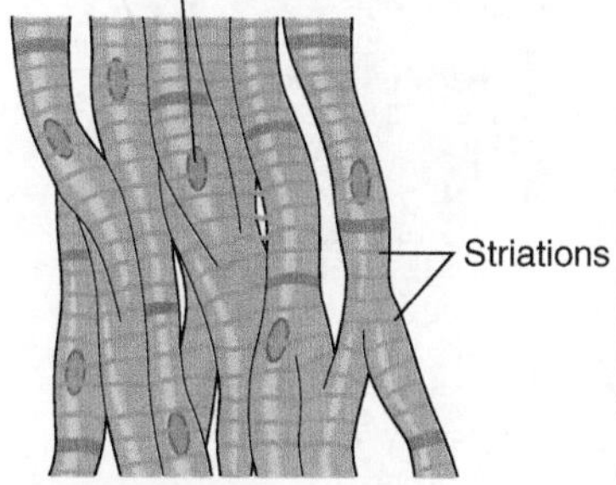

▲ Figure 7–4
Cardiac muscle cells.

nonstriated muscles also known as smooth muscles; muscles that are involuntary and function automatically, without conscious will. These muscles are found in the internal organs of the body, such as the digestive or respiratory systems.

cardiac muscle involuntary muscle that forms the heart. This type of muscle is not found in any other part of the body.

epicranius also known as the occipitofrontalis; a broad muscle that covers the top of the skull and consists of the occipitalis and frontalis.

occipitalis the back (posterior) portion of the epicranius; the muscle that draws the scalp backward.

frontalis the front (anterior) portion of the epicranius; the muscle of the scalp that raises the eyebrows, draws the scalp forward, and causes wrinkles across the forehead.

epicranial aponeurosis the tendon that connects the occipitalis and frontalis muscles.

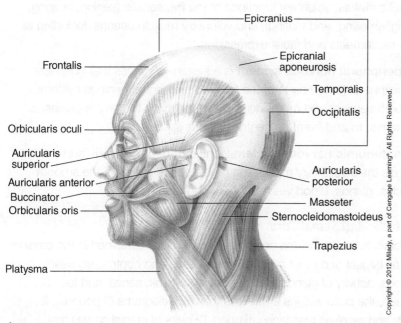

▲ Figure 7–5
Muscles of the head, face, and neck.

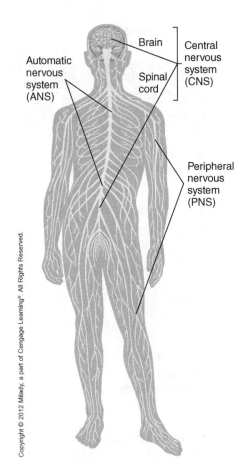

▲ Figure 7–6
Divisions of the nervous system.

nervous system body system that has three main subdivisions: the central, the peripheral, and the automatic nervous system.

central nervous system (CNS) body system made up of the brain, spinal cord, spinal nerves, and cranial nerves. The CNS controls the mental activities; the five senses of seeing, hearing, feeling, smelling, and tasting; and all body movement and facial expression.

peripheral nervous system body system that connects messages from the outer part of the body to the central nervous system. It consists of both sensory and motor nerves.

autonomic nervous system body system that controls the involuntary muscles, such as the glands, blood vessels, heart, and breathing.

Did you know?

Muscular tissue can be stimulated by the following methods:

- Massage (hand, electric vibrator, or water jets)
- Electrical therapy current
- Infrared light
- Dry heat (heating lamps or heating caps)
- Moist heat (steamers or moderately warm steam towels)
- Nerve impulses (through the nervous system)
- Chemicals (certain acids and salts)

Nervous System: Nerves

The **nervous system** is one of the most important systems of the body. It controls and coordinates the functions of all other systems and makes them work harmoniously and efficiently. This system is made up of the brain, spinal cord, and the entire body. These fine fibers (nerves) create a network that covers every square inch of the body. This system is important to the natural stylist to effectively deliver scalp massages during shampoo or treatment services. The nervous system has three main subdivisions: the central nervous system, the peripheral nervous system, and the autonomic nervous system.

Divisions of the Nervous System

The nervous system is divided into three main subdivisions **(Figure 7–6)**.

The **central nervous system (CNS)** consists of the brain, spinal cord, spinal nerves, and cranial nerves. It controls consciousness and many mental activities, voluntary functions of the five senses (seeing, hearing, feeling, smelling, and tasting), and voluntary muscle actions, including all body movements and facial expressions.

The **peripheral nervous system** is a system of nerves that connects the peripheral (outer) parts of the body to the central nervous system; it has both sensory and motor nerves. Its function is to carry impulses, or messages, to and from the central nervous system.

The **autonomic nervous system** is the part of the nervous system that controls the involuntary muscles; it regulates the action of the smooth muscles, glands, blood vessels, heart, and breathing.

The Brain and Spinal Cord

The brain is the part of the central nervous system contained in the cranium. It is the largest and most complex nerve tissue and controls sensation, muscles, activity of glands, and the power to think, sense, and feel. On average, the brain weighs a little less than 1.5 kilograms (3 pounds). It sends and receives messages through 12 pairs of cranial nerves that originate in the brain and reach various parts of the head, face, and neck.

The **spinal cord** is the portion of the central nervous system that originates in the brain and extends down to the lower extremity of the trunk. It is protected by the spinal column. Thirty-one pairs of spinal nerves extending from the spinal cord are distributed to the muscles and skin of the trunk and limbs.

Circulatory System: The Blood Supply

The **circulatory system** is related to the maintenance of good health. The cardiovascular or vascular system controls the steady circulation of the blood through the body by means of the heart and the blood vessels. It is made up of the heart, arteries, veins, and capillaries. The **blood** circulates from the heart through the blood vessels to nourish the entire body. This fluid supplies the body with oxygen and nutrients to the cells and tissues. It also removes **carbon dioxide** toxins and waste from the cells **(Figure 7–7)**.

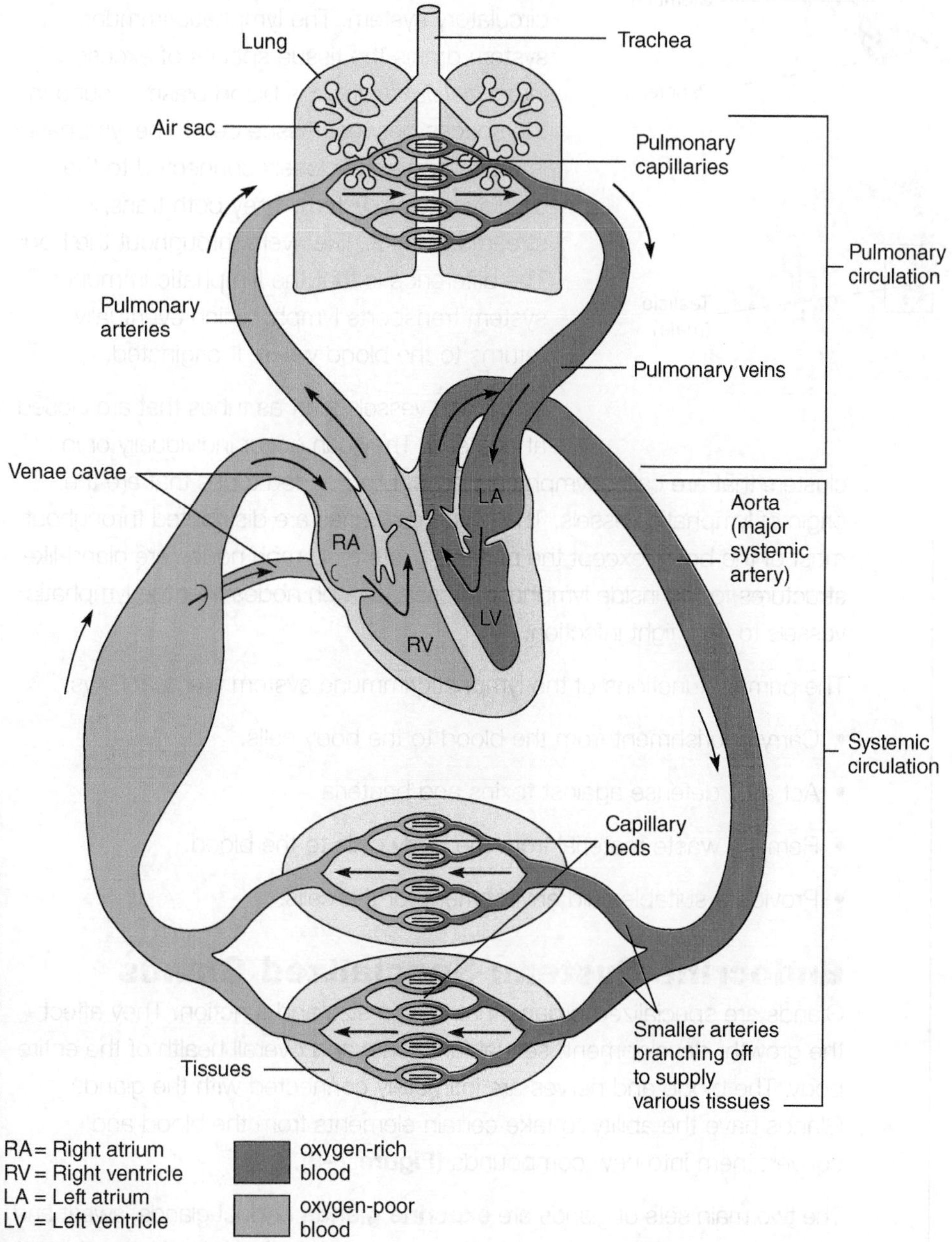

spinal cord portion of the central nervous system that originates in the brain, extends down to the lower extremity of the trunk, and is protected by the spinal column.

circulatory system body system related to maintenance of good health. The cardiovascular or vascular system controls the steady circulation of the blood through the body by means of the heart and the blood vessels. It is made up of the heart, arteries, veins, and capillaries.

blood fluid that supplies the body with oxygen and nutrients to the cells and tissues; circulates from the heart through the blood vessels to nourish the entire body. It also removes carbon dioxide toxins and waste from the cells.

carbon dioxide (CO_2) a colorless, odorless gas produced by burning carbon and organic compounds and by respiration. It is naturally present in air (about 0.03%) and is absorbed by plants in photosynthesis.

RA = Right atrium
RV = Right ventricle
LA = Left atrium
LV = Left ventricle

oxygen-rich blood

oxygen-poor blood

▲ Figure 7–7
Blood flow through the heart.

Copyright © 2012 Milady, a part of Cengage Learning®. All Rights Reserved.

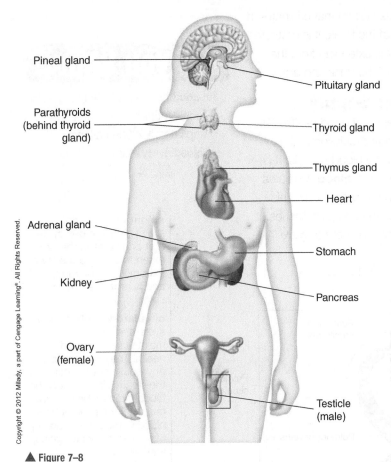

Pineal gland

Pituitary gland

Parathyroids
(behind thyroid
gland)

Thyroid gland

Thymus gland

Heart

Adrenal gland

Stomach

Kidney

Pancreas

Ovary
(female)

Testicle
(male)

▲ Figure 7–8
Endocrine glands.

lymphatic/immune system
body system that is made up
of lymph, lymph nodes, the
thymus gland, the spleen, and
lymph vessels. The lymphatic/
immune system carries waste
and impurities away from the
cells and protects the body from
disease by developing immunities
and destroying disease-causing
microorganisms.

endocrine system body
system that contains eight
types of glands that affect the
growth, development, sexual
functions, and overall health of
the entire body.

**exocrine glands (duct
glands)** glands that produce a
substance that travels through
small, tube-like ducts; sweat
glands and oil glands of the skin
belong to this group.

**endocrine glands (ductless
glands)** glands such as the
thyroid and pituitary gland that
release hormonal secretions
directly into the bloodstream.

The Lymphatic/Immune System

The **lymphatic/immune system** is made up of lymph, lymph nodes, the thymus gland, the spleen, and lymph vessels. The lymphatic/immune system carries waste and impurities away from the cells and protects the body from disease by developing immunities and destroying disease-causing microorganisms. *Lymph* is a clear fluid that circulates in the lymph spaces (lymphatics) of the body. Lymph helps carry wastes and impurities away from the cells before it is routed back to the circulatory system. The lymphatic/immune system drains the tissue spaces of excess *interstitial fluid*, which is blood plasma found in the spaces between tissue cells. The lymphatic/immune system is closely connected to the cardiovascular system. They both transport streams of fluids, like rivers throughout the body. The difference is that the lymphatic/immune system transports lymph, which eventually returns to the blood where it originated.

Lymphatic vessels start as tubes that are closed at one end. They can occur individually or in clusters that are called lymph capillaries, blind-ended tubes that are the origin of lymphatic vessels. The lymph capillaries are distributed throughout most of the body (except the nervous system). Lymph nodes are gland-like structures found inside lymphatic vessels. Lymph nodes filter the lymphatic vessels to help fight infection.

The primary functions of the lymphatic/immune system are as follows:

- Carry nourishment from the blood to the body cells.

- Act as a defense against toxins and bacteria.

- Remove waste material from the body cells to the blood.

- Provide a suitable fluid environment for the cells.

Endocrine System: Specialized Glands

Glands are specialized organs that vary in size and function. They affect the growth, development, sexual functions, and overall health of the entire body. The blood and nerves are intimately connected with the glands. Glands have the ability to take certain elements from the blood and convert them into new compounds (**Figure 7–8**).

The two main sets of glands are **exocrine glands** or duct glands, sweat and oil glands of the skin; and **endocrine glands** or ductless glands, thyroid and pituitary glands, which secrete hormones that are delivered directly into the bloodstream. **Hormones** are cellular secretions that stimulate body functions; they include insulin, adrenaline, estrogen (female), and testosterone (male).

The endocrine system includes eight types of glands: pineal, pituitary, thyroid, parathyroid, pancreas, adrenal, ovarian, and testicular.

Excretory System: Organs of Elimination

The **excretory system** includes the kidneys, liver, skin, large intestines, and lungs. This system purifies the body by eliminating waste matter. Metabolism of the cells of the body forms various toxic substances that, if retained, might poison the body.

Each of the following organs plays a crucial function in the excretory system:

- The kidneys excrete urine (water and waste products).
- The liver discharges toxins produced during digestion.
- The skin eliminates waste through perspiration.
- The large intestine eliminates decomposed and undigested food.
- The lungs exhale carbon dioxide.

The Respiratory System

The **respiratory system** consists of the lungs and air passages; it enables respiration, supplying the body with oxygen and eliminating carbon dioxide. **Respiration**, the act of breathing, is the exchange of carbon dioxide and oxygen in the lungs and within each cell.

The **lungs** are spongy tissues composed of microscopic cells in which inhaled air is exchanged for carbon dioxide during one breathing cycle. They are the organs of respiration. The respiratory system is located within the chest cavity and is protected on both sides by the ribs. The diaphragm is a muscular wall that separates the thorax (chest) from the abdominal region and helps control breathing.

With each breathing cycle, an exchange of gases takes place. During inhalation, or breathing in through the nose or mouth, oxygen is passed into the blood. During exhalation or breathing outward, carbon dioxide (collected from the blood) is expelled from the lungs **(Figure 7–9)**.

The Reproductive System

The **reproductive system** includes the ovaries, uterine tubes, uterus, and vagina in the female and the testes, prostate gland, penis, and urethra in the male. This system performs the function of producing offspring and passing on the genetic code from one generation to another.

The reproductive system produces hormones—primarily estrogen in females and primarily

hormones secretions such as insulin, adrenaline, and estrogen that stimulate functional activity or other secretions in the body. Hormones influence the welfare of the entire body.

excretory system body system that includes the kidneys, liver, skin, large intestines, and lungs. The excretory system purifies the body by eliminating waste matter.

respiratory system body system that consists of the lungs and air passages; it enables respiration, supplying the body with oxygen and eliminating carbon dioxide.

respiration the act of breathing; the exchange of carbon dioxide and oxygen in the lungs and within each cell.

lungs spongy tissues composed of microscopic cells in which inhaled air is exchanged for carbon dioxide during one breathing cycle.

reproductive system body system that includes the ovaries, uterine tubes, uterus, and vagina in the female and the testes, prostate gland, penis, and urethra in the male. The function of the reproductive system is to produce offspring and pass on the genetic code from one generation to another.

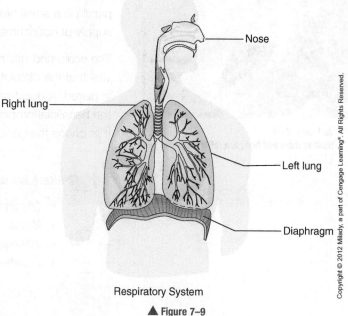

Nose

Right lung

Left lung

Diaphragm

Respiratory System

▲ **Figure 7–9**
The respiratory system.

digestive system (gastrointestinal system) body system responsible for breaking down foods into nutrients and wastes; consists of the mouth, stomach, intestines, salivary and gastric glands, and other organs.

testosterone in males. These hormones affect and change the skin in several ways. Acne, loss of scalp hair, facial hair growth and color, and darker skin pigmentations are some of the results of changing or fluctuating hormones.

Digestive System: Stomach and Intestine

The **digestive system**, also known as the gastrointestinal system, is responsible for breaking down foods into nutrients and waste. The digestive system consists of the mouth, stomach, intestines, salivary and gastric glands, and other organs. Digestion begins in the mouth with digestive enzymes, which are chemicals that change certain types of food into a soluble form that can be used by the body. The process is then completed in the small intestine, where the food, now in soluble form, is transported by the bloodstream and used by the body's cells and tissues[1]. ✓ **LO2** ✓ **LO3**

Nourishment from Within to Produce Healthy Hair

Hair is a wonderful indicator of general good health. It is an extension of the skin. The quality of the hair and skin are reflections of good or poor physical health. Although everyone is aware of the need for proper nutrition to be physically fit, most people do not realize that the same holds true for healthy hair. Healthy hair is the direct result of a healthy body and is mirrored through a person's physical and emotional well-being **(Figure 7–10)**.

Hair receives its nourishment from the foods we eat. At the very bottom of each hair follicle (a tube-like passage for the hair shaft) is the hair bulb. The papilla is a small blood vessel that feeds the bulb. Through the papilla, the supply of nourishment reaches the root and the bulb of the hair shaft.

The scalp and hair receive nourishment from the bloodstream. It is vital that the circulation of the blood in the body is not restricted or impaired. A good balanced diet, exercise, and plenty of water will promote the beneficial properties of the blood and enhance the circulatory system that brings the necessary nutrients to the hair and scalp.

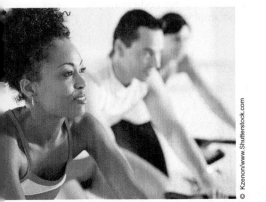

© Kzenon/www.Shutterstock.com

▲ Figure 7–10
Healthy mind and body are reflected in the hair.

FYI

Here are some external and internal sources for healthy hair:

- Oils and fats—add luster, pliability, nutrients, and protection.
- Moisture—keeps hair supple, soft, and hydrated.
- Vitamins and minerals—nourish and fortify hair.
- Protein—restores and strengthens the hair.

Nutrition and Maintaining Healthy Hair

There is a direct link between good health and real beauty. It is the body's way of creating symmetry and balance. This condition is referred to as inside out beauty. The concept of "beauty from within" is not new, yet its direct approach to attaining and maintaining beauty is novel and fresh to the hair industry. Today we are taking a 360-degree approach to hair care. Inside-outside beauty is a proactive approach to maintaining healthy hair. As the natural hair care industry grows, we will see an increase in nutriceuticals (the combination of the words *nutrition* and *pharmaceutical*) in which food and food products provide health, as well as beauty and medical benefits. **Nutriceuticals** come in many forms: natural herbal products and dietary supplements as well as processed foods, such as "hair foods," "beauty drinks," and protein/vitamins with enriched or enhanced formulas. Nutriceuticals offer benefits that include hair manageability, growth, restoration, nourishment, and volume. The world of nutriceuticals and **nutricosmetics** (*nutrition* and *cosmetics*) is growing and will be in the mainstream for many years to come. New dietary products are being engineered to target everything from aging skin to female-pattern baldness. It is important that we as consumers shop wisely; we should buy beauty-enhancing products that are chemically unaltered or that have not been chemically processed. Not all nutriceuticals or nutricosmetics are whole or natural; most are based on processed formulas to enhance their color, taste, or visual appeal. So always read the labels. We want to use products that are compatible to our body systems and that make us feel strong, balanced, and whole. Chemically free products have been noted to have better long-term physical health benefits as well as long-term environmental benefits.

If the products we use are safe for our bodies, then we can assume they are safe for the earth. Herbals, sea botanicals, extracts, essential oils, vegetable and fruit juices, and infusions have been used for thousands of years. These products are sustainable; they are from the earth and return to the earth to replenish and continue the earthly environmental balance. Today this elemental beauty is called "green beauty." Green beauty is the natural alternative for beauty and hair care. Hair products that are "green" are nontoxic; they are free of paraben, formaldehyde, SLSs, and other preservatives; and they generally are eco-friendly. What we put on our hair is just half of our self-care regime. The foods we eat and the supplements we consume influence all our body organs, including our hair, skin, and nails.

As a natural hair care specialist, you must be aware of the general nutritional value of food and its connection to beauty. There is truth in the old adage, "You are what you eat." Healthy, growing hair is interconnected with a healthy body. Specific foods will promote strong, healthy hair. The

nutriceuticals combination of the terms *nutrition* and *pharmaceutical*; refers to food and food products that provide health as well as beauty and medical benefits.

nutricosmetics refers to nutritional supplements that can support the function and structure of the skin.

following foods are considered to be part of a healthy hair and scalp diet that includes various growth-promoting oils, minerals, protein, and iron.[2]

1. Salmon, tuna, halibut, bluefish, catfish, and sardines offer omega-3 fatty acids (oil) that add luster and elasticity to the hair and scalp. These fish are high in protein, vitamin B_{12}, and iron for shaft strength.

2. Dark greens vegetables like kale, collards, and seaweed/kelp are rich in iodine, which is needed for an active thyroid; broccoli, Swiss chard, and spinach are all excellent sources of iron, calcium, carotenoids, and vitamins A and C. These vegetables help produce our natural scalp oil or sebum and slow down aging in the skin. Not only should we consume dark green vegetables, but also red, purple, and blue fruits and vegetables, which contain flavonoids. Flavonoids are antioxidants, which fight internal stressors, diseases, and external stress factors such as pollution, direct sunlight, and cigarette smoke.

3. Beans or legumes are vital to healthy hair because beans are an excellent source of protein, iron, zinc, and biotin.

4. Nuts and seeds from all over the world—for example, Brazil nuts—provide selenium. Walnuts, pecans, almonds, and cashews are excellent sources of essential omega-3 fatty oils and zinc, both of which are antioxidants. Pumpkin seeds and flax seeds also contain zinc and vitamin E, which improves body cells with oxygen and increases circulation to the scalp.

5. Poultry, such as organic chicken or turkey, is high in quality protein to strengthen hair.

6. Eggs are another great source of protein as well as biotin and vitamin B_{12}, which stimulate growth and thicken the cuticle.

7. Whole-grain breads, cereals, and brown rice are fortified with zinc, iron, biotin, and B vitamins.

8. All berries—strawberries, blueberries, goji berries, blackberries, and grapes—offer an excellent source of antioxidants and flavonoids that fight free radicals and diseases as well as increase vitamin C. Black currant has the richest sources of vitamin C, gamma-linoleic acid (GLA), manganese, magnesium, and calcium along with other phenolic compounds that affect the elasticity of the scalp. Acai berry with its rich purple color is filled with flavonoids and is known as a "superfood" and powerful antioxidant **(Figure 7–11)**.

9. Low-fat or skim organic dairy milk, almond milk, soy milk, yogurt, and cottage cheese are great sources of calcium and protein.

10. All vegetables, such as beets and carrots, are great sources of vitamin A, which supports good vision as well as boosts the immune system. Ripe avocados are also high in vitamin B and vitamin E.

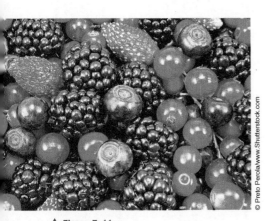

▲ Figure 7–11
Berries are a good source of vitamins.

What Are Free Radicals?

Free radicals are unstable organic cells or molecules responsible for human tissue damage and disease. They attempt to attach themselves to healthy cells and destroy or decay the structure of those cells. Scientists believe that free radicals are the main cause of every disease known, from heart disease to arthritis to cancer. Free radicals are unstable because they have an uneven number of electrons. They float around the body until they find an extra electron to steal and pair with another electron. Once they attach to healthy cells, free radicals create a chain reaction that takes over healthy cells, so that free radicals can multiply. This snowball effect creates disease and a breakdown of the body, aging, and illness. Free radicals are caused by aging, pollution, cigarette smoking, sunlight, harsh chemical cleaners, herbicides, and other poisons. Internal stressors, for example, hormonal changes and extreme exercise, can promote development of free radicals.[3]

What Are Antioxidants?

Antioxidants stop the oxidation or destruction of healthy cell tissues. They are micronutrient molecules found in foods, fruits, vegetables, and vitamins that stop the breakdown of tissue cells and fortify the body. Antioxidants are like "superheroes" that come to rescue the body from the "villain intruders"—free radicals. A balanced diet with four to five servings of fruits and vegetables are the best sources to get antioxidants. However, vitamins are great as supplemental nutrients that we need to stay healthy.

Antioxidant Vitamins

There are three vitamins best known as antioxidants—vitamins A, C, and E.

1. **Vitamin A**, also known as **beta-carotene**, can be found in carrots, sweet potatoes, cantaloupe, broccoli, kale, spinach, green bell peppers, papaya, apricots, skim milk, and eggs.

2. **Vitamin C,** also known as **ascorbic acid**, can be found in citrus fruits and juices, kale, collards, broccoli, potatoes, almonds, blackstrap molasses, all the berries and grapes, and red bell peppers. This vitamin is needed to produce collagen, which makes up protein fibers in the hair.

3. **Vitamin E** is the umbrella term for eight different antioxidants. Vitamin E is usually found in oils or foods with high oil content, including sunflower, olive, canola, soybean, fish oil, nuts, and seeds, as well as, carrots, avocados, wheat germ, and spinach.

It is vital that we eat a variety of fruits, vegetables, grains, and protein and of course that we drink pure, clean water. All our body systems require water to function efficiently. Our bodies are made up of 70 percent water, which is important to healthy hair, nails, and skin. Water also controls our body temperature and aids in our digestion, heart rate, and blood pressure. The more active we are, the more water we will need. Water is a part of our cleansing system to remove toxins from the body. The more water we drink, the easier it is for us to eliminate waste and toxins. It is important to keep the body hydrated with water to avoid headaches and fatigue, and to increase athletic performance. The amount of water required per person may vary, but on average eight (16 oz.) glasses of water will suffice. It is important to keep the body fluids high to detoxify the liver, which filters the blood and

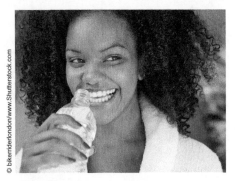

▲ Figure 7–12
Water is important for hydration of the skin, including the scalp.

nourishes the scalp. When clients come into the salon, a cool glass of water with a twist of lemon or lime is the most refreshing beverage to offer them. Water is revitalizing and a great beginning to a hair service **(Figure 7–12)**.

Other Antioxidants

Other antioxidants include the following:

* *Selenium,* which works in conjunction with vitamin E to protect vital organs in the body—like the heart, liver and lungs—against free radicals. Selenium is found in foods like garlic, whole grains, and asparagus.

* *Coenzyme Q10* is a supplement that helps metabolize carbohydrates and fats and has a natural antiaging effect.

Vitamins, Minerals, and Dietary Supplements

In Western culture, we eat more food per person than anywhere else in the world. Our diets are filled with sugar, fast foods, and processed foods. Meats and dairy products clog our system. Due to these high demands for refined or processed foods, we expose ourselves to poisonous chemicals and harmful food additives, which some studies have found to cause illness and degenerative diseases. Herbicides, pesticides, and fungicides as well as some fertilizers, when used in large quantities, are poisonous. In the long term, they are harmful to the earth and to our bodies. Consumption of food additives—such as chemical substances to enhance food flavors and preserve "shelf life," colorants, stabilizers, and bleaching agents—has doubled since the 1950s. Natural food additives do exist, but more than 3,000 synthetic additives are available and are used by many food manufacturers. Growth hormones are additives found in meats and produce. They are used to make plants and animals appear larger, and these additives often reduce the nutritional value of these foods. As a rule, we eat more because our bodies require more food to receive the same nutrients. We take in more calories, but we are still not sufficiently nourished. The vitamins, minerals, plant and vegetable oils, moisturizing products, and protein substances used topically to nurture, protect, and groom the hair are necessary. They are second only to the daily nutritional requirements needed internally to maintain a healthy scalp and hair.

What Are Whole Foods?

Whole foods are foods prepared or eaten in the natural state. They have not been processed or altered to enhance appearance. Nothing has been added or removed nutritionally; as much as possible, these foods are unprocessed and unrefined. Whole foods generally have no added salt, carbohydrates, or fats. They are the foods that grow closest to the ground. There are three main reasons to eat whole foods: (1) a natural source of dietary supplements; (2) a greater source of more complex micronutrients; and (3) an excellent source of dietary fiber, which keeps the colon cleansed and the body systems strong. To stay healthy longer, we need to eat the foods our grandparents used to eat. It is safer and nutritionally more valuable to eat whole foods, and whenever possible to eat organically grown vegetables, fruits, plants, and other food substances.

- Wheatgrass is a powerful detoxifier for the liver and blood; it is a super antioxidant that neutralizes environmental stressors on the body and contains beneficial chlorophyll that is directly absorbed into the circulatory system to nourish the blood.

- Acai berry is an excellent source of flavonoids, which are antioxidants that protect the cells from oxidation and provide protection from free radicals.

What Are Organic Foods?

The word *organic* refers to the way farmers grow and process their food products, which include fruits, vegetables, grains, dairy products, and meat. Organic foods are those grown without chemical treatments like herbicides, pesticides, fungicides, synthetic fertilizers, and chemical food additives or those that contain no genetically modified organisms. Organic farming is designed to encourage soil and water conservation and protect the environment by reducing toxic pollution. Are organic foods better for us? The more organic foods we eat, the less exposure we have to harmful chemicals. Conventional foods are treated with hundreds of chemicals to preserve and enhance their appearance. The **U.S. Department of Agriculture (USDA)** has provided a certification program with strict guidelines for all organic foods to meet government standards. If the food bears a USDA label, that means that it is 95 to 100 percent organic. The terms *natural, free range,* and *hormone free,* are not interchangeable with the word *organic*. Although they all may be what they say they are, do not confuse them with being organic. Only foods that are grown by the USDA standards for organic food can make that claim and display that label.[4]

United States Department of Agriculture (USDA) federal organization that provides a certification program with strict guidelines for all organic foods to meet government standards. If the food bears a USDA label, that means it is 95 to 100 percent organic.

B-Complex: The Stress Fighter/Balancer

B-complex vitamins provide the body with energy by converting carbohydrates into glucose (sugar), which the body needs to burn to produce energy. They are essential to the breakdown of fats and proteins. In addition, B vitamins are vital in the normal processing of the nervous system and may be the single most important factor for healthy nerves.

One of the richest sources of B-complex vitamins is brewer's yeast. Brewer's yeast is also high in protein, biotin, B_{12}, selenium, lecithin, chromium, potassium, and 18 amino acids. It can be added to cereals, yogurt, and other foods, yet is most popular in drinks, juices, and shakes **(Figure 7–13)**. The need for B-complex vitamins increases when the body is under stress or infection. Alcohol and sugars deplete the B-complex vitamins. There are supplemental forms of B complex. Premature gray hair, hair breakage or loss—including types of baldness such as alopecia areata—and other skin problems such as eczema and acne are indications of a lack of B vitamins.[5]

Biotin: "The Hair Vitamin"

Biotin, which is part of the B-complex supplements (B_7), helps increase the body's immune system. It is also known as vitamin H. Deficiencies in

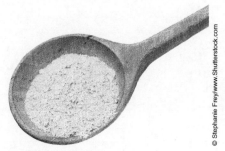

▲ Figure 7–13
Brewer's yeast is a good source of vitamin B.

© Stephanie Frey/www.Shutterstock.com

this vitamin are linked to hair thinning, hair loss, and alopecia. Biotin is a vital component in cell production. When digested, biotin reacts to **cell enzymes** that help produce **amino acids**, which are the building blocks for protein. Protein cells are the principal components of keratin. Biotin boosts the renewal of the keratin protein and helps increase the anagen (growth) phase of the hair growth process. It has been said that biotin prolongs the anagen phase and allows the hair to stay in the growth phase longer, thereby creating longer, thicker hair. Biotin topical products like shampoos or conditioners can only make the hair appear thicker. Biotin is water soluble; it coats the hair, making the shaft feel thicker temporarily. Biotin food sources are retrieved from peanuts, almonds, fish, brewer's yeast, beans, avocados, raspberries, and wheat products.

Silica

Silica is a mineral found in the earth and in the human body. Silica is a main building block of the body. It is found in stones and rocks in a form known as silicon. It acts to stabilize calcium and magnesium, which assist in hormonal balance; it strengthens bones, tendons, tissues, muscles, cartilage, hair, and nails; and it boosts the immune system. Silica is a major factor in the production of collagen protein, which gives the skin and scalp strength, elasticity, and balance. As we age, we lose the ability to produce silica on our own. As we lose collagen, we lose elasticity in our skin, moisture in our hair, and strength in our bones. Silica food sources are wheat bran, soybeans, beets, green vegetables, cucumbers, mango, and brown rice.

Sulfur Supplement: MSM (methylsulfonylmethane)

Sulfur is one of the major elements in the chain of amino acids that make protein in hair and skin. It is vital to formulation and production of collagen and keratin protein. Sulfur works with biotin to keep hair in the anagen growth phase. It strengthens hair by fortifying keratin protein.

MSM is a sulfur-based by-product of dimethyl sulfoxide (DMSO; see next paragraph). It is not a natural product, nor is it a pharmaceutical. It is a by-product of wood. When used topically, it has been known to address the issues of different types of inflammation surrounding alopecia. It is often recommended by dermatologists to reduce inflammation of the scalp.

Sulfur Supplement: DMSO (dimethyl sulfoxide)

When used topically, DMSO is an amazing healing agent. It is an anti-inflammatory agent used to reduce joint inflammation, rheumatoid arthritis, and herpes 1 and 2. It is a super antioxidant that fights free radicals, which attack the body when it is scared or injured. It aids in speeding up the healing process.

Zinc

A zinc deficiency will lead to thinning hair or diffuse alopecia. Zinc helps the body process B-complex vitamins, biotin, and vitamin E. Zinc is a vital mineral in the cellar activity of more than 100 enzymes that help in the healing process and the autoimmune system. Zinc controls the oil production in our skin and scalp. Zinc is found in food sources such as poultry, red meat, lobster, crab, beans, pumpkin seeds, nuts, wheat grain products, dairy products, and oysters.

Omega-3 and Omega-6

Omega-3 and omega-6 fatty acids help in the development of oils in the skin and scalp. They keep the scalp moist and flexible. Food sources for omega-3 and omega-6 are flax seeds, walnuts, salmon, sardines, soybeans, avocados, whole-grain breads, cottonseed oil, hemp oil, and sunflower seed oil.

Vitamina A, C, D, and E

The following are some benefits of vitamins A, C, D, and E:

- Vitamin A regulates cell production of **retinoic acid** in the hair follicle. It can be applied to the hair shaft and used internally to stimulate hair growth.

- Vitamin C regulates the absorption of iron, which is vital to the growth of healthy hair. The body cannot produce its own vitamin C; we can get it only from fruits, vegetables, or supplements.

- Vitamin D is made by the body. It is called the "sunshine vitamin" because when the body is directly in the sun, it produces vitamin D. This vitamin is necessary to metabolize calcium. Just 10 minutes a few times a week can produce vitamin D. Calcium strengthens bones, teeth, and hair.

- Vitamin E is a powerful antioxidant that works with vitamin A to strengthen and add elasticity to hair. Food sources that produce vitamin E are avocados, spinach, nuts, peaches, sunflower seeds, and tomatoes.

retinoic acid a nutrient that the body needs in small amounts to function and stay healthy. All-trans retinoic acid is made in the body from vitamin A and helps cells to grow and develop, especially in the embryo.

As a natural hair care specialist, the diets just recommended are also important to your well-being and health. As a role model for a healthy approach to life, you should increase your intake of wholesome and healthy foods and supplements to help increase your stamina and allow you to work and be creative. If you adhere to basic nutritional eating habits, you will gain credibility as a professional natural hair care specialist (Figure 7–14). ☑ **LO4**

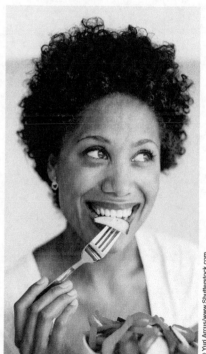

▲ Figure 7–14
Happy and healthy woman.

© Yuri Arcus/www.Shutterstock.com

Myth: For Lock Grooming, Beeswax Is Better Than Gel

Textured coily hair locks naturally without the need to apply any products. Cultivated or groomed locks require butters and water-soluble gels to give them a neat finish, while organic or free-flowing locks do not require any gel at all. The curl or coil pattern determines how and when hair locks. Beeswax, clay, mud, and even honey have been used to lock hair. All of these substances have their drawbacks; they leave a residue or lock debris, which eventually breaks the lock.

Review Questions

1. List the 11 main body systems and their functions.
2. Describe the three main subdivisions of the nervous system.
3. The scalp and skin receive nourishment from where?
4. List and describe three vitamins that are antioxidants.
5. What vitamin is part of the B-complex supplements (B_7), also known as vitamin H, and helps strengthen the body's immune system?
6. Name two fatty acids that help in the development of oils in the skin and scalp.
7. What are whole foods?
8. Describe the meaning of organic foods.

Chapter References

1. (2012). *Milady standard cosmetology.* Clifton Park, NY: Milady, a part of Cengage Learning.
2. Simpson, P. M. Nutricosmetics: A new way of delivering beauty: Nutricosmetics are causing a paradigm shift in the way beauty is achieved and maintained. *Nutraceuticals World* (September 1, 2010).
3. (2013) *Milady standard esthetics: Advanced* (2nd ed.). Clifton Park, NY: Milady, a part of Cengage Learning.
4. Gabriel, J. (2008). *The green beauty guide.* Deerfield Beach, FL: Health Communications, Inc.
5. McKeith, G. (2009). *Gillian McKeith's food bible: How to use food to cure what ails you.* New York: Penguin.

CHAPTER 8

Shampoos, Conditioners, Herbal Treatments, and Rinses

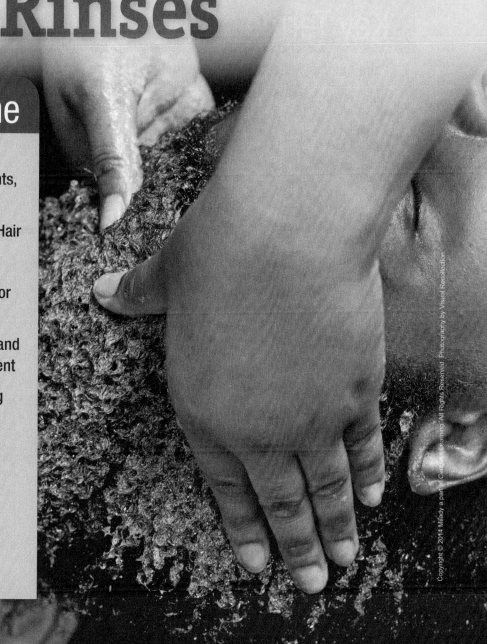

Learning Objectives

After completing this chapter, you should be able to:

☑ **LO1** Shampoo braids and natural hair.

☑ **LO2** Remove braids before shampooing for touch-ups.

☑ **LO3** Describe nurturing shampoo techniques for textured hair.

☑ **LO4** Explain the different types of shampoos.

☑ **LO5** Discuss types of herbal rinses, essential oils, and conditioners.

Key Terms

Page number indicates where in the chapter the term is used.

acidic rinse
p. 159

ampholytes (amphoterics)
p. 165

anionic
p. 164

botanical
p. 171

braid sediment
p. 157

cationics
p. 165

co-washing
p. 172

cold water conditioning
p. 173

crown
p. 155

deionized water
p. 163

detangling
p. 156

detergent
p. 163

emollients
p. 169

essential fatty acids
p. 167

hard water
p. 166

humectants
p. 169

medicated shampoo
p. 168

moisturizer
p. 164

monionics
p. 165

pustules
p. 158

soft water
p. 166

surfactants
p. 163

Many people in the natural hair care profession believe that the head is the most sacred part of the human body. It is the place where thoughts dwell, the imagination is born, and the connection between spirituality and earth are created. For this reason, natural hair care specialists believe that the head is the most charged part of the body. The soft center of the head, called the **crown**, is sensitive to touch and rhythmic motion. Natural stylists believe that the crown of the head transmits and receives life's energy forces; it is the essence of our spiritual well-being. This view is not so far-fetched when you recognize that all human functions are engineered from the head. The head protects the brain, which is the command center for what you taste, see, hear, think, and feel. Emotional and physical well-being are rooted in the head.

In traditional African culture, the head is glorified and adorned because it is treated as the spiritual center of the body. It houses the brain, which controls thoughts and emotions. All human functions stem from the head—heartbeat, breathing, digestion, and body movement. If the head is the conduit of life's energy force, then so is the hair, rooted in the head and extending outward. Notice that when you are under physical or emotional stress, your hair may shed or break. Such hair loss may result in balding. The Rastafarian culture (mainly in the Caribbean) believes that locked hair is an antenna to God, that locks are spiritually connected to the creator, and this link keeps people emotionally strong and vital.

Therefore, most natural hair care specialists recognize that hair is more than just protein and keratin. To the natural hair care specialist, hair is the outer manifestation of the inner being. When hair is properly cleaned and groomed, the mind, body, and spirit are renewed and revived. During a shampoo treatment, the braid specialist wants to create a relaxing, soothing, and meditative experience for the client. It is a treatment that addresses the condition of the hair and scalp as well as the client's well-being. Proper hair care should be a positive, transforming experience. Clients come to a salon expecting to be changed for the better. The shampoo experience is the initial service that promotes sharing between the client and stylist. Through the sense of touch, it creates the emotional and physical bond between the two people so that ideas and conversation can flow. With every shampoo/treatment experience, the braid stylist must provide a "healing" or therapeutic process. This healing process begins with scalp manipulation or massage during the shampoo. The hands-on healing and soothing shampoo/treatment will transmit energy from the stylist to the client, and vice versa. Hands are our creative tools. They are the medium by which our intuitive creative abilities are executed or demonstrated.

| **crown** the soft center of the head.

Why Study Shampoos, Conditioners, Herbal Treatments, and Rinses?

Natural stylists should study and have a thorough understanding of shampoos, conditioners, herbal treatments, and rinses for these reasons:

- The shampoo service is the first opportunity to reinforce your position as a professional while making a connection with your client.

- You will be able to identify any hair conditions that were not revealed in the initial consultation.

- A thorough knowledge of hair care products will assist you in determining the best preparation for other services to be performed.

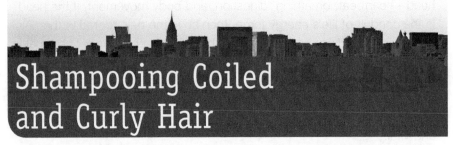

Shampooing Coiled and Curly Hair

detangling the process of removing all knots and tangles from the hair.

When cleansing the scalp of the client with naturally curly hair, it is important to **detangle** the hair thoroughly. All tangles must be removed before the service, to prevent the hair from matting or fusing. Hair that has a curly or coil-patterned texture requires a gentle, detangling comb-out before shampooing (see Chapter 9, Textured Hair Is Manageable). Depending on the texture of the client's hair, it may be best to coat the hair with a conditioning agent rather than combing out the hair while it is dry. Coating the hair with a conditioner first will prevent breakage and be gentler on the hair. You might also work with clients who are transitioning from chemically processed hair to natural hair. Therefore, not all of their hair will have a coiled/curly texture. The hair closest to the scalp will be natural, and the hair that has been chemically processed will be straight. It is equally important to look out for the possibility of chemically processed hair becoming matted if left in braided styles for an extended period of time. Chemically processed hair will also benefit from a coating of conditioner before combing it through when removing braids. The comb-out will stretch, elongate, and separate the coil-patterned strands, giving the hair a fuller look.

Combing Out Recently Braided Hair

If the hair has been braided recently, be aware of debris and loose hair. During the average braided period (two to three months), the natural process of daily combing or brushing causes the hair to shed about 50 to 100 strands per day. This hair shedding is normal when wearing braided styles. The longer the client wears a braided style, the more loose hair will be seen during the pre-shampoo comb-out. For this reason, many professional braiders recommend that clients maintain one style no longer than two to three months. After three or four months, braid sediment collects between the scalp base and the extensions. **Braid sediment** refers to the sediment and debris that accumulate or "build up" over time on the hair and scalp from oils, creams, dirt, and debris from improper cleansing and care. Braid sediment becomes imbedded between the hairs and hardens. It will lead to atrophy (weakening) of the braided strands. An excessive amount of hair comb-out may occur at this point. Hair has a life force. If the braids are not removed periodically, the hair loses its vitality. During this period, atrophy will occur and lead to thinning and hair breakage.

braid sediment debris that accumulates on the hair and scalp over time; sediment from oils, creams, dirt, and debris resulting from improper cleansing and care.

Why Braids Appear to Damage Hair

As natural stylists, we recognize that proper care of the braided style can promote growth and protect the hair and scalp. However, the stylist must educate the client that braids kept in for an excessive amount of time will adversely affect the hair strand. The one comment most often heard in the salon is, "The braids took my hair out." This is a misconception. Braids, with or without extension, done properly do not take the hair out. Hair becomes weakened and damaged when:

- The braids are put in improperly.

- The braid is put in too tightly.

- An excessive amount of extension hair was added to the client's hair.

Throughout this chapter, the term *braids* is used interchangeably with the term *twists*. Braids are typically a three-strand, soft-binding method of styling the hair; twists are a two-strand, soft-binding method. Each method allows the hair to be styled in a manner that enables the client's own hair to rest unhampered, because these techniques do not require combing, brushing, or other types of grooming.

When Done Properly, Braids Do Not Damage Hair

Clients and stylists sometimes use improper braiding techniques and make mistakes that ultimately weaken hair and cause breakage. The following is a list of techniques for the natural stylist to avoid when braiding hair.

- **An imbalance between the extensions and natural hair.** Too often, braiders use too much hair in the extension. The extension material (synthetic/human hair or yarns) should not be too heavy for the natural hair texture. A proportionate amount of extension material must be placed into the braid.

- **Too much tension.** Braids often are put in too tight, and so they cut off circulation to the scalp. Overly tight braiding eventually causes hair breakage, can pull the hair completely out of the follicle, and can even

pustules raised, inflamed papules with a white or yellow head or center containing pus.

permanently damage the follicle. Excessive tension on the scalp has been known to leave inflamed bumps containing pus, or **pustules**, around the hair line or on the nape of the neck.

- **Leaving braid styles and extensions in the hair too long.** Braids should not be kept for more than two to three months, because the individual strands of hair will become thin and weak. The natural texture of the hair will also determine how long the client should continue to wear a braided style. Fine, soft, coily hair is most fragile. The hair will intertwine around the braid, making the separation of the hair from the extensions difficult and laborious.

- **Improper shampooing and conditioning of braided styles.** Without proper care, oil and cream residue as well as dirt will "build up" and clog hair follicles. Residue is referred to as braid sediment or debris.

- **Braiding chemically treated hair right after treatment.** The hair should be properly conditioned and braided at least a week or two after a chemical treatment. Ideally, a braided style is best when the hair is all natural. Hair in transition can be braided; however, breakage is unavoidable. When a client is growing out a relaxer, the hair is in transition. The shaft has two textures, and breakage often occurs at the point where the textures meet.

Shampooing textured hair does not require scrubbing. The object of a shampoo is to effectively remove dirt and oil residue from the scalp. The service should be, as mentioned earlier, soothing and emotionally relaxing. A scrubbing motion can be agitating and harsh. Due to the properties of textured hair, scrubbing can also cause damage. Textured hair is curly, coiled, or wire-like. It also tends to be dry, fragile, and easily tangled. It often wraps around itself. Scrubbing of textured hair can cause matting and intertwining of the strands as well as breakage when untangling the hair.

When cleaning textured hair, concentrate on cleaning the entire scalp in a rhythmic, soothing motion. You want to massage the scalp to circulate the blood as well as clean the scalp. Good blood flow provides the hair follicles with the nutrients needed to stay healthy. A relaxing touch and stimulating movements can invigorate the scalp to produce its own natural oil, sebum. Sebum is the scalp's natural moisturizer.

With curly hair, the natural oil does not always reach the end of the hair follicle, unlike the case with straight or slightly wavy hair. This limited amount of sebum is why textured hair tends to feel dry and can be brittle. On textured hair, the sebum must travel around the twists and bends in the hair and often coats only a small portion of the hair strand. That portion is generally closer to the scalp, leaving the ends of textured hair the least coated. Brushing repeatedly may be productive for straight hair or slightly wavy hair; however, coiled hair/textured hair is too fragile. Bending coils in and out can cause breakage at the curves of the coil where the hair strand is weakest.

When shampooing coiled hair and braided styles, *your aim is to cleanse the scalp.* The shampoo will remove dirt and oil on the hair when it is rinsed.

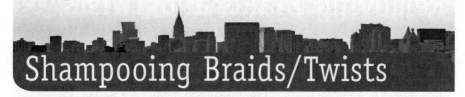

Shampooing Braids/Twists

Unique Steps for Proper Cleansing of Braids

When shampooing braided styles, avoid using heavy cream shampoos. No matter how much water you use to rinse cream shampoos, a residue will still remain, attracting dirt and weakening the braid.

To avoid or reduce braid sediment, follow these guidelines:

- Avoid heavy cream shampoos that will coat the braid shaft. (These are usually the products that claim to condition and shampoo in one step.)

- Use clear gel shampoos that rinse thoroughly. Also available in today's market are many daily shampoos that don't include harsh detergents. These shampoos are also easy to rinse out of the hair. Cream-based shampoos are a trend on the market today, and many believe these shampoos are gentler. Whether the shampoo is cream based or gel based matters less than the actual ingredients in the shampoo and the effect they will have on your client's hair and scalp.

- Avoid using any petroleum-based product on braids and scalp. Petroleum-based products only lacquer the hair and scalp; they do not allow moisture to enter or leave the hair.

- Avoid heavy, waxy gels or pomades that attract dust and dirt from the environment.

- Use a clarifying or cleansing shampoo as the first shampoo. Dilute cream shampoos to avoid braid sediment.

- Commercial dandruff shampoos are not recommended for braided or locked hair. They are made with harsh chemicals that strip too much sebum from the scalp. If a client has been using dandruff shampoos, a deep conditioning treatment is required to moisten the hair.

- Always rinse with warm or tepid water after shampooing. Water spray should be forceful.

- An **acidic rinse** (lemon juice, lime, apple cider vinegar, and water) can be used to reduce sediments and close cuticles. Any acidic rinse should be diluted with 95 percent water and 5 percent acid ingredient. Always follow up any acid rinse process by using a leave-in conditioner for the hair.

acidic rinse a product used to reduce sediments and close cuticles. Contains 95 percent water and 5 percent acid ingredient.

- Squeeze braids downward without pulling them when rinsing. This motion may bring sediment that has not been properly rinsed to the surface. ✔ **LO1**

Removing Braids and Twists for Cleansing Hair and Scalp

After extended wear, to give hair a thorough cleansing and conditioning, the braid style must be removed professionally. Taking out braids is a special skill and can be a separate service that a salon provides. Many clients dread the thought of taking out their own braids. For a client, it is a long and tedious job. If not done properly, it can be painful and cause excessive hair breakage. The old adage, "It's a dirty job, but somebody has to do it," certainly applies to removing braid extensions. A salon can provide the service separately, and an assistant can be trained for the task.

A Unique Skill That Prevents Damaging the Hair

What is the big deal about removing braids? It is a service that requires skill and practice. The braid removal service is as important as the service of creating braids. The smaller the braids, the more time and skill are required to remove them. Also, the more fragile and smaller the base of the braid is, the more likely it is to be covered with scalp and dirt residue. The average head of medium-sized braids can take one client four to six hours to remove. The braids must be removed one at a time (or at the most a few at a time) and combed gently to avoid breakage and scalp irritation. Clients who have tried to remove their own braids know how awkward this task is, because they cannot seem to position themselves properly. Some clients report feeling as though they should be contortionists to do this job, and they often miss a few braids they are unable to reach.

Comb-Out

The comb-out is the process of brushing the hair after the braids are out. This is the part of braid removal that can cause the most damage to clients' hair, because the hair debris is hardened and sebum is crusted at the base of the natural hair. This condition can create knots or hair that is tangled into a ball, usually at the ends of tightly coiled hair. The knots have to be unraveled gently to ensure a smooth, loose comb-out. When clients attempt to do this task themselves, they become frustrated and anxious. They rush, ripping through the hair, generally using improper tools. In haste, they wash their hair without thoroughly combing it out and make the problem worse for themselves due to hair fusing or matting. Often, because this task is so daunting, many clients delay the process and wear the braid style longer than recommended. By offering clients a braid removal service, you ensure the optimum care and health of the hair, which is the goal of a professional natural hair care specialist.

Reasons for Providing Braid Removal Service

Here are six excellent reasons to provide your clients with a braid removal service:

- Ensures safe removal with minimal breakage
- Saves time
- Helps maintain proper hair care
- Allows for partial removal for braid/weave touch-ups
- Prevents prolonged periods of wearing braid styles
- Helps save the integrity of the client's hairline ✓ **LO2**

Selecting the Best Cleansing and Nurturing Options for Your Client

As a natural hair care professional, it is your responsibility to understand and choose the appropriate shampoo for varying hair types and conditions. Whether the client's hair is natural or chemically treated, dry, oily, fine, or coarse, a shampoo is available to best address the needs of the hair type. The market offers literally thousands of shampoos professing to make hair more manageable, bouncy, and well-behaved. Other shampoos promise to condition the scalp and hair as well as cleanse. Some even promise to aid highlighting and brighten hair color.

For the natural hair care specialist, less is definitely more. With the growing industry of natural, gentler shampoos that are free from preservatives and not tested on animals, options for more wholesome and nurturing products exist. Using shampoos made from herbal extracts and essential oils is effective in creating healthy hair for harmonious hairstyling.

Thousands of shampoo types fill the beauty supply stores. They vary in colors, fragrances, and descriptions for proper hair care. A braid stylist must be aware of and knowledgeable about the ingredients listed on every product label.

Since 1976, the Food and Drug Administration (FDA) has required by law that all hair manufacturers list product ingredients to ensure consumer safety. The labeling regulation requires that ingredients are listed prominently in their decreasing order of prevalence. In other words, the product contains the greatest amount of the ingredient that is listed first on the label. For example, if water is listed first, then that shampoo is largely water with other ingredients included. The last item is the smallest amount contained in the product. If the label is not large enough to list all ingredients, then a tag must be attached to the product.

Today, many brands state that their products are natural and/or that they have organic ingredients. Not all products making this claim are telling the truth, so read the labels and make certain that product contains organic ingredients and is certified organic. The bottle or container should have a label stating "certified organic," meaning that the U.S. Department of Agriculture (USDA) has ensured that the product was organically produced.[1]

Commercial shampoos are designed to cleanse the hair and scalp. However, too much use of a cleansing agent can strip the natural oil (sebum) that coats the hair. Sebum protects the hair strand and contributes to its luster and manageability. Textured hair is extremely vulnerable because sebum is not evenly distributed on the hair strand, and often the hair is drier, more fragile, and less protected. Oil and moisture have to be replaced manually to keep the hair shaft sealed, moist, and radiant. Basic shampoos usually clean well, but they also remove all the natural oils. Textured hair needs mild (or low-pH) shampoos that gently cleanse but do not strip the hair of natural oils. To remove braid debris from hair braided with extensions requires cleansing shampoos with slightly more cleansing or clarifying action to remove debris from the braid and scalp. It is important to use a moisturizing shampoo and conditioner after clarifying to neutralize and soften the hair shaft.

Frequent shampooing of textured, coily, kinky hair can result in extreme dryness and brittleness. The hair must be adequately moisturized and then conditioned after each shampoo. Braided hair should be shampooed about every two to three weeks. Lint, oil, and dust (debris, braid sediment) become embedded in the braid and remain on the scalp. This sediment must be removed in order to maintain healthy braided styles. More cleansing shampoos should be used for the first wash. The second or third shampoo, if necessary, should be a milder, pH balanced clear-type conditioning shampoo to moisturize the hair.

For locked hair or hair that is in braids or twisted styles, avoid heavy cream shampoos. Heavy creams can leave a sticky residue buildup on the hair that attracts more dirt and makes the hair look dull. Creams become embedded in the hair locks or braids and do not rinse thoroughly. If the cream residue is allowed to build up, it also can harm the hair. The residue can harden and cause breakage. It can also clog hair follicles and block sebum, which will result in a condition that eventually has a drying effect on the hair. Lock sediment actually becomes a part of the lock. Once sediment becomes a part of the lock, it is almost impossible to remove without picking apart or weakening the lock. ✔ **LO3**

The Five Classifications of Shampoos

Shampoos have five very distinctive classifications. These include detergents, mild pH shampoos, medicated shampoos, protein/conditioning shampoos, and herbal/organic shampoos.

Basic or commercial shampoos are generally made with synthetic products. Today, many companies are removing harsh chemicals and seeking to include healthier ingredients in their products. Many "daily shampoos" now on the market are phosphate free and contain little to no sodium lauryl sulfate. These shampoos are gentle on the hair and highly recommended for those who must shampoo their hair daily or more than once a week. However, if you really need your hair cleansed because of sweating in your scalp, chlorine, or other prominent reasons, a product considered a daily shampoo may not properly cleanse your hair. An ever-expanding cottage industry is also making natural hair care products available to the general market today.

The first ingredient in most shampoos is water, either purified or deionized. The second most prominent ingredient is the base detergent or base surfactant, which can be used interchangeably to mean the cleansing or "surface active" agent. **Surfactants** are chemical compounds designed to create the wetting, emulsifying, dispersing, and liquefying properties of a shampoo. The third most common agent in shampoos counteracts or complements the negative characteristics of the original base detergent, because the base is generally the harshest chemical. These are the basic types of detergent bases that actually clean the hair. They differ in intensity and removal of hair oil and debris.

surfactants chemical compounds designed to create the wetting, emulsifying, dispersing, and liquefying properties of a shampoo.

detergent a soap that is usually high in pH (potential hydrogen) or alkaline.

deionized water water that has had impurities such as calcium and magnesium and other metal ions that would make a product unstable removed.

Detergents and Understanding pH (Potential Hydrogen)

Detergents are usually high in pH (potential hydrogen) or alkaline, which kills bacteria. However, high-alkaline products strip the hair's natural oils. In a shampoo, the pH refers to the strength of the cleansing agent only. The ideal pH of hair and skin is usually about 4.5 to 5.5 on the pH scale. The neutral level is 7.0, which is equivalent to pure water containing no minerals.

To determine which shampoo will leave your client's hair in the best condition for the intended service, you need to understand the chemical and botanical ingredients regularly found in shampoos. Many shampoos have ingredients in common. It is often the small differences in formulation that make one shampoo better than another for a particular hair texture or condition.

Water is the main ingredient in most shampoos. Generally it is not just plain water, but purified or **deionized water**: water that has had impurities such as calcium and magnesium and other metal ions that would make a product unstable removed. Water is usually the first ingredient listed, which indicates that the shampoo contains more water than anything else. From there on, as mentioned earlier, ingredients are listed in descending order, according to the percentage of each ingredient in the shampoo.

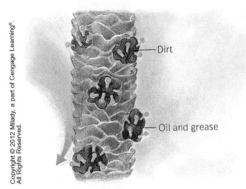

▲ Figure 8–1
The tail of the shampoo molecule is attracted to oil and dirt.

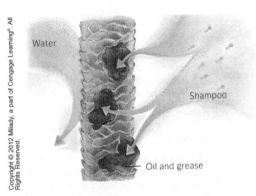

▲ Figure 8–2
Shampoo causes oil to roll up in small globules.

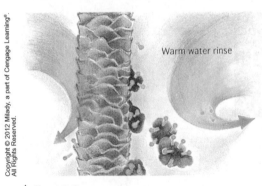

▲ Figure 8–3
The heads of the shampoo molecules attach to the water molecules.

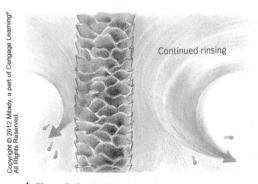

▲ Figure 8–4
Thorough rinsing washes away debris and excess shampoo.

Surfactants

The second ingredient that most shampoos have in common is the primary surfactant (or base detergent). Surfactants are cleansing or surface-active agents. A surfactant molecule has two ends: a hydrophilic or water-attracting head, and a lipophilic or oil-attracting tail (**Figure 8–1**). During the shampooing process, the hydrophilic head attracts water and the lipophilic tail attracts oil (**Figure 8–2**). This combination creates a push-pull process that causes the oils, dirt, and deposits to roll up into little balls (**Figure 8–3**) that can be lifted off in the water and rinsed from the hair (**Figure 8–4**).

Other ingredients are added to base surfactants to create a wide variety of shampoo formulas. **Moisturizer**, which is a product formulated to add moisture to dry hair or promote the retention of moisture, is a common additive along with oil, protein, preservatives, foam enhancer, and perfume.

Basic Detergent Agents

Detergent shampoos typically contain the following agents:

- **Anionic**—Anionic shampoo is high-foaming and has lots of suds. It tends to strip the hair of natural oil. A strong cleansing agent, sodium lauryl sulfate, is used to produce thick lather that rinses well in soft or hard water. According to Dr. Marianne Nelson O'Donoghue, dermatologist and author, "These [anionics] occasionally can be too strong and irritating. This could be because of the pH, or because there is too much detergent action on the hair, which causes too much sebum to be removed."[2]

  Here are some other anionics to be aware of in commercial shampoos:

  - triethanolamine lauryl sulfate (TEA)
  - ammonium laureth sulfate
  - lauroyl sarcosine
  - cocoyl sarcosine
  - laureth sulfate (TEA)
  - sodium lauroyl sarcosinate
  - sodium cocoyl sarcosinate
  - sodium lauroyl isoethionate
  - sodium dioctyl sulfosuccinate
  - coconut sulfated monoglycerides
  - disodium oleamide sulfosuccinate
  - magnesium salt
  - potassium salt

- **Cationics**—These detergents or surfactants are made of quaternary ammonium compounds, or quats. Quats have antibacterial characteristics usually found in dandruff shampoos and also found in cleaning disinfectants.

  The following are cationics in commercial shampoos:

  - quaternary ammonium

  - benzalkonium chloride

  - N-2 ethylaminoformy, methylopyridinium

- **Monionics**—These are detergents that emulsify well and usually have a mild cleansing action. They are gentle to the skin and cause little irritation to the scalp or eyes. However, these products are boosted with ethonylated compounds to increase lather. These compounds also increase thickness and solubility. The conditioning agent in these monionics is sorbitol ester, also known as tweens. They are emulsifiers (or softeners).

  Monionics found in commercial shampoos are as follows:

  - diethanolamide

  - polysorbate 20 and 40

  - palmitate

  - monoethanolamide 5

  - sorbitan laurate

  - stearate

  - ethoxylated fatty alcohols

  - ethoxylated alkylphenols

  - ethoxylated fatty amines

  - ethoxylated fatty amides

- **Ampholytes** or **amphoterics**—These detergents cling to the hair, making it appear more manageable. They contain germicidal or antiseptic characteristics and are often used in baby shampoos because they do not irritate the eyes or skin. They are the mildest of detergents and claim not to strip the natural oils from the hair and scalp, because of their gentle moisturizing effect.

  These ampholytes are found in most commercial products:

  - sodium lauraminodipropionate

  - triethanolmine lauraminodipropionate

  - cocamide betaine

  - amphoteric 1 through 20

The natural hair care specialist must realize that detergents are found in all hair cleansing products, whether they claim to be natural or not. Even

moisturizer a product formulated to add moisture to dry hair or promote the retention of moisture.

anionic a classification of detergent; *anionic* means "neutral ions."

cationics detergents or surfactants made of quaternary ammonium compounds, or quats.

monionics detergents that emulsify well and usually have a mild cleansing action. They are gentle to the skin and cause little irritation to the scalp or eyes.

ampholytes (amphoterics) the mildest detergents that cling to the hair, making it appear more manageable. They contain germicidal or antiseptic characteristics, but do not strip natural oils from the hair and scalp. They are often used in baby shampoos and have a gentle moisturizing effect.

in health food stores, 1 out of 10 cosmetic shampoos claiming to be organic and herbal had one or more surfactants listed. This means that for most products to be user friendly and have a longer shelf life, many chemicals must be used.

You are not limited to commercial products. It depends on the specialists' philosophy as to how natural their products must be. The goal, however, is for natural hair care specialists to be in balance with their environment and the demands of their businesses. Find products that can satisfy both.

The Chemistry of Water

Water is the most abundant and important element on earth. It is classified as a universal solvent because it is capable of dissolving more substances than any other solvent known to science.

Fresh water from lakes and streams is purified by sedimentation (matter sinking to the bottom) and filtration (water passing through a porous substance, such as a filter paper or charcoal) to remove suspended clay, sand, and organic material. Before the water enters public water pipelines, small amounts of chlorine are added to kill bacteria. Boiling water at a temperature of 212 degrees Fahrenheit (100 degrees Celsius) will also destroy most microbes. Water can be further treated by distillation, a process of heating water so that it becomes a vapor and then condensing the purified vapor so that it collects as a liquid. Distillation is often used in the manufacturing of cosmetics.

Water is of crucial importance in the natural hair care and braiding industry. It is used for shampooing, mixing solutions, and many other functions. Depending on the kinds and amounts of minerals present in water, water can be classified as either hard or soft. You will be able to make a more professional shampoo selection if you know whether the water in your salon and area is hard or soft. Most water-softener companies can supply you with a water-testing kit to determine how hard or soft your water is (soft, slightly hard, moderately hard, hard, or extremely hard).

soft water rainwater or chemically softened water; contains only small amounts of minerals and thus allows soap and shampoo to lather freely.

hard water often in well water; contains minerals that reduce the ability of soap or shampoo to lather.

Soft water is rainwater or chemically softened water that contains only small amounts of minerals and, therefore, allows soap and shampoo to lather freely. For this reason, it is preferred for shampooing. **Hard water** is often in well water and contains minerals that reduce the ability of soap or shampoo to lather.

The pH Scale

Understanding pH levels will help you select the proper shampoo for your client. The amount of hydrogen in a solution, which determines whether it is alkaline or acid, is measured on a pH scale that has a range from 0 to 14. The pH of a neutral solution, one that is neither acidic nor alkaline, is 7. A shampoo that is acidic will have a pH ranging from 0 to 6.9; a shampoo that is alkaline will have a pH rating of 7.1 or higher. The more alkaline the shampoo, the stronger and harsher it is. A high-pH shampoo can leave the hair dry, brittle, and porous. A slightly acidic shampoo more closely matches the ideal pH of hair (**Figure 8–5**).

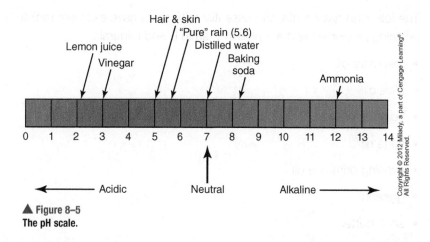

Lemon juice
Vinegar
Hair & skin
"Pure" rain (5.6)
Distilled water
Baking soda
Ammonia

0 1 2 3 4 5 6 7 8 9 10 11 12 13 14

◄─────── Acidic   Neutral   Alkaline ───────►

▲ Figure 8–5
The pH scale.

At the optimum pH level, the shampoo should have a low enough acidity to retain the hair's natural fatty acids or sebum, which protects the hair shaft and retains moisture.

The list of ingredients is your key to determining which shampoo will leave a client's hair shiny and manageable, which will treat a scalp or hair condition, and which will prepare the hair for a chemical treatment. Now that you are familiar with pH and the chemistry of water and shampoo, the following paragraphs describe some of the different types of shampoos.

Low-pH Shampoos

Commercial low-pH shampoos are designed for the consumer who has dry, brittle, damaged hair. They contain milder cleansing agents that do not strip all natural sebum. However, in most cases, pH-balanced products are difficult to measure (nobody walks around with litmus paper to test the acidity of a product).

On a pH chart, lemon juice and hydrogen peroxide rate as having a low pH or low acidity. However, if used when applying permanent color, hydrogen peroxide can dry and damage hair. Diluted lemon juice, on the other hand, is an excellent conditioner for removing shampoo residue and debris from braided and locked hair. It too has a low pH, but it helps maintain the **essential fatty acids** and sebum that protect the hair and scalp. Pure lemon juice can irritate the scalp and dry the hair.

Natural hair care specialists must educate themselves on the different products that claim to offer pH-balanced ingredients. These products can leave the hair and scalp dry and itchy because of the additives, preservatives, and fragrances.

For textured hair, the natural stylist should consider products that offer the most natural ingredients with essential fatty acids (essential organic oils). Essential fatty acids cannot be produced. The human body must be supplied through diet and application of organic oils found in seeds, extract of vegetables, and animal fats. These fatty acids are labeled as "essential" because they are so necessary for life. The hair and scalp need the organic oils for normal growth and natural luster.

essential fatty acids the fats needed to complete biological processes.

The following natural oils with essential fatty acids have excellent moisture-retaining properties and are high in vitamin E and minerals:

- rosemary oil

- olive oil

- coconut oil

- sage oil

- evening primrose oil

- glycerin

- shea butter

- linseed oil

- flaxseed oil

- cod liver oil

Medicated Shampoos

medicated shampoo contains special ingredients that are effective in reducing dandruff or relieving other scalp conditions.

Medicated shampoo contains special ingredients that are effective in reducing dandruff or relieving other scalp conditions. Some medicated shampoos have to be prescribed by a physician. They can be quite strong and could affect the color of color-treated or lightened hair. In some cases, the shampoo must remain on the scalp for a longer period of time than other shampoos in order for the active ingredient to work. Always read and follow the manufacturer's instructions carefully.

Medicated shampoos contain active ingredients that help control scalp flaking or scalp disorders like seborrhea dermatitis or psoriasis. Most anti-dandruff shampoos are basic detergent shampoos with harsh, drying ingredients. They not only treat the problem of the scalp but also remove too much of the natural oils that protect the hair.

The following are some of the ingredients added to dandruff shampoos that address and treat scalp flaking, seborrhea and psoriasis:

- tar

- selenium disulfide (most effective and harsh)

- zinc pyrithione (least drying)

- salicylic acid

- sulfur

- kekoconazole

Most of these ingredients are added to moisturizing shampoos (particularly zinc pyrithione, tar, and salicylic acid) so that you can shampoo more frequently without stripping the scalp. A study provided by the University of Pennsylvania adequately demonstrated that there is "an increased epidermal cell turnover in seborrheic dermatitis" when using shampoos with these additives.

For textured hair types, these anti-dandruff and anti-seborrheic shampoos, such as selenium sulfide shampoos, are extremely damaging. The natural stylist must take extra care when serving clients who have these scalp conditions.

Esthetic Shampoos

Protein, conditioning, and moisturizing additives: These are shampoos with little to no stripping effect on natural hair oils. With the advances in natural product development, these shampoos cleanse as well as any other commercial shampoo, just in a gentler way. It was once believed that these shampoos were not a sufficient alternative to a "real" cleansing shampoo, but they have proven that more natural can be just as effective.

Esthetic shampoos are usually composed of some of the milder anionic, monionic, and amphoteric surfactants. Hydrolyzed animal proteins are added to the basic shampoo to address split ends and damaged cuticles and increase hair elasticity. But most protein shampoos coat the shaft, fill in the cuticle, and give the hair strand more bulk or body. Many aesthetic shampoos have conditioners and moisturizers to make the hair more manageable. These shampoos are often designed so that they do not rinse out thoroughly. Instead, they leave a deposit of film to add and seal moisture into the hair. The additive fills in the gaps on the hair cuticle that has been raised from excessive chemical, heat, mechanical damage.

You will also find that many of these milder shampoos are designed with sunscreen agents to protect color-treated or permed hair from the damaging rays of the sun. They can be useful products to protect virgin hair from harmful environmental elements and do not strip natural oils. But they are also so mild that they have very little cleansing action. Shampoos that contain honey or honey shampoos provide **emollients** to seal in moisture and contain **humectants** or moisture retainers. These esthetic shampoos work effectively as products used on the second or third shampoo to detangle and soften textured hair.

Herbal or Organic Shampoos

A real herbal or organic shampoo is not made with detergents or surfactants. The more basic herbal shampoos contain castile soap or black soap. Soaps were used before detergent shampoos were marketed in the 1930s. Soaps can be mixed with a variety of excellent herbal infusions that will address the needs of individual clients. A moisturizing or emollient herb as well as herbs that add an aromatic quality to the product should be a major component of a natural shampoo. There are also optional ingredients for enhancing color, stimulating growth, reducing hair thinning, and solving dandruff problems.

Here's a Tip.........

As an alternative to anti-dandruff or anti-seborrheic shampoo, the following procedure can be used to avoid the harsh effects of these additives. This procedure can be done on all hair types.

1. For the first shampoo, combine black soap, tea tree, peppermint, or eucalyptus oil and shampoo in an applicator bottle with a small nozzle top. Part the wet hair in ½-inch (1.3-cm) sections, and apply the product until the entire scalp is covered.

2. With small circular motions, massage the scalp until the lather covers the scalp. Avoid vigorous motions to limit the shampoo to the hair.

3. Shampoo thoroughly and allow the lather to remain on the scalp for five to ten minutes so that the active ingredients can work. The client's scalp will feel invigorated and refreshed.

4. Rinse; apply a second shampoo application. Use a mild moisturizing, herbal, or conditioning shampoo to soften hair.

emollients oily or fatty ingredients that coat the hair, aid in its elasticity, and prevent moisture loss.

humectants water-binding agents or substances that promote moisture retention.

When looking for products that offer natural ingredients, the natural hair care stylist should ask several questions. The stylist will need more than one kind of shampoo. Consider the many different hair types, overall conditions, and required results as well as the finished look for braids, extensions or locks, loose hair, and weaves of your many clients.

For the natural stylist, herbal or organic shampoos offer the best alternative to commercial shampoo products. After an extensive study comparing natural extracts to their synthetic copy, Aubrey Hampton says, "There was invariably a difference between the synthetic and the natural extract. The difference was that the body responded differently to the real substance than to the synthetic substance. Using the synthetic copy of a natural extract on the skin or hair in cosmetic formulas gave me an inferior product every time from every standpoint. Pure vegetable glycerin, for example, is a thicker, richer, and a far better emollient than synthetic propylene glycol (the petrochemical replacement usually found in moisturizers). The synthetic chemical is usually substituted for a natural extract. Most product manufacturers will endorse the scientific hype around the synthetic substitute. In the process they reveal little knowledge to the market, of the amount used or how the body will react."[3]

As mentioned previously in Chapter 3, cultivating harmony is a vital part of the natural hair care service. Using healthy, wholesome products is very important in developing a relationship with your client. The all-natural hair client will have greater results with organic or herbal products. Clients who have consciously decided to wear their hair naturally need to have quality products to groom, protect, and complement the body's healing ability. Herbalist Adio Akil of Praises Enterprises and Master Pioneer believes that shea butter is one of the best restorative and healing moisturizers of those that have become popular in the last decade. With shea butter, people experience the beneficial properties immediately, they receive the subtle health effects that replenish their bodies as well as make them feel safe from synthetic chemicals. Akil states, "To know that the product that you are using on the client is wholesome, not physically damaging or creates the wrong body condition is the reason why the natural hair industry has been brought forth and is growing. There is no end to it. Now that we know about the effectiveness of using natural hair products there is no unknowing."[4]

Herbal and organic products do not mask the problem like many commercial products do. Instead, they enhance the hair and scalp and increase their ability to heal. With natural products, there is no quick-fix solution. Natural products can be altered or designed to address each client's needs. Herbal rinses can be added to commercial shampoos to enhance and assist in the cleansing and moisturizing process. Herbal shampoos and rinses should be designed to address each client's specific needs. These treatments are easy to incorporate simply by adding several drops of an infusion or herbal extract to an existing product. With this understanding, the natural hair stylist can create a new "recipe" that will address particular hair care needs. You will see the improvements in the hair over the long term. The stylist must make the client aware of the long-term effect of organic products on the body and in their lives.

It is useful to know that some synthetic products can also be helpful in the servicing of natural hair. The stylist must be conscious of the long-term effects of that product. Natural and synthetic products can be high in toxicity and can cause some skin reaction. Read and understand all product labels before using the product. It will allow you to educate yourself and the client.

Dry Shampoos

At the beginning of the natural hair movement, many women wore their hair in braided, twisted, or weave hairstyles with extensions for up to three months at a time. And many of these women would not shampoo or cleanse their hair for the entire duration of their hairstyle, for fear of ruining the styles or lessening the life span of the hairstyle. These were not good practices and often led to a buildup of debris and a rank smell on the hair and scalp. Fortunately, today women are more aware of the importance of regularly cleansing the hair and scalp and the option of alternative solutions to cleansing the hair and scalp.

One popular way of cleansing the scalp is with what is known as a dry shampoo. Not all dry shampoos are actually dry, but they are an alternative to having your scalp and hair saturated with water. The "home care" type of dry shampoo consists of simply going through the scalp with a clean, wet cloth and gently rubbing the scalp to remove dirt and debris. This process can be repeated for several rounds. Once you have studied the use of botanicals, you will learn that botanical oils such as rosemary, sage, lemon, essential oils, tea tree, and other astringent hair and scalp botanicals can be used to address scalp issues your clients may have. These botanicals can be and should be diluted by adding them to water for a more effective and invigorating dry-shampoo experience.

Some home care dry-shampoo techniques make use of items that can be found in your kitchen—things like baking soda, baking powder, cornstarch, cornmeal, salt, and dry oatmeal. These items can be ground down and mixed together and then combed or brushed through the hair to remove dirt, debris, and oils. These types of dry cleansing items are not for the scalp, but for the hair only, and typically for hair that is straight or has a long curl pattern. Contrary to popular belief, clients with straighter textures also wear their hair natural or are transitioning to natural, and they too are looking for natural styling, cleansing, and nurturing regimens for their hair.

Some of the dry-shampoo products on the market today offer scalp-cleansing products with all that you need in one bottle. Many of these products have **botanical** (plant matter) ingredients that cleanse the scalp while invigorating and nourishing it.

CAUTION

Herbal and aromatherapy applications should not be taken lightly. Clients can have mild to severe reactions to herbs as well as to synthetic compounds. Therefore, it is recommended that you embark on a study of the power and nature of herbs before using (testing) them on clients. You must obtain a client history before any application.

| **botanical** term relating to plants.

Daily Shampoos

Since the start of the natural hair movement, an evolutionary process has occurred. Young women in their early twenties are discovering their natural textures for the first time. Many of these women have had chemical straighteners in their hair since they were children and now seek a change with their hair. In addition to no longer wanting to put chemical straighteners in their hair, many of these newbies to natural hair also do not want braids, twists, weaves, or any type of extensions. They prefer to wear their hair loose, free, and unrestrained by braid styles.

Loose and free textured hairstyles, also known as the Afro, require daily grooming and maintenance, which requires products to cleanse, condition, and groom this type of styling option. These loose and free textured styles are referred to as "wash 'n' go" styling. Many of these women are seeking to enhance the natural curl pattern of their hair and in some cases are looking to emulate a curl pattern that is longer and looser than their own natural texture.

Loose Afro hair is exposed to the elements, causing it to become especially dry in the extreme seasons of winter and summer. In addition, after sleeping with your hair out and loose, this style choice can pose a challenge in the morning for those with tightly coiled hair. They may find it hard to re-create that same hairstyle; not only has it been smashed by lying on it all night, but the curl pattern has shrunk and the hair is no longer as hydrated. These types of styles can call for daily hydration. For the do-it-yourself (DIY) community, one technique for keeping textured Afros hydrated is to use a gentle, sulfate-free, low-suds shampoo. Daily shampoos and moisturizing conditioners gently moisturize and enhance the curl pattern. This wash 'n' go hair care regime is practiced often by many clients who have wavy/curly hair; however, for those with coily, kinky/wiry hair, this practice can change the acid balance of textured hair and create dry, brittle hair. With textured natural hair, "less is more." The less combing, brushing, and general manipulation, the better it is for the hair. ☑ **LO4**

Other Techniques for Cleansing Hair

Co-Washing

A technique that has become quite popular is called **co-washing**. Many women believe that using any type of shampoo more than once a week is drying or strips their hair, leaving it dry and brittle. Instead, they use the technique called co-washing: "shampooing" their hair using conditioner instead of shampoo.

This co-washing technique, while adding moisture, does not really cleanse the hair. It does add moisture, conditions, and leaves the natural oils and sebum in place.

Co-washing the hair consists of the following steps: First rinse the hair with warm water for about three minutes. While running the water

co-washing using conditioner rather than shampoo to cleanse the hair.

through the hair, massage the scalp to loosen any buildup on the scalp before adding the conditioner to the hair. After adding conditioner, finger the product thoroughly through the hair. The conditioner can be left on for three minutes or more before being rinsed out with cool water. A client using the co-washing technique may require a clarifying shampoo to release some of the buildup of conditioner on the hair.

Cold Water Conditioning

Another cleansing technique is known as cold water conditioning. **Cold water conditioning** is just a matter of rinsing the conditioner out of the hair using cool to cold water instead of hot water. Some clients believe that they should have their hair shampooed with cold water, but it is not really possible to cleanse the hair properly when shampooing with cold water. You need warm water to loosen up and release the dirt and oils that have accumulated on the hair and scalp. Warm water opens the pores of the scalp and opens the scales of the hair shaft to release, lift, and remove dirt, old oils, and debris. The water should not be piping hot, but instead nice and warm during the shampoo process.

Instead of cold washing or using the technique of shampooing with cold water, rinsing out the conditioner with cool water is best for closing the pores and hair cuticle (since coldness contracts). Cool water seals in moisture, which in turn prevents frizz. Rinsing your hair with hot water can completely remove all the conditioner from your hair and literally wash it down the drain.

To summarize, you should ask yourself the following questions before using a new product:

- What are the main ingredients the product contains? (Remember: The first few ingredients listed on the label are more prevalent in the product than any other ingredient.)

- Does the product contain synthetic or natural ingredients that should be avoided? Beware of the toxicity in all products.

- Does the product have enough of the desired ingredients that will benefit the client's hair and scalp needs? Many manufacturers add natural ingredients to attract the consumer but do not add enough to benefit the hair.

- Do the benefits of the product outweigh the disadvantages? Most natural products still contain a number of preservatives, surfactants, and fillers to enhance color or fragrance.

- Is the packaging much more attractive than the product itself? Some of the highly commercial products look more attractive,

Here's a Tip..........

Exposing natural hair to water with conditioning agents on a regular basis (at least once or twice a week) helps to moisturize the hair and create curl definition. It also helps keep natural hair hydrated. Hydration is the key to length retention and healthy textured hair.

cold water conditioning practice of rinsing the conditioner out of the hair using cool to cold water instead of hot water.

Here's a Tip..........

Some natural stylists often use shampoo that is based in black soap or castile soap.

serious, and medicinal than they really are. Do not be fooled by packaging; read the labels carefully.

- Although many clients like to mix and match product lines, sticking to one product line at a time will offer better insight as to how well a particular line suits that particular client's hair. Recommend that your clients use one product line at a time, so that they can properly gauge the results of the line. Most product lines are formulated so that each product in the line works in tandem with the other products in the line for a better overall hair experience.

The earth has produced natural botanical medicines that address every symptom the body can experience. The body has natural healing ability, and herbs can enhance that process. The vitamins, minerals, and nurturing properties of the herbs can condition, stimulate, and strengthen textured hair.

Common Chemicals Found in Hair Products

When you are choosing hair care products, always read the back of the label. Look before you leap. If you want natural products, you will need to invest time to search for them. The product may say "herbal" on the front portion of the container, but the back label contains a list of named ingredients that the product is actually made of. There are also "semi-natural" hair products that offer you a lot of natural ingredients but may have synthetic colors, fragrances, or preservatives for greater appeal or a longer shelf life. The following are just a few of the most common toxic ingredients found in hair products:

- **Sodium lauryl sulfates/Sodium laureth sulfate (SLS/SLES)**—derived and processed from coconuts. Found in most shampoos as a detergent that emulsifies to make foam or bubbles. May be present in scalp treatments, hair color, liquid soap, laundry detergents, body wash, and toothpastes.

- **Parabens**—often listed as **methyl paraben, ethyl paraben, propyl paraben, butyl paraben.** preservatives for products; used to stop the growth of bacteria and microbes. Linked to breast cancer.

- **Propylene glycol**—a conditioning agent or humectant that softens and provides moisture to the hair and scalp; associated with eye, skin, and lung irritation. Fragrance ingredient. Linked to allergic skin reaction.

- **1,4 Dioxane**—used in shampoos for babies and adults as a preservative solvent; added to products to make harsh chemicals mild. Found in hair dyes; considered to have high carcinogenic effects.

- **Selenium sulfide**—used in all dandruff shampoos; considered very toxic. Reported to have some link to kidney, respiratory, heart, liver and blood toxicity; considered a carcinogen.

- **Acrylamide**—found in hair products, tobacco smoke, and other items. Known to cause eye, skin, and lung irritation. Very toxic and also known to be a carcinogen.

- **Formaldehyde**—a by-product of and released by a number of cosmetic preservatives. Highly toxic to human immune and respiratory systems; found in cigarette smoke. Linked to cancer.

- **Resorcinol**—common ingredient in hair color and bleaching products; a high skin, eye, and lung irritant. Toxic to the immune system.

- **Paraffin**, also known as crystalline petroleum wax—a synthetic wax made from petroleum or natural gas. Acts as a binder, emulsion/foam stabilizer, emollient, and water repellent. Low toxicity to organ systems; skin irritant.

- **Phthalates**—a type of plastic used in hair products to moisturize and soften; found in nail polish. Linked to toxins that affect male reproductive and developmental abilities.[5]

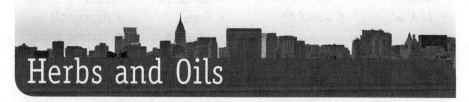

Herbs and Oils

Natural Hair Care Applications

In the natural hair care profession, it is common for natural stylists to use "recipes" that they have created themselves. Many will use common herbs, botanicals, vegetable oils, and essential oils to create natural hair solutions for their clients.

The botanicals presented in the table on page 176 give the natural hair care specialist a working knowledge of how to enhance any service you provide to your clients (**Figure 8–6**). Whether the specialist adds several drops of an essential oil or extract to a commercial product or is inspired to create a customized blend of conditioning treatments, the innate properties of these botanicals can enhance the quality and condition of the hair and scalp. As the public demands more environmentally safe products and "back-to-basics" hair care, hair care specialists will be required to know more about alternative chemical-free products and treatments.

These oils can be used in combination or singularly. Again, try them only after you have studied the uses of herbs and oils. It is best for the head and hair to be wet and warm. Warming of the essential oils can kill their healing properties and is not required in order for

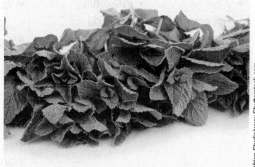

▲ Figure 8–6
Mint is an example of a natural botanical.

© Africa Studio/www.Shutterstock.com

HERBS, PLANTS, AND OILS USED IN NATURAL HAIR CARE

OILY SCALP

- Peppermint
- Bergamot
- Witch hazel
- Basil
- Yarrow
- Eucalyptus
- Lemongrass
- Rosemary
- Thyme

ANTISEPTIC

- Thyme
- Chamomile
- Comfrey
- Lemongrass
- Tea tree oil
- Camphor
- Citrus rinses
- Eucalyptus
- Myrrh
- Sage
- Lemon juice

MOISTURIZER

- Almond oil
- Chamomile
- Basil
- Cocoa butter
- Glycerine
- Lecithin
- Castor oil
- Extra virgin olive oil (EVOO)
- Avocado oil
- Comfrey
- Aloe vera
- Shea butter
- Lanolin
- Apricot oil
- Jojoba oil

HAIR LOSS

- Jojoba oil
- Nettle
- Emu oil
- Calendula
- Horsetail
- Kelp
- Rosemary
- Thyme
- Black seed oil
- Olive oil
- Hemp seed oil
- Coltsfoot
- Sage
- Rose hip seed oil

HAIR GROWTH

- Camphor
- Coltsfoot
- Nettle
- Sage
- Dandelion
- Lavender
- Aloe vera
- Basil
- Black seed oil
- Rose hip seed oil
- Horsetail
- Kelp
- Rosemary
- Jaborandi
- Thyme
- Burdock root
- Avocado oil

SCALP SOOTHERS

- Chamomile
- Comfrey
- Aloe vera
- Olive oil/EVOO
- Sage
- Emu oil
- Camphor
- Jasmine
- Almond oil
- Avocado
- Eucalyptus
- Carrot oil

ANTI-DANDRUFF

- Sage
- Eucalyptus
- Rosemary
- Horsetail
- Calendula
- Tea tree oil
- Jojoba oil
- Neroli oil
- Olive oil
- Peppermint
- Goldenseal
- Hysop
- Evening primrose oil
- Garlic
- Patchouli
- Burdock root

CELL REJUVENATION

- Echinacea
- Comfrey
- Lavender
- Emu oil
- Rose hip seed oil

- Calendula
- Aloe
- Papaya
- Black seed oil

SOFTENER

- Lavender
- Rose hip seed oil
- Ginseng
- Coltsfoot
- Rosemary
- Jojoba oil
- Hemp seed oil
- Avocado
- Grapeseed oil
- Papaya
- Castor oil
- Evening primrose oil
- Coconut oil
- Olive oil
- Glycerin
- Sandalwood
- Borage
- Shea butter

CONDITIONER

- Jojoba oil
- Sage
- Burdock root
- Thyme
- Nettle
- Lavender
- Kelp
- Almond oil
- Evening primrose oil
- Rosemary
- Eucalyptus
- Shea butter

ASTRINGENT

- Lemon juice
- Peppermint
- Rosemary
- Sandalwood
- Witch hazel
- Sage
- Apple cider vinegar
- Tea tree oil
- Yarrow
- Nettle
- Chamomile
- Lavender
- Balsams

Table 8–1 Herbs, Plants, and Oils Used in Natural Hair Care.

them to be effective. Always dilute botanical oils in a base oil. The ratio of the botanical oil should be no more than 5 to 10 percent. This means that your base oil would make up 90 to 95 percent of the formulation. Initially, the herbal oil may not be as easy to detect. But if the mixture sits overnight or for a couple of days, the oils marry and it becomes easier to detect the smell of the essential oil (**Table 8–1**).

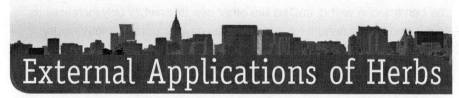

External Applications of Herbs

Many of the herbs listed include information about the scalp and skin. It is important to understand that the scalp is skin. The health of the scalp determines the health of hair. When the body is stressed, the scalp is the barometer of its health status.

Almond Oil

Almond oil is often used as a base oil in treatments, lotions, and creams. It acts as an emollient and moisturizer and is soothing to the scalp. It contains protein, copper, zinc, vitamin E, and essential fatty acids (stearic, lauric, oleic, and linoleic) that have excellent moisture-retaining properties similar to those of natural sebum. Apricot and peach oils can often be substituted because they, too, are great moisturizers. Many people are allergic to all types of nuts. If a client has nut allergies, he should avoid using any oils derived from nuts.

Aloe Vera

For centuries, the aloe plant has been known for its first-aid value. Aloe vera is a member of the Lily family. It feels and looks very much like cactus. This "medicinal" plant cleans and relieves burns, soothes sunburns, and heals minor cuts and abrasions. It is also used on cold sores. It helps promote new growth of living cells, can help stop stinging pain, reduce infection, and alleviate scarring. It contains antibiotic properties (polysaccharides), healing hormones, and dozens of amino acids, enzymes, vitamins, and minerals such as calcium, potassium, sodium, manganese, magnesium, iron, lecithin, and zinc. The gel within the plant is 95 percent water, filled with properties that stimulate the scalp. The gel is excellent for African locks and is useful during the locking service to nurture hair. It can be added to creams and lotions to use directly on the scalp as a moisturizer. It softens and has a soothing, cool, refreshing quality. The gel may have a mild drying effect when used alone, but acts as a great emollient when vitamin E oil is added.

For best results, use fresh aloe gel. The plant is very easy to care for. Remove a thick leaf, rinse it clean, and then slice it in the middle. Scrape the gel from the leaf with a spoon and add to any moisturizing treatment for grooming gels or lotions for locks. Dermatologists have used aloe to treat oily scalp and dandruff. Pure gel from the aloe plant is often used during the cultivation of locks, to accelerate the locking process.

Argan Oil

Argan oil, also known as Moroccan oil, is derived from the kernels of the argan tree. Argan oil has been around for centuries but has recently become a highly sought-after commodity. The harsh conditions under which this tree grows are difficult to duplicate, and so this rare oil cannot be harvested in vast quantities like other oils. Its scarcity only increases its value and the demand for it. Argan oil has a high content of fatty acids, including omega-6 and vitamin E, and its revitalizing and moisturizing properties make it a wonderful source for antiaging products. It is also very silky and smooth to the touch. It is great for all kinds of skin problems, including wrinkles, psoriasis, acne, eczema, and so forth. It also is known to increase the elasticity and tension of the skin.

Due to its high content of unsaturated fatty acids, argan oil provides excellent results on repairing damaged hair, making hair smooth and manageable, and repairing spilt ends. It easily penetrates the skin and scalp. In other words, argan oil is known as liquid gold. Thanks to the popularity of argan oil, some advertisements regarding the amount contained in products can be exaggerated. Also due to the high demand of argan oil, it is now under government protection. Fair trade practices are in place to ensure its sustainability and the financial well-being of the women who harvest this precious commodity.

Avocado Oil

Avocado is a carrier oil used to stimulate hair growth. It is a rich oil that works well with other carrier oil and is excellent for restoring dehydrated, aging, sun-damaged hair. Pulp from this edible fruit can be used in facial and scalp packs for concentrated and penetrating treatments. It is filled with vitamins A, D, and E as well as potassium, sulfur, chlorine, fatty acids, and amino acids. It also moistens and softens.

Balsam

Balsam is a very special aromatic flower and bark. It contains mild antiseptic properties and kills parasites (such as ringworm) and their eggs. Balsam aids in the regeneration of skin cells and is used in shampoos, conditioners, and perfumes for its fragrance. It is a disinfectant and stimulant and contains benzoic and cinnamic acid esters, which are natural preservatives.

Basil

Basil is considered a sacred herb in India, and in certain parts of the country it is dedicated to the gods. It is called the love herb because of its aromatic qualities. This herb can be used in rinses or tonics to bring shine and luster to the hair. For dark hair, basil can be mixed with rosemary as a rinse; for blonde or light brown hair, it can be added to chamomile rinses. Basil stimulates hair growth and reduces snarls and tangles when it is mixed with oil of lavender as a grooming aid. Some Arabian women use this mixture as a hair perfume. In general, the fragrance stimulates and invigorates the senses, promoting growth. Basil contains high amounts of calcium, phosphorous, iron, magnesium, and vitamins A, D, and B_2.

Beeswax

Beeswax is derived from the honeycomb and smells like honey. It is used in hair lotions and creams as a thickener and stiffener. It is also used as an emulsifier to keep products from separating. It contains 71 percent fatty acid esters and is used on locks to keep them in a cylindrical shape. However, beeswax also leaves a very heavy coating and attracts dirt and debris from the environment when used as a grooming agent for locks. Beeswax is not recommended for this application unless it is greatly diluted with other emollient ingredients. The dilution can be as small as 1 percent.

Bergamot (Also Called Bee Balm)

Bergamot herb is an essential oil used in hair products, toilet water, colognes, and floral and heavy perfumes as well as in soaps for its scent. Because it is so fragrant, it is a soothing aromatic that helps clear the head and relieve tension. Bergamot oil (derived from a citrus fruit) is used on the scalp as a preparation for greasy hair. When used in a rinse, the herb can stimulate the scalp. It builds resiliency in hair after it has been damaged. As a facial treatment ingredient, it may cause skin sensitivities or redness. It is a remedy for such skin problems as acne, boils, cold sores, eczema, and oily complexions.

Black Seed Oil

Black seed oil is considered a multi-nutrient. Black seed oil is rich in the essential fatty acids omega-3, -6, and -9. These omega fatty acids work to strengthen and regenerate the hair and scalp.[6] Black seed oil contains nutrients that fortify the body with A, B_2, C, zinc, iron, potassium, magnesium, selenium, linoleic acid, oleic acid, calcium, and niacin.

Burdock Root

Burdock, when taken internally, is a great blood purifier. It helps promote kidney function and nourishes poorly functioning pituitary glands (responsible for hormone balance). Externally, burdock root is extremely cleansing and soothing for skin problems such as acne, canker sores, dandruff, and eczema. When used as a rinse, burdock root addresses flaking and scaly scalp problems, and will restore tones. It helps dark hair tones maintain their color. It can strengthen follicles that have been stressed from poor grooming. Nutrients found in burdock are large amounts of vitamin C and iron, 12 percent protein, and 70 percent carbohydrate. It also contains some vitamin A and B complex, vitamin E, PABA, sulfur, and small amounts of silicon copper, iodine, and zinc.

Calendula (Marigold)

Calendula has a mild astringent quality. When flowers are used in an infusion, it can be effective in washing cold sores and irritated skin. It cleans and soothes cuts, abrasions, eczema, and acne as well as scalp disorders such as dandruff. It helps in healing and relieves minor pain. Calendula is also effective in rejuvenating skin cells. As a moisturizer, it can soften hair and scalp. When used with vinegar as a rinse, calendula can enhance natural highlights in dark brown and blond hair. It contains a large amount of phosphorous and some amounts of vitamins A and C. It can also aid in the slow healing of cuts, scratches, and burns.

Carrot Oil

Many people are aware of the great benefits of eating carrots and the high content of vitamins A, C, and K, and potassium found in them. However, many are still unaware of the great benefits derived from using carrot oil for the hair. Carrot oil is great in relieving itching, dryness, psoriasis, and eczema. Carrot oil also assists in rejuvenating the skin and scalp and reducing scarring. Like all essential oils, carrot oil should not be used directly on the skin, but instead diluted in a base oil.

Castor Oil

Castor oil, from castor beans (seeds), has been found in Egyptian tombs that were more than 4,000 years old. Used internally, it is a laxative. Externally, it is a moisturizer used as a base oil to moisten or soften skin. It is often found in transparent soap and shampoos for dry hair. Castor oil is rich in essential fatty acids and can be used to nourish hair and scalp. It can be used as an emulsifier in ointments, grooming products, creams, and lotions. It is a humectant and emollient that moisturizes, smooths, and seals the cuticle. Castor oil has healing properties, and it is great as a hot-oil treatment for dry hair and scalp.[7]

Chamomile (Gold and Blue)

Chamomile is one of the most popular herbs in the world. Its aromatic essence of apple is sweet and wonderful for potpourris. Internally, chamomile acts as a sedative to relax the nerves; it can also settle an upset stomach. It soothes and calms without harmful side effects, and it induces sleep. Externally, chamomile is excellent for relieving eczema and skin inflammation. In shampoos and rinses, it cleanses as well as moisturizes to soften hair gently. When combined with neutral henna as an infusion and rinse, it can give dark hair golden highlights. It has a penetrating quality, so it is great to use as a facial or herbal hair treatment. Chamomile stimulates the natural hormone thyroxine, which influences and rejuvenates the texture of the skin and hair. Chamomile contains calcium, magnesium, potassium, iron, manganese, zinc, and vitamin A.

Cocoa Butter

Cocoa butter is a derivative of the cocoa plant and the cocoa bean that gives us chocolate. This thick, fatty oil has the fragrance of chocolate. In the form of cocoa butter, it is an excellent lubricant and skin softener. It is often used as a base to mix with other vegetable oils and coconut oil to protect the scalp from flaking. Cocoa butter adds firmness to bar soap; it also works well in the making of pomades, balms, and massage and scalp butters. Food-grade cocoa butter adds great flavor to every dish.

Coconut Oil

Coconut oil comes from India, the Caribbean, Asia, and the South Pacific islands. This oil has a soft, solid texture in room temperature, but it will liquefy with heat. The key nutritional ingredient in coconut oil is lauric acid—a fatty acid that is antiviral and antibacterial. Coconut oil is often used in soaps, shampoos, and conditioners to give the hair a brilliant shine and luster. The oil has great regenerative and soothing effects on the hair and scalp. It also moisturizes brittle hair, seals split ends, reduces frizz, and lessens scalp inflammation caused by seborrheic dermatitis (dandruff). Coconut oil contains vitamin E, which helps to strengthen protein.[8]

Coltsfoot

Coltsfoot contains large amounts of cystine and silica, which are excellent for the hair and are important foods for the hair root. Cystine is an essential amino acid, which is a protein (keratin) derivative of the hair. Cystine acts to restore and repair protein in the hair. Coltsfoot helps prevent hair loss due to overprocessing and overmanipulation. As an extract added to hot-oil treatments, rinses, or tonics, coltsfoot renews and stimulates growth. The sulfur in the herbal extract is absorbed into the scalp and aids in correcting dry scalp or seborrhea (oily scalp) and hair loss due to stress. Coltsfoot also contains high levels of vitamins A and C, potassium, vitamin D, zinc, and vitamins B_{12} and B_6.

Comfrey

Comfrey is a powerful healing herb and an excellent emollient. As a healing agent, comfrey is an astringent that helps clean and destroy bacteria. It can aid in healing cuts, abrasions, and sores. It softens and soothes skin and scalp, which is vital for regenerating cells and tissue. Comfrey contains a natural hormone called allantoin, which helps strengthen bones and produce healthy skin cells. It can be used in an herbal rinse and tonic because of its amino acid and protein content; it is useful for dry, damaged, and overprocessed hair. Comfrey can retard hair loss.

Dandelion

Dandelion is an excellent stimulant to promote circulation. It is also a mild astringent that cleans and aids in healing. Dandelion is a great source of protein, which helps strengthen the hair. It also can help regenerate skin cells and soothe an oversensitive scalp. As a refreshing rinse or tonic, it can invigorate a dull scalp.

Echinacea

Echinacea is considered the "king of blood purifiers." It stimulates the body's ability to fight against infection and builds up the immune response. It regenerates skin cells to promote healing. When used topically, the antibiotic form of echinacea neutralizes healing. Internally, it is a natural cleanser that benefits the skin. It contains vitamins A, E, and C, iron, copper, sulfur, and potassium.

Emu Oil

Emu oil is an oil derived from the fat of the emu bird, which is indigenous to Australia. Emu oil easily penetrates the skin and is rich in essential fatty acids omega-3, -6, and -9. The fatty acids found in emu oil aid in this oil's ability to penetrate the skin easily, making it a great anti-inflammatory agent. Emu oil can address any number of skin issues, including thinning/balding and scalp inflammation problems. This oil is similar to the human sebum. It has been reported to have "reactive properties" and reduces hair loss by blocking the dehydrotestosterone (DHT) male hormone that shrinks the hair follicle and causes male pattern baldness in men and women. Emu oil helps to increase hair cell growth and supports the follicle growth stages. It is said to be able to revert the follicle back to its healthy state, increase hair growth and fullness, and support the prevention of future hair loss.[9]

Eucalyptus

Eucalyptus is a common herb in Australia, where over 500 species comprise more than three-quarters of the vegetation on the continent. Eucalyptus oil has an extremely antiseptic and antibacterial quality. The active germicide agents it contains prevent infection. It has a very aromatic and stimulating scent. It cools and soothes the scalp and is usually found in products that address dandruff and flaky scalp conditions. Eucalyptus is an effective herb for shampoos because of its cleansing properties, but it must be used in small amounts to avoid irritation and toxicity.

Evening Primrose Oil

Evening primrose oil is an excellent moisturizer and softener. It is high in fatty acids, which is good for many body functions as well as for hair follicles. It is used in creams and lotions to allow a product to safely coat and protect the hair strands and scalp. This coating is not greasy and increases absorption when mixed with other oils. Evening primrose oil is often used for dry hair and in herbal rinses. It must be used in small amounts to avoid sensitivity or irritation. Also be aware that like many oils, evening primrose oil easily can become rancid once it has been opened and exposed to oxygen and or heat. Always check to make sure oils are fresh.

Fennel

Fennel is a very sweet and aromatic herb that tastes like licorice. It is excellent for herbal steams and rinses as well as facial and/or scalp treatments. It opens and medicates pores. It is an effective cleansing and rejuvenating herb for skin cells. Fennel is often found in creams and lotions and contains sulfur, potassium, and sodium.

Frankincense

Frankincense is known to Christians as one of the gifts offered by the three wise men to the baby Jesus. It is extremely aromatic and used mostly in incense. When used as an oil, it can be a warm, soothing stimulant. It removes dead skin cells and relieves flaking from severe dermatitis; it promotes healing of minor cuts and burns. Frankincense is also a great oil to soothe and relax the mind and quiet unsettling thoughts. It is said to be an oil that carries spiritual properties.

Garlic

Garlic is a natural antibiotic (**Figure 8–7**). Its strange odor destroys bacteria, fungi, and yeast. It stimulates cell growth and rejuvenates the healing process. It is high in essential fatty acids, which protect and strengthen the hair strand. The sulfur compounds reduce microorganisms and repair damaged hair follicles. Garlic is excellent for treating dermatitis and skin inflammation. Garlic contains vitamins A and C, selenium, sulfur, calcium, manganese, iron, copper, and vitamin B. It is high in potassium and zinc.

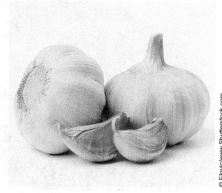

▲ Figure 8–7
Garlic.

Ginseng

Ginseng is known as the king of herbs. Internally, ginseng stimulates the entire body by increasing resistance. Ginseng improves the heart as well as circulation and reduces blood pressure and cholesterol. Externally, its silica content strengthens and repairs protein bonds in hair, and it soothes the scalp as well as stimulates growth. It can reduce scalp flaking. Natural glycerides contained in ginseng moisten and soften hair. Ginseng contains vitamins A and E, thiamine, riboflavin, B_{12}, niacin, calcium, iron, phosphorus, sodium, silicon, potassium, manganese, magnesium, sulfur, and tin.

Glycerin

Glycerin is a thick, transparent liquid that easily dissolves in water and alcohol. Glycerin is a great humectant, absorbing moisture from the environment and restoring it back to the hair. Glycerin seals in moisture, conditions, and reduces frizzy brittle hair. It is extremely beneficial for fine tight coily/kinky/wiry hair, which a moisture sealant to coat the shaft and protect the cuticle. Glycerin gives hair elasticity while reducing split ends, and mixes well with honey, essential oils, base/carrier oil, and herb extracts. It is a great ingredient to add when making a detangling or leave-in "cocktail."[10]

Goldenseal

Goldenseal is used primarily by Cherokee Native Americans in a mixture to stain their faces and dye clothing. As used by the Native Americans, goldenseal is a natural insect repellent. Cosmetically, goldenseal is an astringent, cleaning tonic used to reduce bacteria, fungi, and cold or canker sores. It has anti-dandruff properties and is excellent when used in shampoos, rinses, and tonics. Goldenseal contains vitamins A, C, E, F, and B complex, calcium, copper, potassium, phosphorus, manganese, iron, zinc, and sodium.

Grapeseed Oil

Grapeseed oil, also known as grape oil, is a by-product of pressing the seed for wine making. This light, thin, colorless, and odorless oil is full of essential fatty acids such as antioxidants, omega-6, and vitamin E. It absorbs into the scalp, is great for hot-oil treatments, and reduces flaking caused by seborrheic dermatitis. Grapeseed oil can be mixed with other oil or used as a base oil. It has good moisturizing effects on dry, brittle hair and gives hair a light luster while strengthening cuticle.[11]

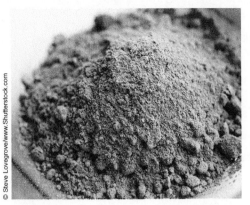

▲ Figure 8–8
Raw henna dye.

Hemp Seed Oil

Hemp seed oil, also known as Indian hemp seed oil, is filled with essential fatty acids omega-3 and omega-6, which play an important part in fortifying protein and strengthening the hair. It is a great source of amino acids, which also help to build protein. This heavy oil is a good sealant to reduce split ends and frizz.[12]

Henna

Henna is an herb generally made into a powder. In a clay form, it has been used in Egypt for more than 4,000 years to color the hair, palms of hands, feet, and nails (**Figure 8–8**). It is an excellent source for coloring oily hair. As a colorant, the powdered herb coats the hair with a thin, filmy stain that leaves hues or highlights and shine. Commercial henna colors vary in shades from neutral for brightening to deep blues and blacks that cover grey hair. Paprika can be mixed with henna as a hair rinse to color hair reddish bronze. The film residue henna leaves on thin hair gives hair the appearance of thickness and adds body. Henna has an astringent quality that can control an oily scalp. However, it can be very drying to dry hair types. Neutral henna is often used in shampoo and rinses to neutralize pH and bring hair back to a stable pH state. Please be aware that because henna coats the hair, clients who recently have had a henna treatment are not good candidates to have their hair dyed. The dye will be unable to penetrate the henna.

Hibiscus

Hibiscus is a beautiful flower, native to North America and the Caribbean, that can be used as a gentle colorant to give the hair a reddish tone when used in a rinse. Hibiscus must be used repeatedly in order to intensify color. Hibiscus can be mixed with other herbs to add a reddish hue. Also, hibiscus acts as an emollient for moisturizing and softening most hair types.

Honeysuckle

Honeysuckle is known for its aromatic, sedative fragrance. As a hot-oil treatment, it soothes and calms the scalp. It is often used in shampoos and soap because of its cleaning properties. Topically, it is an emollient, moisturizer, and softener. Natural honeysuckle oil is very rare and extremely expensive. So if you see it listed on a product label, that ingredient is typically not real honeysuckle. Instead, it is either a synthetic version of the scent (which would provide no benefits of true honeysuckle) or a combination of balsamic and other botanical, natural oils that approximate the smell of true honeysuckle.

Hops

The oil of hops is best known for its sedative quality. When used topically, it has a calming and soothing effect on the scalp. It is used as a mild antiseptic and astringent. It has a very strong aroma and helps reduce stress. It is excellent when used as a rinse or hot-oil treatment to reduce dermatitis. As a colorant, hops oil can give hair a brown hue. As an infusion with chamomile, it reduces swelling.

Horsetail

Horsetail is said to heal ulcers and stop bleeding wounds when used externally. Typically, horsetail oil or extract is mixed with coltsfoot to stimulate the scalp for hair growth and repair. It is rich in both silicon and cystine acid, found in the sulfur compound of hair protein, which are essential to creating a healthy infrastructure for hair. Shampoos and conditioners that offer proteins mixed with sulfur-containing amino acids (silica or cystine) are said to be excellent products to promote growth and stimulate follicles to prevent hair loss. Horsetail in shampoo curtails dandruff because it is a cleansing astringent that increases scalp circulation, reducing seborrheic conditions. As a hair rinse (horsetail, coltsfoot, rosemary, and sage combined), it promotes the general health of hair and scalp. Use horsetail after chemical damage or episodes of alopecia. Rich in silicon and selenium (which helps the scalp but can be drying to hair), it contains vitamin E, pantothenic acid, PABA, copper, manganese, sodium, cobalt, iron, and iodine.

Jaborandi

Jaborandi is considered an essential oil that stimulates hair growth. As an herbal rinse or tonic, it opens pores and extracts impurities. As a steam or bath, jaborandi removes excess water from skin tissue. It is a mild antiseptic and can induce perspiration.

Jasmine

Jasmine is most famous for its aromatic, sultry fragrance. In shampoos, creams, and lotions, it is primarily used as an aromatic because of its variety of fragrances. Topically, jasmine soothes and helps cleanse the scalp. Jasmine oil can be used in rinses, hot-oil treatments, or simply massaged into the scalp to sedate and calm. The olfactory reaction produces a feeling of euphoria and optimism and is used as an antidepressant, according to researchers. Jasmine as a tea, or in some German wines, is said to be an aphrodisiac. It is generally nonirritating and can be used on sensitive skin. It is claimed to rejuvenate aging skin by improving elasticity, and it reduces inflammation and itching. True jasmine is extremely expensive and used primarily in natural perfumes. It is well-known that it takes one million pounds of jasmine flowers to produce one pound of jasmine oil. So beware of hair products claiming to include jasmine as an ingredient.

Jojoba Oil

Jojoba oil is known as liquid wax. It is an extract from the cactus-like plant. It is used by Native Americans for cooking and for hair and body grooming. It has an extensive history of promoting hair growth because it is extremely rich in nutrients that restore, protect, and moisturize the hair. It is a vegetable-based oil that mixes well with other herbal extracts while resisting rancidity and extending shelf life. It is an expensive oil that is said to replace sebum. Hot-oil treatments and conditioners with this oil will address hair loss problems due to extreme dryness. This "liquid gold" also aids oily scalps by removing embedded sebum, making the scalp less acidic. It contains amino acid, silica, B complex, vitamin E, chromium, iodine, copper, and zinc.

Kelp

Kelp is an algae derived from the sea, rivers, and ponds. It is a popular food that is high in nutritional value. Kelp is filled with vitamins A, C, F, and B complex, calcium, and sulfur. The sulfur contains silicon (a strengthener). Kelp stimulates metabolism and nourishes hair. It contains 30 minerals, including cobalt, nickel, silver, and titanium. The plant extract contains phosphorous, iron, sodium, potassium, chlorine, copper, zinc, manganese, and small amounts of lecithin.

Lavender

Lavender is cultivated throughout the world and is native to the Mediterranean. More than 28 species have been cultivated. Because of its popular aromatic fragrance, lavender is often found in perfumes. As an essential oil, it is an antibiotic, antiseptic, detoxifier, and antidepressant (its fragrance uplifts the emotions). It is useful in healing burns and cuts because it rejuvenates skin cells. Lavender stimulates the scalp while acting as a calming agent. Lavender, like aloe, will quickly soothe a burn and aid in its complete recovery. Due to its beautiful aroma and great benefits, the cost of true lavender oil continues to rise.

Lemongrass

This botanical ingredient originated in Central America and Sri Lanka. Lemongrass is an essential oil used to normalize oil production for dry and oily scalp conditions. It is fragrant, light, and antiseptic. In a hot-oil treatment for both dry and oily scalp, lemongrass is very effective. It is an excellent source of vitamin A, which helps heal and soothe dry skin. It can be used for all skin types and can be found in most perfumes, deodorizers, and antifungal products.

Lemon Juice

The lemon is native to southern Europe and North America, and it is cultivated worldwide. Lemon juice is a strong astringent, antibiotic, and disinfectant. It is very aromatic, with a sharp, clean, light fragrance. In a rinse, it restores the acid mantle of the hair and scalp (natural pH) and stimulates the scalp. It can act as a bleaching agent or highlighter. It is helpful in the removal of stale smells and odors from the hair. It is full of vitamin C. When diluted and used as a rinse, it can soften debris in locked hair. Lemon can also be used during the locking process to lift cuticles and help coils to spiral. It can tingle or irritate the scalp if not diluted properly.

Myrrh

Myrrh is an ancient botanical—at least 2,000 years old. Ancient Egyptians often used myrrh in the embalming process and valued it spiritually for its perfume. Its medicinal uses include antiseptics, astringents, and disinfectants. Myrrh has antifungal properties and is known to kill ringworm. It can also be a preservative in other oil mixtures. Myrrh is commonly used in toothpaste, chewing gum, and mouthwashes. Because of its strong fragrance, it is relaxing and soothing to the nervous system. On the scalp, myrrh soothes, dries, and fortifies hair.

Neroli Oil

Neroli oil is derived from the bitter orange blossom and has a delicate scent. Its fragrance is said to be an antidepressant that counteracts shock and fatigue, nervousness, and insomnia. Neroli oil is also an antibacterial agent and antiseptic to the skin. On the scalp, its regenerative properties promote the new growth of skin cells. It also reduces inflammation and soothes irritated skin. Neroli is an expensive oil that is typically used in very small quantities for natural perfumes or high-end skin care products.

Nettle

Nettle is commonly used in hair and skin products because of its stimulating effect on circulation. Rich in silicon, which helps restore protein, nettle is used in herbal rinses, tonics, and treatments to promote hair growth. Often it is used with horsetail, coltsfoot, rosemary, and sage—other hair-growing botanicals. This botanical is rich in chlorophyll, which gives it a green color. Nettle also provides essential trace minerals needed for healthy hair and skin. It is an important food for the hair root and follicle. It is mildly astringent and a natural cleanser and tonic. As a rinse, it softens and soothes dry skin; it can also neutralize an overly acidic scalp mantle. Nettle contains vitamins A, C, E, F, and P, calcium, sulfur, sodium, copper, manganese, chromium, and zinc and is high in protein.

Olive Oil

The olive tree is one of the oldest trees on record. Often referred to as liquid gold, olive oil has become the go-to oil for every hair texture for its health benefits. Olive oil is an excellent emollient used in all types of cosmetics, shampoos, soaps, lotions, and creams. It is an excellent base oil to mix with other essential oils, rinses, and tonics. Olive oil gives moisture, elasticity, and shine to hair, and it is rich in vitamin E and fatty acids omega-3, -6, and -9, which nourish the follicle. Olive oil is oleic acid: an antioxidant that is the source for restoring, fortifying, and rejuvenating the hair and scalp. As a deep conditioner, it softens hair and reduces frizz. As a deep treatment, it provides the scalp with moisture to reduce flaking. It is very effective as a hot-oil treatment for dry hair and scalp when mixed with coconut oil. Combining lemon juice and olive oil results in a soothing rinse. Olive oil and chamomile can be used as an infusion to moisturize and soften dry hair. Extra virgin olive oil (EVOO) is considered the best because of its higher concentration of antioxidants and vitamins.[13]

Parsley

Used as a hair rinse, parsley is excellent for all hair types. It is especially soothing and healing in cases of eczema and psoriasis. It is highly nutritious for the hair. It is often found in shampoos, perfumes, soaps, and other natural cosmetics. It is an excellent hot-oil treatment for an overall healthy scalp. It contains high levels of iron, chlorophyll, vitamins A and C, sodium, copper, thiamine, riboflavin, and small amounts of silicon, sulfur, calcium, and cobalt.

Patchouli Oil

Patchouli oil is an essential oil that is anti-inflammatory, antibacterial, antifungal, and antiseptic. It cleans as it helps to remove flaking in eczema and dandruff. Patchouli oil is very aromatic, often used in perfumes, and can be found in mouthwashes.

Peppermint

Peppermint, as well as other mints such as bergamot, spearmint, pennyroyal, and pineapple mint, is excellent for the digestive system. Peppermint relieves cramps, nausea, hangovers, and motion sickness. It is also an excellent decongestant. Even when used topically, peppermint as a hot-oil treatment opens breathing passages. Menthols in herbal mints are stimulants to the scalp and have a cooling effect. It can improve dry, lifeless hair. With its antiseptic properties, it cleans and removes embedded oils and can be wonderfully refreshing when added to vinegar rinses or herbal rinses. It can leave the scalp feeling tingly and restores balance to an oily scalp. Avoid using peppermint on clients during pregnancy because of its antispasmodic properties. Peppermint contains vitamins A and C, magnesium, potassium, inositol, niacin, copper, iodine, silicon, iron, and sulfur.

Rose

The rose is native to the Middle East and is cultivated worldwide. It symbolizes love and passion, which is one reason that it is used so often in perfumes, oils, and soaps. The petal from the flower is a mild astringent; as a rinse, such as rosewater, it is great for a dry, flaky scalp. True rose oil is considered the queen of botanical oils. And as such, real/true rose oil is extremely expensive and not typically found in hair products unless it is a by-product of the extraction process, like the wax that is left over from the oil-extraction process or water from the distillation process (known as rose water). The wax is also known as concrete—that is, rose concrete. If true rose oil is being used in a hair product, it would be in minute amounts, which means it is very unlikely that you would detect the smell or gain the benefits of using true rose oil. None of the aforementioned substitutes have the potency and effects of a true essential oil. But because most people have not been exposed to true essential oils, they prefer the smell of synthetics. Our noses have become adulterated and are more familiar with and accustomed to synthetic fragrances.

Rose Hip

Rose hip refers to the fruit of the rose plant and is an excellent source of vitamin C, more so than oranges. It is very nourishing to the scalp and helps fight infections.

Rose Hip Seed Oil

Rose hip oil is derived from the rose seed. It is potent and concentrated with vitamin C. It is also high in fatty acids (similar to the properties of horsetail and coltsfoot) and aids in the production of collagen—a protein that is helpful to the skin because it rejuvenates skin cells. Rose hip seed oil has large amounts of silicon—an amino acid that is necessary for protein metabolism. It adds elasticity and strength to the hair strand. When mixed with other oils, it helps prevent hair loss and balding. Rose oil is generally very expensive. It is effective when treating different types of alopecia. It contains vitamins A, C, E, and D, as well as high levels of vitamin B complex, flavonoids, some iron, calcium, potassium, and sulfur.

Rosemary

Rosemary should be a staple herb in every natural hair care salon (**Figure 8–9**). Whether it is used as an herbal rinse or an oil, rosemary has a long history as a strong stimulant for hair growth. It feeds the hair root. It makes a great conditioner for all hair types. Rosemary oil has an aromatic fragrance that stimulates the olfactory senses. As a mild astringent mixed with lavender, basil, and nettle, it cleanses and aids in the healing process. It is known as the herb of remembrance—good for the memory and mental clarity.

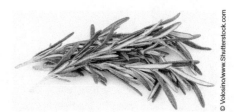

▲ Figure 8–9
A twig of rosemary.

Sea Salt

Sea salt can be used as a rinse and can be useful in the locking process. It changes the acid mantle of the hair. It affects the pH factor of the hair, opens the hair cuticles, and gives the strand a rough, dry touch. The open cuticle is layered and allows the hair to coil around itself easily. Sea salt as a rinse has a healing effect but may be irritating to a dry, sensitive scalp.

Shea Butter

African shea butter, as it is also known, comes from the nuts or seeds of the Kotschy tree (*Vitellaria paradoxa*). This light, nongreasy butter is an excellent pomade for dry, damaged hair. It is often found in shampoos and natural hair products as a moisturizer and softener. The plant oil or fat has the ability to protect the skin and hair from ultraviolet rays that cause sunburn and dry the hair. Shea butter is a great humectant and emollient for the hair and scalp. It provides moisture and a protective barrier of oil that seals weathered ends. Shea butter contains vitamins A, E, F, and cinnamic acid—a natural sunscreen. This thick butter allows the scalp and hair to breathe without clogging the pores or follicles. Shea butter is effective because it is low in acidity and high in fat and waxy substances that protect and coat. In its natural state, shea butter is used by vegetarians as a cooking substitute for dairy butter. In West Africa and Ghana, shea butter is used as a cream and moisturizer for the skin and hair, but it is also used to fry foods.[14]

Tea Tree Oil

Tea tree oil has been used by the Aborigines for hundreds of years as a gentle but highly effective antifungal disinfectant. The volatile oils in tea tree oil create a powerful soothing and cleansing agent. When used in shampoos, rinses, and conditioners, tea tree oil stimulates and irrigates the scalp. The oil is similar to peppermint and eucalyptus and should be warm when applied but cool after it is rinsed. It is a great additive for shampoos to fight dandruff and flaking.

Thyme

Thyme is a powerful herbal antiseptic with healing properties. It can be an antifungal as well as a rinse to remove crabs and head lice. It is excellent as a general tonic for all hair types. As a stimulant, thyme can accelerate skin cell growth because it contains sulfur and silicon. It is often used in a mixture of herbs with similar or compound properties such as sage, lavender, comfrey, rosemary, and peppermint.

Witch Hazel

Witch hazel extract is distilled from the bark of common trees. It is commonly found in hair and skin products as a mild astringent. It is popular in aftershave products because it helps stop external bleeding. It is used as a massage liquid and body lotion. In hair rinses, witch hazel is a cleansing astringent that leaves vital oils and amino acids, which condition and stimulate the hair and scalp. Witch hazel contains 15 percent alcohol and should not be used regularly on a dry scalp.

Add an emollient to witch hazel rinses to moisturize and counteract the alcohol's drying action. Witch hazel helps fight dandruff and soothe inflamed skin. It closes pores, tones skin, and refreshes. It is often used to cleanse the scalp between touch-ups while wearing braided styles. To freshen the scalp, witch hazel can be applied with cotton balls or swabs between parts. Rub lightly and avoid saturating the hair.

Ylang-Ylang

Ylang-ylang essential oil is often found in cosmetics to groom the hair. It is a mild stimulant, which helps blood circulation in the scalp. It has a mild menthol component that cools and helps regulate the sebaceous gland. Very aromatic, it relaxes and soothes nervous energy and acts as an emollient on dry hair. Because of its cleansing and detoxifying properties, it makes a great additive in shampoos and rinses. Ylang-ylang is good for all hair and skin types, especially overactive sebaceous glands or seborrhea.

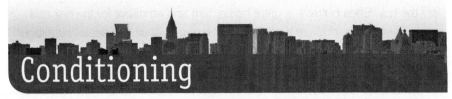

Conditioning

After a mild shampoo, the hair still needs a conditioning agent to give it manageability, strength, and luster and to further cleanse the hair or scalp. Rinses are usually a mixture of distilled water with a mild acid, herbal, or oil base designed to benefit the hair in a particular way.

Types of Hair Rinses

Rinses can be customized to address any hair problem. Generally, rinses provide hair with a protective coating or nutrients.

Acid Rinses

Acid rinses neutralize or restore the pH balance (acid mantle) to the hair. They remove soap residue and braid and lock debris. They remove buildup from heavy cream shampoos. Hair coated with debris and soap scum can break hair and make hair look dull. Acid rinses are great for textured and locked hair. Acid rinses seal in nutrients by closing the cuticle layers of the hair shaft.

Acid rinses can be made of citric acids, such as lemon juice, lime juice, orange juice, grapefruit juice, and cactus juice. Acidic aids are apple cider vinegar or distilled white vinegar. A tartaric acid can be wine, champagne, or beer (but these ingredients can leave an odor that must be rinsed out). Lactic acid is derived from a lactose or sugar of milk.

Cream Rinses

Cream rinses are temporary conditioning commercial products. Cream rinses are applied after the shampoo to soften, detangle, and add luster to the hair. Most are very fragrant, having a creamy or pearlized appearance. The creamy appearance is esthetic but can cause problems if used improperly. Cream rinses are great to use when detangling textured hair after a shampoo. Wet, coily hair is very fragile. Cream rinses coat the hair and allow the large-toothed comb to glide through the hair. A cream rinse actually makes the hair temporarily manageable. To avoid a heavy buildup of these topical cream rinses, dilute them. They will still be effective.

Heavy cream rinses should be avoided when conditioning hair with braid extensions or locks. The heavy coating never rinses out thoroughly; a thin film will remain and become embedded in the braid or lock. It leaves the hair dull and unsightly with clumps of cream residue. Avoid cream rinses for clients with human hair extensions. Cream rinses will soften the entire braid and cause it to slip away from the base. However, some stylists use the cream rinse to give the braid extension a fuller hair effect. If you must use a cream rinse, apply it to the ends of the braid extension only. Though cream rinses appear to solve many hair problems, use them selectively and in moderation on all hair types. They can be harmful to the hair over time, because of residue and coating buildup.

Leave-in Conditioners

Leave-in conditioners can be use as an alternative to and/or supplement for your standard conditioner. Many leave-in conditioners are water-based, liquid conditioners that are typically sprayed directly on the hair whether it is braided, twisted, locked, or loose. The purpose of the leave-in conditioner is to moisten and protect, and it can also assist with detangling. Cream-based leave-in conditioners are usually richer and more moisturizing than water-based leave-in conditioners. These cream-based leave-in conditioners work well for people with extremely dry hair and are typically preferred by those with loose curl patterns to control frizzy hair and seal split ends. Cream-based leave-in conditioners are not recommended for use on locks, but can be used on loose human hair in weaves.

Herbal Rinses

The best hair conditioners on the market do enhance the esthetic beauty of hair and make it easier to manage. They are also nutritional for the hair and scalp. They can help eliminate hair problems or correct the source of the problem.

Natural hair care specialists approach hair conditioning from two perspectives: internal replenishing and external treatment. Internal replenishing means to restore and replace nutrients the body needs to survive and maintain health. As a part of the service, the natural stylist wants to replenish nutrients and help the client maintain healthy hair and scalp. It is not enough to camouflage the problem. To keep the hair in its healthy and natural state, a variety of conditioning agents are required. Detergents and synthetic shampoos often strip the natural oils and properties that protect hair. Herbal rinses restore natural hair properties.

External uses of herbal rinses can aid in coloring, enhancing, and conditioning hair while replenishing essential oils, vitamins, and minerals. They can stimulate the vitality of hair to help it grow. Some herbal rinses are used as treatments for severe hair problems; others are more fragrant and cosmetic. But all give back something beneficial to the hair.

To prepare an infusion, use a nonmetal electric pot to boil water. Thoroughly mix herbs in a separate bowl. Pour boiled water over the herbs and cover. Do not allow the herbs to boil, because boiling them destroys their properties. Steeping herbs extracts the active ingredients. Steep for 20 to 30 minutes—the longer, the better. (The client can be serviced with a hot-oil treatment or deep conditioner while awaiting the infusion.)

Strain the herbs from the pot or bowl. Add 1½ cups of cool water to make the solution comfortable. Add oils, shake, and pour cooled mixture over clean wet hair. Gently rub into scalp and down the hair shaft. Use an infusion as a final rinse on dry hair and locks.

This type of infusion can be sprayed through the hair daily to correct or resolve hair and scalp problems. It is great for thinning, breaking, or overprocessed hair and is excellent for use on braided and locked hair. As a spray, the solution is easier to use. Hair will absorb only what it needs. You can massage the solution and rub it down the hair shaft. Spray locks directly.

Botanical Colors and Herbal Rinses

For natural hair care treatments, most state regulations forbid chemical altering of colorants. Check and follow your state regulations regarding color or dyes.

Conditioners that enhance hair color are available for the natural stylist to use. They are not reactive or structurally altering chemicals but are clays, powders, and/or liquid mixtures that highlight, condition, and bring out the natural hue of the hair.

For thousands of years, henna has been used in many parts of the world. Egypt, parts of West Africa, Arabia, Persia, and India, to name a few, have used henna to add highlights to the hair and as a cosmetic stain to the palms of the hands, nails, and soles of the feet. The wonderful thing about henna is that it is nontoxic to the scalp and skin. Pure henna compounds are generally soothing and do not irritate the scalp. Hennas are offered in a variety of semipermanent hair stains.

Henna stains can be mixed with an herbal rinse to condition and highlight. For a more effective shade of color, henna can be mixed with boiling water, made into a paste, and applied directly to the hair. Adding heat or moisture aids the processing time. Staining the hair with henna may take several applications because the colors are subtle and, in some cases, unpredictable in intensity. The average time frame for a staining service is 1 to 1½ hours.

Henna works best on oily hair or on dry hair that gets oily by the end of the day. It also aids in the removal of dead skin cells or dandruff flaking. When using henna on dry hair, always re-moisturize as a final step.

Hues range from neutral, which has no hue, to hues such as marigold, copper, dark brown, blue, and black. The botanical powders also give thickness and body to hair.

There are other botanicals that can be used to enhance color. Herbs such as hibiscus, for example, add red tones to hair; chamomile adds a gold hue to light colored hair; burdock and black walnut darken hair. Staining or highlighting hair takes longer to see true results, but the process is safer and nonabrasive to the scalp.

Instant Conditioners

Instant conditioners are quick, temporary treatments. They generally coat the hair in order to make it more manageable and give sheen and fullness to the hair. Instant conditioners are useful to protect the hair from the sun and blowdrying. Some contain vitamins and botanicals. These ingredients can be good for the hair but are often combined with waxes and detergents that can damage hair. Therefore, most instant conditioners have only cosmetic value. They coat and soften hair but provide very little deep conditioner to repair damaged hair.

Protein Conditioners

Protein conditioners usually contain polymers, which are small molecular combinations of any of 23 amino acids. These amino acids are what make up the keratin protein in hair and skin. They are used to recondition and strengthen hair strands. Protein conditioners are more concentrated and are meant to stay on the hair for at least 20 minutes, during which time the treatment may include a heat or steam application. Heat helps break down the protein molecule and allows it to pass through the cuticle of the hair and directly into the cortex. Deep protein conditioners can help close split ends. They increase the elasticity of the hair and reduce breakage. They also improve porosity as well as soften and lubricate the hair strand.

Moisturizers

Moisturizing conditioners are formulated to penetrate the hair. They have many of the same properties as instant conditioners. However, with the application of heat or steam, these conditioners are more effective and longer lasting. Deep conditioning with these products requires a 15- to 20-minute application.

Many moisturizers contain quaternary ammonium compounds (quats). Some moisturizers have an antibacterial action (often found in dandruff shampoos). Quats are also used as an environmental disinfectant. Quats are included in the moisturizing solution of conditioners because they counteract the drying effects of anionic (harsh) detergents. Quats, such as stearalkonium chloride, enable the cream moisturizer to adhere to the hair strand and protect the hair longer than instant conditioners can.

Moisturizers contain humectants that attract and seal water in the hair shaft. Oils protect, add shine, and seal in water, allowing for easy combing and styling. Moisturizers can generally be used without any problems; however, some active ingredients can cause acne on the forehead and stimulate scalp disorders, such as seborrheic dermatitis, which is common among African Americans.

According to some dermatologists, some ingredients may aggravate seborrheic dermatitis, or induce inflammation or folliculitis. These include lanolin, castor oil, wheat germ oil, and soybean oil.

The most effective conditioning moisturizers offer natural vegetable glycerine, instead of propylene glycola synthetic that can be irritating to skin and mucous membranes when found in spray form. According to Aubrey Hampton, author of *Natural Organic Hair and Skin Care,* the vegetable glycerine is "extremely superior."[15] It was found that pure vegetable glycerine is a thicker, richer, and far better emollient than the chemical replacement. Still, manufacturers prefer the synthetic product over the natural extract because they believe it is difficult to tell the difference.

Petrolatum (such as Vaseline™) and mineral oils are also emollient conditioners, but they can cause irritation to the skin and actually dry the skin. They absorb poorly and inhibit the occurrence of natural moisturizing.

Natural Moisturizers

Sebum is the most natural lubricant (emollient) produced by the body. It protects and softens the hair and scalp. Essential fatty acids are nature's replacement for sebum. *Essential fatty acids* is the chemical term for organic oils found in vegetable or amino fats. They are absorbed into the skin to soften and lubricate. The body cannot manufacture these organic oils or fats. They must be supplied through diet and external application. Be aware that hair loss, dullness, and drying due to water loss result when the body is deficient in essential fatty acids.

Fatty acids act as natural agents, sealants, or barrier substances that leave a thin coat on the surface of the hair and skin and protect the hair and skin from drying conditions. They help the body conserve water (moisture) on the skin.

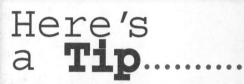

Here's a Tip.........

An effective lock moisturizer is a light rose water and glycerine spray.

Some moisturizers (or humectants) commonly listed on product labels are

- propylene glycol (synthetic)
- glycerol (natural or synthetic)
- glycerine (natural or synthetic)
- sorbitol (natural)

The unsaturated compounds of organic oils found in products include

- linoleic acid
- linolenic acid
- arachidonic acid
- oleic acid

Saturated compounds include

- palmitic acid
- stearic acid

These organic oils have excellent moisture retention properties. They are effective nurturing emollients that have high penetration on the hair and scalp. However, these organic herbal oils and extracts should be added to base oils to enhance their therapeutic value.

Many of the essential oils in their pure form are very concentrated. It is highly recommended that all essential oils be diluted in base oil before being used on the skin or scalp. The base oil not only protects the skin from the potency of the oil, which can burn or cause severe reactions, it also serves as a carrier of the essential oils (aka botanicals), assisting in their even distribution and smooth absorption into the skin and scalp.

Base Oils
The following is a list of carrier or base oils used to mix with other essential oils. Base oils, also known as carrier oils, are used to dilute essential oils that provide nutrients to the hair and scalp.

- Sweet almond—Soothing to the skin; contains minerals and vitamins and is rich in protein. It relieves dryness, reduces itching, and reduces inflammation.
- Apricot—Contains minerals and vitamins. Apricot is good for all hair and skin types and is an excellent emollient to soften dry hair.

- Avocado—Enriched with vitamins, protein, and lecithin (which is an antioxidant), avocado is an excellent emollient and natural emulsifier. Avocado is great on all skin types. It is an effective remedy for eczema, and it absorbs well into the skin.

- Borage seed—High in amino acid (linolenic), vitamins, and minerals, it has excellent rejuvenating and stimulating properties.

- Coconut oil—An emollient for all hair types; coconut softens hair.

- Jojoba—A waxy substance, similar to natural sebum, that replaces collagen. Jojoba has high penetration to hair and scalp and controls flaking.

- Extra virgin olive oil (EVOO)—Absorbs well, is soothing to the scalp, and contains vitamins and minerals.

- Peanut oil—Contains protein as well as amino acids. Peanut oil is good for all hair types.

- Safflower oil—High in lecithin and is a good base for nonmixing substances. It contains amino acids, protein, minerals, and vitamins.

- Sesame oil—Contains lecithin, amino acids, protein, minerals, and vitamins. Sesame oil fights psoriasis and eczema.

- Soybean oil—Contains proteins, minerals, and vitamins. Soybean oil can be used on all hair types.

- Sunflower oil—Contains vitamins and minerals. Sunflower oil can be used on all hair types.

- Shea butter—An excellent emollient that prevents dryness, regenerates skin cells, helps healing, and absorbs into hair and scalp. Shea butter strengthens hair by re-moisturizing.

- Castor oil—Has excellent absorption properties; is soothing and lubricating to the skin. Castor oil contains hydroxy acid. ✓ **LO5**

Myth: If I Don't Like My Locks, I Can Just Comb Them Out

Yes, some hair types when locked can be combed or picked out. The wavier or softer the curl pattern, the easier it is to comb or pick locs out. This process is not traditionally recommended, because almost half the amount of hair is lost with the comb-out and a good amount of the locked hair is the hair that was not shed naturally.

PROCEDURE 8-1 How to Remove Braids Professionally

This is a simple method for removing braids professionally. Use a detangling solution to make the procedure less difficult.

Synthetic and human hair removal may be handled using the following 12-step technique:

1 Section hair. The smaller the braid, the more sections are needed.

2 Each section can be handled or divided into subsections, gathering three to four braids at a time.

3 Open up braids by cutting off the finished or extended ends. In most cases, look for where the client's natural hair ends and the extension continues. Then cut about 2 to 3 inches (5 to 7 cm) below the natural length. Avoid cutting the client's real hair.

4 With a small to medium tail or cutting comb, in a picking motion, comb upward on braid shafts. The motion should be rapid and in a circular pattern. Stay close to the unbraided portion of the braids. Your finger should be positioned on top of the sectioned braids to control the unraveling and support braids to avoid pulling the hair while the comb is working through the braided stitch.

5 Comb down the braids after several picking motions to unravel the loose ends.

6 As the comb gets closer to the base of the scalp, drop the subsections and work on one braid at a time. Comb up the braid shaft until the teeth reach the scalp base, then use the tail end of the comb to open the braided hair at the base.

7 Braid debris must be loosened and removed at this point or once the subsection is unbraided. Do not try to comb all braid debris after the entire head of braids is removed. For best results, remove lint and oil residue section by section.

8 If braid debris is extremely heavy or crusted, spray on a combination of water, cream rinse, and oil to soften hair and detangle.

9 Once one subsection is completed, go to the next subsection and work your way through each braid separately.

10 Use a large-toothed comb to detangle the entire section.

11 Twist ends to separate one section from the next.

12 Proceed to the next section. Once the entire head is completed, check hair for any residual debris, lint, oil deposits, and tangles. Prepare to shampoo.

8-2 Shampooing Techniques for Curly, Coiled, and Braided Hair

A proper shampooing technique is essential for both the client's comfort and to maintain healthy hair.

To properly wash and help put the client at ease, use the following shampoo techniques:

1 Properly drape the client.

2 Remove clips, pins, bands, and so on.

3 Remove braid debris and excess extended material, if necessary, by combing and detangling with a large-toothed comb.

4 Examine scalp and hair for breakage, bald spots, sores, flaking, and general condition.

5 If any braid extensions are hanging from thin strands of hair, cut tips of the extension and remove. Avoid pulling to prevent hair from snapping off.

6 If there is no need to remove braids, seat the client at the shampoo bowl.

7 Drape a towel around the client's neck to absorb excess water from extensions if needed.

8 Check water pressure and temperature. Water should be comfortably warm and pressure moderate to strong. Ask the client if the water temperature is comfortable. (It is appropriate to ask clients to close their eyes to avoid splashing in them.)

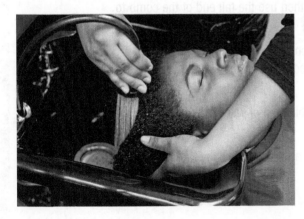

9 Saturate hair, braids, or hair extensions. The thicker the braid, the more water is needed to penetrate.

10 Protect the client's face with a free hand when wetting the hairline with the spray nozzle. Use your thumb and pointer finger to create a shield for the face.

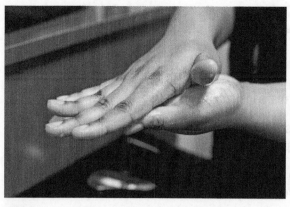

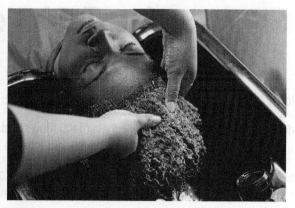

11 Once the hair is wet, pour a small amount of shampoo into the palm of your hand. Create an emulsion by rubbing hands and distributing shampoo to the fingertips before applying it.

12 Begin at the hairline and apply shampoo to the scalp as well. Apply a moderate amount to the crown of the head, moving and massaging the shampoo toward the back or nape of the head. If necessary, add more shampoo.

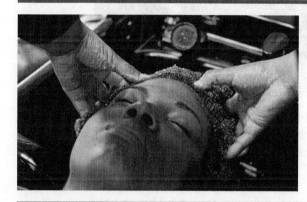

13 When the shampoo is evenly distributed, work it into a lather with the pads of your fingers.

14 As the lather increases, use circular massaging motions and smooth the shampoo downward into the sink. Do not apply much pressure to the braids.

15 Pressure applied to the scalp massage should be firm but not painful or intense. Avoid putting pressure on sensitive or abused areas of the scalp. Do not rub areas where there are open sores or cuts.

Shampoo Massage

A shampoo massage helps to relax the client while stimulating the scalp and promoting healthy hair.

The following steps are an effective method of administering a shampoo massage:

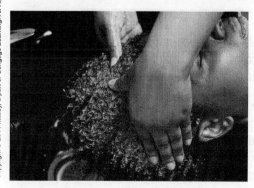

1 With pads of the fingertips, firmly start at the hairline right above the temple and work the scalp in small circular motions toward the crown of the head. Move around the scalp clockwise, using the thumbs around the hairline.

Shampooing Techniques for Curly, Coiled, and Braided Hair continued

2 Move toward the center of the head, palming the head as you massage around the crown.

3 Move down toward the ears in a rotary movement. Movements should be small and slow, moving about ½ inch (1.3 cm) at a time. If the hair is braided, work into the parts of the braid.

4 In some cases, a back-and-forth movement must be applied to the scalp in order to effectively cleanse the scalp. For braided styles, shampoo the parts between braids to avoid loosening the braid style.

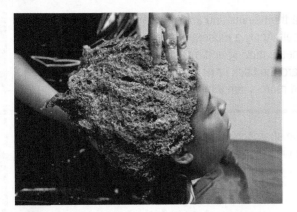 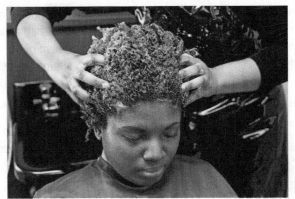

5 Moving toward the nape of the neck, lift the client's head gently from the sink with one hand. With the other hand, strategically place fingers under and around braids and then massage the nape area back and forth.

6 Repeat this circular shampoo pattern at least two times. This motion will effectively clean and stimulate blood circulation to the scalp.

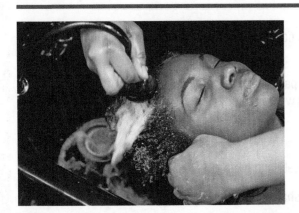

7 Rinse thoroughly. First rinse the scalp where most of the lather is located. Bring the spray nozzle close to the scalp to give it added pressure and to remove lather from braids. For braided styles, hold the nozzle directly on the braid. Sink water should be cleared of lather to complete the rinse.

8 Once water is totally clear, repeat application of shampoo. Shampoo at least two times. The first shampoo just loosens the dirt and oil; the second shampoo actually cleanses. If a third or fourth shampoo is required, then the scalp may have a disorder or a problem of excess sebum dandruff. The client may need a special shampoo to address the problem.

9 With braid extensions, hold water, so gently wring hair downward with both hands to remove excess water before towel drying. Use the towel ends to remove all moisture around hairline, forehead, and ears. Drape the front of the head with towel, pat gently, and wipe. Hold the hair or braid with the towel a few seconds to squeeze out any excess water. The scalp is now prepared for treatment rinse and conditioning.

Review Questions

1. Is there a difference between shampooing straight hair and shampooing tightly coiled or textured hair?
2. Are all shampoos created equal?
3. What is the difference between different types of shampoos and their effects on the hair?
4. What is the purpose of always using a conditioner after you shampoo the hair?
5. Is using henna to color the hair the same as coloring the hair?
6. What effects do base oils have on the hair?
7. Why is performing a scalp massage so important in a natural hair care shampoo service?
8. Why is it important to understand the proper use and application of essential oils and conditioning preparations?

Chapter References

1. USDA. U.S. Department of Agriculture. Retrieved from www.usda.gov/wps/portal/usda /usdahome?navid=ORGANIC_CERTIFICATION
2. Wilborn, W. S. (1994). Disorders of hair growth in African Americans. In E. A. Olsen (Ed.), *Disorders of hair growth: Diagnosis and treatment* (p. 395). New York: McGraw-Hill.
3. Hampton, Aubrey. *Natural Organic Hair and Skin Care*. Tampa, Florida: Organica Press, 1984.
4. Adio, A. (2012, April 1). Personal interview.
5. United States Food and Drug Administration. (2013). Retrieved from www.fda.gov/Cosmetics /ProductandIngredientSafety/default.htm
6. The American Remedies.com. (2012) Retrieved from www.theamericanremedies.com/oils/details/black -seed-hair-oil/
7. Hupston F. (2011,October 7) NaturalNews.com, Castor oil helps hair breakage, helps to grow and darken hair. Retrieved from www.naturalnews.com/033797_castor_oil_hair.html
8. Environmental Working Group's Skin Deep Cosmetic Database. Coconut Oil. (2013) Retrieved from www.ewg.org/skindeep/ingredient/701566/COCOS_NUCIFERA_%28COCONUT%29_OIL/#jumptohere
9. MPB Research. (2013) MPB Research 1999–2013 Emu Oil Hairloss and Frontal Regrowth. Retrieved from www.ewg.org/skindeep/ingredient/702248/EMU_OIL/
10. Laschinsky, T. (2011, June, 14) Livestrong.com, Glycerin for Dry Hair. Retrieved from www.livestrong.com /article/278889-glycerin-for-dry-hair-
11. Thompson, C. (2011, November, 21) Livestrong.com, Benefits of grapeseed oil for hair. Retrieved from www.livestrong.com/article/177894-benefits-of-grapeseed-oil-for-hair/
12. Pietroluongo, L. (2013) eHow.com, Hemp Oil & Hair. Retrieved from www.ehow.com/about_6319974 _hemp-oil-hair.html
13. Allen, D. (2011, Jan 27) Livestrong.com, Does Olive Oil Stimulate Hair Growth? Retrieved from http://www.livestrong.com/article/367409-does-olive-oil-stimulate-hair-growth/
14. Environmental Working Group's Skin Deep Cosmetic Database. Shea Butter. (2012) Retrieved from www.ewg.org/skindeep/sheabutter
15. Hampton, Aubrey. *Natural organic hair and skin care*. Tampa, Florida: Organica Press, 1984.

Textured Hair Is Manageable

Chapter Outline

Learning Objectives

After completing this chapter, you should be able to:

☑ **LO1** Explain the importance of regular hair cutting and trimming.

☑ **LO2** Describe how to brush and comb out textured hair safely, and how to section hair to prepare for various braiding designs and natural texturizing techniques.

☑ **LO3** Describe shampoo and massaging techniques.

☑ **LO4** Identify hair crafters' tools and know how to handle them to create braiding and other natural styling techniques.

☑ **LO5** Explain how to straighten natural hair without the use of chemicals.

☑ **LO6** Describe how to apply and use various hair oils and conditioning preparations.

Key Terms

Page number indicates where in the chapter the term is used.

Afro
p. 205

Bantu knots (Nubian knots)
p. 209

braid-out
p. 206

diffuser
p. 211

dusting
p. 206

finger combing
p. 209

flat twist-out
p. 206

flexi-rod set
p. 208

grooming
p. 204

knots
p. 207

locks
p. 210

straw set
p. 208

texture on texture
p. 206

twist-outs
p. 211

two-strand twist
p. 206

Natural hair is virgin hair, not altered by chemical or thermal services. Natural hair care, in turn, is the process by which the hair service enhances that natural state.

Natural hair care takes a holistic approach to hair care. This approach recognizes the integrated balance between the body, mind, and spirit. The services provided are generally gentle, wholesome, corrective, and nurturing to the hair—all of which have a positive effect on the mind and body. Environmentally safe products or nontoxic products are often a part of the service. Products that include the essences of plants, fruits, vegetables, herbs, or essential oils are ingredients in these products and are therefore a positive by-product of these therapeutic services.

Most important, natural hair care protects and preserves the original state of textured hair and makes it manageable through shampooing, grooming, braiding, extending, twisting, weaving, cutting, and setting the hair.

Why Study Textured Hair?

A natural hair stylist should study and have a thorough understanding of textured hair because:

- You need to know grooming techniques in order to guide your clients for proper home care.

- You need to understand the different care that goes into each texture type in order to easily and successfully service each client.

- Having a thorough knowledge of the tools will improve your ability to perform flawless natural hair and braiding styles.

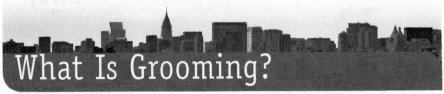

What Is Grooming?

grooming the process by which the natural stylist nurtures the client's hair by cleansing, conditioning, and styling in order to enhance or improve the client's personal appearance.

The proper **grooming** of textured hair is a nurturing experience. Regular hair care and grooming will encourage new growth, nourish weakened or damaged hair, and enhance the overall aesthetics of your client's hair.

Often, a client comes to the natural hair care specialist looking for nurturing of the hair and seeking creativity and professionalism in hairstyling options. Many are interested in natural styling as a chemical-free approach to hair care. The natural hair specialist, through various natural hair and braiding techniques, is in a unique position not only to correct hair problems, but also to promote the cultural aesthetics of natural hairstyling without altering its texture through chemicals.

When the natural hair care movement was started, many clients were serviced in the homes of natural hair care providers but did not receive some preliminary grooming services such as shampooing, conditioning, deep conditioning treatments, and haircutting services. In a professional setting, however, these preliminary services are part of the requirement and expectation of the client. Always start by providing the basics of grooming services to your client's hair. Then you can express your creativity—styling your client's hair.

A New Natural: A Paradigm Shift in Beauty

As the concepts and practices of natural hair care evolved, so did the client's needs and desires. The new millennium ushered in a whole new generation of *neo-naturals,* or those clients who are new to and just discovering natural hair. Many of these clients have been receiving chemical services since they were children. Now they are seeking something new. At this stage in their lives, they want to know what their true texture is—without the use of chemicals. Many of these new clients of natural hair techniques do not wish to have their hair bound up in braids, twists, or weaves. Often, even if they do desire braided or twisted services, they prefer to have no extensions added to their hair. Newcomers to natural hair want every freedom of exploring and working with their newly discovered texture. Many novices want to wear their hair loosely styled, in an updated, snazzy version of the **Afro**. Neo-naturals are also looking to accentuate and enhance their natural curly texture with the use of products and proper grooming. Many are looking for ways to define and/or elongate the curl pattern of their hair without the use of chemical relaxers. For the neo-naturals, it's all about the "curl": how to create healthy curly/coily hair and how to encourage length retention.

There are three different goal aspirations for the neo-naturals:

1. To achieve healthy, soft, manageable hair

2. To accomplish and retain longer hair

3. To repair, correct, or camouflage pervious damage or breakage

In the twenty-first century, the "new natural" is a more carefree and organic look. Everyone's hair looks different, unique to their own hair texture, hair shape, and length. Newbies do not seek uniformity, nor do they want the perfect shape. Instead, they seek freedom and self-expression.

Products for the Neo-Natural

The concept of the neo-natural has spawned a plethora of natural hair care products in the marketplace. Today's natural client is highly focused on either defining or creating better-defined curl to their hair texture. The many products on the market today profess to be able to assist these clients in achieving the curl definition they seek. These products can be

---

A New Approach to Hair Care Is "Natural" Hair Care

- All textures are good, and all textures have their own intrinsic beauty.
- Enhance and define client's texture, instead of altering it with heat or caustic chemicals.
- If you want to offer heat services, be sure you know the correct way to do so.

Afro a style made popular in the 1960s and 1970s of wearing your hair natural but having it perfectly shaped in a mostly round fashion.

Did you know?

The Afro style gained popularity in the 1960s and 1970s. It allowed you to wear your hair natural, but the natural hair was shaped in a mostly round fashion. The Afro of the 1960s and 1970s was expected to have a perfect look, achieved with a precision cut; this style gave the "natural" a very symmetrical look. The bigger your Afro was, the better. Those who could not grow the big Afro started wearing big Afro wigs that soon became popular.

texture on texture a general term used to describe the set of styling techniques on naturally textured hair that alter, elongate, or enhance the original curl patterns. Hair is set or manipulated. Then it is dried and the curl opened to create a uniformed textured finish. These set styling techniques include twist-out, braid-out, flat twist-out and knot-out.

braid-out the technique of using a single braid as a set to enhance, elongate, or define a client's texture. Hair is braided wet or dry and then opened to enhance original texture.

flat twist-out styling technique using a flat twist as a set to enhance and define a client's texture such as the two strand flat twist. Hair is flat twisted wet or dry and then opened to enhance and define a client's texture.

dusting an at-home technique that would-be clients practice by putting their hair in several two-strand twists and then cutting the tips of those two-strand twists.

two-strand twist created by overlapping equal sections over one another.

found not only in salons and beauty supply stores but also in national retailers, on-line, and at beauty trade shows. The effects of a product on hair last only a couple of days before wearing off and needing to be replenished. For clients who are seeking longer-term results of achieving better definition to their curly texture, another option is texture on texture setting, or outing the hair. **Texture on texture** setting, or outing the hair, has more of a lasting effect that can range from a few days to a few weeks, depending on the hair texture.

You will want to learn how to create these texture on texture hairstyles by twisting, twirling, palm rolling, braiding, knotting or flat twisting and then opening or "outing" the set (for example, **braid-out** or **flat twist-out**).

Another unique characteristic of this new generation of clients is that many do not remember what their natural texture looks and feels like, or how to care for it. Most of those in the new generation have not seen their natural texture since before they began chemically straightening their hair as small children. Consequently, they have no idea how to manage or ensure the growth and health of their natural texture as they move toward transitioning from chemically relaxed hair to their original texture. In other words, these clients are coming to you, seeking professional advice on how to move into this new territory of discovering, grooming, and styling their natural hair.

Therefore, as a professional, you must be able to execute the styles that you offer your clients in a professional and proficient manner. Your hairstyling will allow the client to realize the expertise and knowledge you offer them, and to see that it is superior to what they can do for themselves at home.

The Importance of Cutting and Trimming Natural Hair

Once the shampoo is complete, the next step for growing healthy hair is a haircut. One of the most basic ways to ensure the health of the hair is by regularly removing dead and split ends. A client who is transitioning from chemically altered to natural hair can assume that once the hair is natural, it is no longer necessary to cut the ends. As a natural stylist, you must educate your client that avoiding cutting their hair or practicing **dusting** does not foster longer lengths but encourages damage. Dusting is an at-home technique that would-be clients practice by putting their hair in several **two-strand twists** and then cutting the tips of those two-strand twists. When your clients visit, it is essential to educate them on the drawbacks of the practice of dusting or avoiding regular trims. They should be having their hair properly cut by you, the professional.

Recommending a trim (at least once a season—four times a year), at a minimum, would be a great way to get clients on a hair regime. The haircutting service will prevent split ends, allowing the hair to grow healthy and thus longer. Haircutting is also a great way to prevent tangling of the ends. Regular trims will prevent what is known as

knots from forming on the ends of the client's hair. When the dead ends of the hair are allowed to thrive and curl up, they form knotted balls at the ends of the hair. This type of damage is found more often in tightly coiled or kinky hair types. Trying to comb through these knotted balls invariably breaks and tears off the ends of the hair, resulting in split and uneven ends. Offering your clients regular hair-trimming services will ensure a healthier head of hair as you begin your natural hair care services with them. ☑ **LO1**

knots the condition that takes place when damaged split hair ends are allowed to thrive and over time, curl up, forming knotted balls. Combing through knotted balls invariably breaks and tears off the ends of the hair, resulting in damage.

Texture on Texture: Natural Texturizing Techniques

There are many hair-setting options for defining the curl pattern of your client's hair. Each client's hair and hair texture are as unique as their fingerprints. However, you will find similarities in textures that can help you identify which setting technique would be best for a particular texture. The following paragraphs describe some of the techniques used for setting different types of textures.

Tightly Coiled Textured Hair/Two-Strand Twist

Tightly coiled textured hair tends to be quite dry and can tangle easily if it is not taken care of properly and not routinely moisturized. One of the easiest methods of defining the curl pattern of tightly curled or coiled hair is to set it using the two-strand twist method.

After shampooing the hair and giving it a deep conditioning treatment and while the hair is still wet, add natural hair oil to the hair and scalp. Then part the hair in small, symmetrical sections. Using a moisturizing curling cream or light setting solution, two-strand twist each small section of the hair. Once the entire head has been set, place the client under the dryer until the hair is completely dry. When the hair is dry, untwist the two sections of each two-strand twist. Then separate the two sections, one at a time, at least once more. Untwist each section over the entire head until each section has been opened and twice separated. Depending on the hair texture, you could open and separate each section a third time. If the hair is really coily, two much separating will result in a fuzzy look, which is not the desired outcome. Instead, if this method is done properly, the results are a full head of a uniform curl pattern that has been elongated.

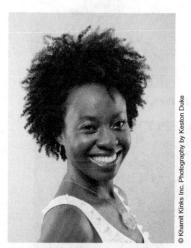

▲ **Tight curled texture.**

Coily/Curly Hair: Two-Strand Flat Twist Method

Coily or curly hair with a longer curl pattern can show definition more readily. You can use the two-strand twist method and open each section more times than you can with a tightly coiled pattern. Another option for hair with a looser curl is the two-strand flat twist method. Depending on how much definition your client desires, you can decide how many flat twists to make. The average number is 10 to 15 flat twists. This technique for setting the hair really works best on clients who have naturally thick hair that is at least 5 inches (12.5 cm) long.

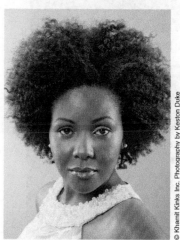

▲ **Coily/curly hair.**

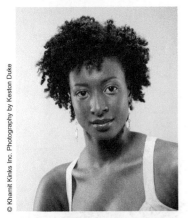

▲ Short, coily hair.

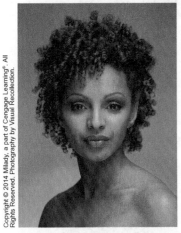

▲ Thick, long, coily hair.

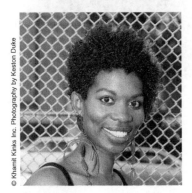

▲ Rod set.

▲ Straw set.

Short, Coily Hair: "Comb Twist" or Single-Strand Twist

For short, coily hair, an effective technique is the comb twist, or single-strand twist method. For this method, the hair should be prepped with a shampoo and conditioner and then treated with natural oil. While the hair is still wet, begin parting the hair into small, symmetrical sections. Use a fine-toothed comb to twist each section of the hair into small, cylindrical curls. After the setting has been completed, apply a gentle holding solution, such as a natural holding gel or cream to help keep this style in place for a longer time. Then place the client under the drier until the hair is completely dried. After the hair has dried, you can leave the style as is, or you have the option of separating each curl until you have made each curl multiply two to three times.

Thick, Long, Coily Hair with Slightly Elongated Curl Pattern: "The Chubby Twist"

For thick, long, coily hair with a slightly elongated curl pattern, you can create a style like the chubby twist. First prep the hair by cleansing, conditioning, and oiling the hair and scalp. Then set hair in the two-strand twist method, using a setting cream or solution. Place the client under the dryer. Once the set hair has completely dried, begin separating each two-strand twist. Keep in mind that to get the right effect for this technique, you will separate the twists only once. This style is not recommended for clients with fine or thin hair. It looks best on those with really thick hair that is at least 6 inches (15 cm) long.

All Textures, Chemically Relaxed Hair, and Those Who Are Transitioning: Flexi-Rod Set

Another effective way of achieving natural curls is to set the hair on rods. To begin the process, shampoo and condition the client's hair. Next, decide on a holding product that is best for the texture of that particular client's hair. Put the rods in on an angle and roll the hair in a spiral formation so that it resembles an elongated curl. This means that the hair should be rolled into a spiral formation. Ensure that each section of hair is wet and prepped with a holding solution before rolling it onto the rod. This technique also works well on chemically relaxed hair, on natural hair, and on those who are transitioning and are working with two distinct textures. The **flexi-rod set** styling option can last for a couple of weeks and allows the hair to rest, because it does not require daily grooming. The great thing about rods is that they come in different diameters to accommodate different thicknesses and lengths of hair.

Transitioning/Straw Sets

Another popular option for naturally texturizing the hair is a style known as a **straw set**. Clients transitioning to natural hair from chemically processed hair often gravitate to this style. They like not having their hair in braids or twists. Instead, the hair is loose and has a curly, textured look. Straw sets are very much like rod sets. The difference is that the straw set offers a tighter, more solid set than you get with the flexi-rods. The straw set has a better hold because the straws are smaller and more defined than flexi-rods. The downside is that the client's hair should be no longer than 5 inches (12.5 cm); otherwise, you will not be able to fit the client's head under a hooded dryer.

The process is the same as for a rod set except that instead of using rods, you will be using new, clean plastic straws on each client. The straws can be purchased wholesale from a straw supplier. You can cut the straws to size either before or after rolling the hair onto the straws. Use bobby pins to hold the hair onto the straw. Once the hair is set on the straws, cut each straw just a little below the client's hair on the straw. For precision, cut each straw individually. Once you move the client from under the dryer, remove the hairpins from the straws. Gently and carefully slide the straws from the hair. When you have finished, the client's head will be covered with cylindrical curls. Gently separate each curl two or three times to create a lush look of beautiful curls over the entire head.

Bantu Knots

Bantu knots, or **Nubian knots**, can be worn as a style or as a way of setting the hair. When wearing knots as a style, clients can have geometric designs parted into the head to separate each section. To create the Bantu knot, part the hair and make a small, symmetrical section. Take that section of hair and twirl the hair while twining it around the base of the section. Tuck the end of the hair at the base to complete the section. Continue this technique over the entire head. You can choose the type of holding product to use on the hair as you create the sections. The hair does not have to be wet when creating this set. But if the hair is wet, seat the client under the dryer until the hair is completely dry for a more defined curl. Once the hair has dried, release the ends if the client desires a hairstyle with spiral curls. Otherwise, leave the hair in Bantu knots.

Finger Combing

Another popular technique used today is known as **finger combing** or shingling. First, shampoo and condition the client's hair. While it is still wet, apply a desired hair product by evenly distributing it throughout each strand and using your fingers like you would use a comb. Use the fingers of both hands in a steady, gliding fashion to spread and distribute the product. The end result of this technique is to create more definition of the client's natural curl pattern. After distributing the product throughout the hair, finger combing is complete. For best results, have the client sit under a hooded dryer, or use a blowdryer with a diffuser to dry the hair. If the weather is warm, clients may prefer to air-dry their hair. However, using the hooded dryer creates more definition and overall consistency in the finished look. ☑ **LO2**

Summary of Natural Texturizing Techniques

For all of the techniques described so far, it is recommended that you use a setting cream, gel, or solution. Remember *not* to use setting

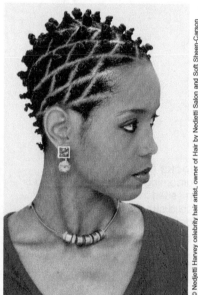

▲ **Bantu knots.**

products that are high in alcohol content or that have synthetic products that offer a hard hold. Instead, use products that will not dry out the client's hair. We recommend that you use soft holding, moisturizing setting solutions in all cases for the long-term health of your client's hair.

As a natural hair care specialist, your touch must be therapeutic. You will use additional gentle massaging techniques when shampooing or rinsing. The recommended products are natural, aromatic, and soothing—not caustic. Be sure that your approach to serving every client is one that attends to that person's emotional and physical health.

For clients with highly textured hair, the natural hair care specialist provides an essential service: helping both men and women embrace their distinctive hair types. The astute stylist can redefine what is beautiful or "acceptable." And, by educating clients on how to take better care of their hair, the natural hair care specialist is an important catalyst in helping them develop a healthier approach to self-image and self-acceptance. ✔ **LO3**

Grooming Locks

Depending on whether the specialist is a barber, hair braider, or loctician, the term *grooming* can refer to different techniques and services. The person who specializes in locking techniques is often referred to as a loctician.

locks (locs) a technique of grooming hair that is interlaced or meshed in symmetrical, cylindrical, solid strands that are never combed or brushed.

What are **locks**? Locks—also known as **locs**—are a technique of grooming the hair in symmetrical, cylindrical, solid strands that are never combed or brushed. Instead, each individual lock is either twisted or interlaced at the base of the forming lock as the new growth comes in. This grooming or training of the new growth continues throughout the life of this hairstyle, which can be worn for a few years or indefinitely. The locks continue growing, so if they are not cut from time to time, they can grow far beyond even the length of the client's body. Locks worn very long are typically heavy and cause stress at the shoulders, back, neck, and scalp, which can lead to the loss of hair. Therefore, it is recommended that clients have their locks trimmed from time to time to maintain a "reasonable" length that does not damage their particular hair strength and texture.

Depending on the hair type, texture, density, and length, locks can be combed out, but they are typically cut off because it takes weeks to comb them out. Dismantling or combing out locks is a very tedious and time-consuming service. Be sure to have a lengthy consultation before providing any service. A loctician not only grooms locks, but should also be adept at refining, mending, repairing and elaborately styling locks. Locticians should also concern themselves with the health of their clients' hair and scalp and be conscious of when the lock style may be causing stress and damage to the hair and hair follicles. Designer-styled updos are very creative and beautiful; however, the client should not wear tightly wound, braided, or twisted lock styles for long periods of time. Some styles may last for several weeks. It is advise to unravel and release the tension from intricate lock styling to avoid tension-stress, and thinning. Additionally, a great loctician is generally well-versed in herbal rinses and natural hair conditioners that embellish and strengthen the hair. The professional loctician often provides the client with a holistic approach to hair care that address the needs of the hair, as well as nutritional and dietary suggestions that promote healthy hair and well-being.

Locked hair is groomed differently than hair that is being prepared for braiding, weaving, **twist-out** styles, or cutting. A loctician, like most natural hair stylists, refers to grooming as "cultivating" locks for starting, maintaining, nurturing, and finishing natural hair and locks to enhance the overall beauty of the style. Chapter 10 discusses the proper maintenance and grooming of locked hair.

Further, to groom safely and prevent breakage, a stylist must be able to identify the variety of coil patterns in textured hair. Once these patterns are identified—through professional consultation, client information, observation, shampoo, and rinse preparations—the stylist must then choose the proper tools.

twist-outs the technique of using a double-strand twist as a set to enhance and define a client's current texture. A setting solution or curl enhancer is applied. Hair is twisted wet and dried until set; then each twist is unraveled or opened to create a defined textured pattern.

diffuser blowdryer attachment that causes air to flow more softly and helps accentuate or keep textural definition.

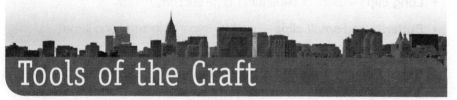

Tools of the Craft

A natural hairstylist is an artist, and like any other artist, the stylist creates the art with implements that are necessary to execute the finished product **(Figure 9–1)**. The tools the stylist chooses are essential to this profession, as they are to any other. To complete beautiful, lasting, natural styles such as braids, twists, weaves, and twist-out styles, you should use only the best and proper tools to assist in the service.

A list of your tools should include the following:

- **Blowdryer with pick nozzle**—loosens the wave pattern in textured hair for braiding and weave styles. It dries, elongates, and softens textured hair. Use hard plastic pick nozzles (metal attachments become too hot).

- **Diffuser**—dries hair without disturbing the finished look, and avoids the use of direct heat, which removes moisture. Blowdryer attachment that causes the air to flow more softly and helps accentuate or keep textural definition.

- **Finishing comb**—usually 8 to 10 inches (20.5 to 25.5 cm) in length; great on fine or straight hair, also used while cutting hair.

- **Wide-toothed comb**—available in many different shapes and designs. The teeth of wide-toothed combs should have long, rounded tips to avoid scratching the scalp. In widths, the teeth can range from medium to large. The distance between the teeth, however, is the most important feature of this comb. Wider spacing allows curly, kinky hair

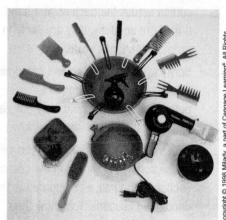

▲ Figure 9–1
Some of the tools you will use to execute the finished look.

Did you know?

Unlike working with relaxed or straightened hair, styling of textured hair requires you to use different tools. Any item that creates discomfort, snags, or pulls out hair must be discarded. All tools, including clips, should be easy to use and must be clean.

to move easily between the rows of teeth. Wide-toothed combs can be drawn through hair with less snarling than when using smaller combs.

- **Tail comb**—ideal for parting hair to prepare for braiding styles. A tail comb is excellent for design parting and weaving, easy to use for sectioning large segments of hair, and excellent for aiding the opening and removal of braids.

- **Plastic pick with rounded teeth**—used for lifting and separating textured and curly hair, such as Afros and human hair extensions. Teeth are long and widely spaced. They can be made of metal, plastic, or wood and are great for separating and lifting textured hair.

- **Double-toothed comb**—excellent on wet, curly hair, this comb is designed to limit tangling and snarling.

- **Curved needle**—for weaving thread and used for braid weave styles and weaves. Curved needles are excellent for getting close to the scalp without harming it.

- **Spray bottle container**—used for combing out and finishing a look, and to hold detangling solutions.

- **Long clips**—used for separating large sections of hair.

- **Butterfly and small clips**—used for separating small and large sections of hair.

- **Cutting comb**—used for cutting small sections, only after hair has been softened and elongated with a blowdryer.

  - **Hands**—please take care of them, because they are one of your most important tools.

  - **Mannequin**—used for practicing styles and braid techniques.

  - **Vent brush**—a wide-bristled plastic brush to be used on wet, wavy hair or on dry, curly hair. It is excellent on human hair extensions. Vent brushes may have either a single or a double row of teeth. This brush helps to detangle hair, but use it gently to keep its teeth from snarling or snagging in kinky hair.

  - **Cutting Shears**—necessary for a finished look and to trim fringes and excess extension material; used to create shape.

  - **Hackle**—a board of fine, upright nails; used for combing through human hair to detangle or blend colors and highlights.

  - **Drawing board**—used to help control human hair while braiding. Drawing boards are flat leather pads with very close, fine teeth that sandwich the human hair. The sandwich is weighted down to secure the hair so braids can be pulled (drawn) from the board in the required proportion without losing and disturbing the rest of the hair.

  - **Hood dryer**—a hair dryer mounted on a stand; provides dry heat, used to remove excess moisture before blowdrying hair

Here's a Tip.........

- When choosing your tools, run your combs across the back of your hand. If they are scratchy, they are likely to irritate the client's scalp.

- Spray with moisturizing and detangling solution as often as needed for detangling and softening. Very porous hair may absorb the water quickly.

- With very coiled or kinky hair, you will notice some springiness in the combed section of the hair, as compared to the uncombed sections. You know then that the curl has been stretched and separated.

by hand. The hood dryer eliminates excessive use of hand blowdrying and reduces the amount of direct heat on the hair.

- **Steamer**—looks like a hairdryer, but provides moist heat; great tool to provide extreme moisturizing benefits of a deep conditioning treatment. Warm heat opens cuticles of the hair shaft as well as the follicles to allow any vitamin and nutrients the hair product will offer. Soothing relaxing steam provides a spa-like treatment for the scalp. Warm moist heat softens and liquefies product as it smooth cuticles and reduces frizz.

- **Other accessories**—cloth towels, professional paper towels to protect the neck from touching the capes, cloth capes, and water-repellent capes for water services. ✓ **LO4**

Combing and Sectioning: The Proper Way to Handle and Detangle the Hair

Contrary to what many people may believe, kinky hair is not tough. This textured hair is very fragile when dry. It is more elastic when wet. However, the best way to work with textured hair is when it is wet and conditioned. This preparation makes it easier to stretch textured hair for detangling, parting, combing through, and managing tight coils. The structure of most textured hair has varying formations of curls or coils. At each bend in the coil, the hair strand is thinner, so each strand has several potential breakage points. The closer the curl/coil pattern, the more fragile the hair. It is important to understand that combing wet, textured hair is very meticulous work that takes lots of patience. Remember: The more coil in the hair, the more fragile it is when dry; Remember: For hair with more coil, if it hasn't already been shampooed, conditioned, detangled, and blowdried, then it will be more fragile when dry. (Procedure 9-1).

Blowdrying Textured Hair

Why blowdry textured hair? Because it dries the hair quickly and also softens the hair, making it manageable for easy combing. Blowdrying loosens the wave patterns in the hair while stretching the shaft length. This excellent technique can be used on all lengths of hair. For short hair, blowdrying the hair stretches it out and enables the client to wear longer braiding styles with the use of extensions (Procedure 9-2).

Thermal Heat Services; An Alternative Look for "Natural" Hair

The art of natural hair styling is to provide healthy hair services that do not diminish or permanently alter the original virgin hair texture. On occasion, some of your clients may prefer to straighten their hair without using chemical services.

There is an ongoing debate about thermal straightening in the natural hair industry. Although thermal straightening temporarily alters the natural hair texture, some people consider it less damaging than chemical straightening services. Most natural hair professionals do not provide thermal services because over a period of time, extreme heat can permanently damage and diminish texture. The debate continues. In the meantime, you will want to know that mastering this skill can set you apart in the natural hair care industry. You will be able to offer something that most natural hair care stylists do not offer. It is up to you to determine whether or not you want to offer your clients this service. Many natural hair care specialists do not offer it. If you decide to offer this service, be properly prepared. Know that these clients will also expect you to have exceptional cutting skills, because they will want the same styling options available to those with chemically straightened hair.

Thermal heat services such as hair straightening, or pressing, is a popular service that is very profitable in the salon. When textured hair is properly thermal straightened or curled, the service can offer the client a variety of silky and sleek styling options. A light thermal straightening leaves the hair manageable and temporarily elongated, and may cause minimal damage to the texture. A light heat service with the proper tool and skill set will last from several days to a full week before returning to its original spiraled texture. A heat protectant must be applied before using or providing any thermal application.

When used at higher temperatures, these thermal tools can actually damage and alter the molecular structure of the hair. Often, hair will not return to its natural texture. The client's hair has become permanently altered and will remain that way until it is cut off. The new hair will grow out in its natural texture, of course. ☑ **LO5**

Analysis of Hair and Scalp

Before performing any thermal heat service on a client's hair, you will need to analyze the condition of the hair and scalp. As a professional, you want to provide services that address the clients needs, to resolve and

CAUTION

When the pressing is done improperly with excessive heat, the protein bonds of the hair can be broken. Once the bonds are broken, the hair texture is diminished and can promote severe breakage.

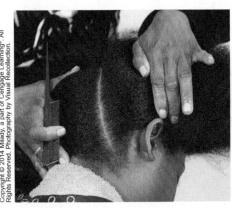

▲ Analysis.

diminish the varying scalp disorders that may affect the finished style. If your client appears to have a severe skin disease of the scalp, it is not your job to diagnose the condition, but rather to advise the client to see a dermatologist.

If the hair shows signs of neglect or abuse caused by faulty pressing, chemical damage, or damage from styling tools, recommend a series of conditioning treatments. Failure to correct dry and brittle hair can result in hair breakage during hair pressing.

Remember to check your client's hair for elasticity and porosity. If the porosity is normal, the hair will return to its natural wave pattern when it is wet or moistened.

A careful analysis of the client's hair and scalp should cover these points:

- Wave pattern or curl configuration

- Length

- Texture or hair type (coarse, medium, or fine)

- Density

- Feel (wiry, soft, or silky)

- Elasticity

- Color (natural, faded, streaked, gray, tinted, or lightened)

- Condition of hair (normal, brittle, dry, oily, damaged, or chemically treated)

- Condition of scalp (normal, flexible, or tight)

Thermal Straightening Heat Service

Before you offer any thermal or heat service, it is important to cleanse and condition the client's hair. Products such as leave-in conditioners or thermal sprays are also recommended to coat and protect the hair from the heat before using a flat iron to straighten your client's hair. Apply the leave-in conditioner or thermal spray to the client's hair after you shampoo and condition the hair while it is still wet. Then blowdry the hair to elongate the texture. When the hair is completely dry, the client is ready for thermal heat services. To avoid damaging client's hair and scalp, always consider the texture of the hair and the condition of the scalp. The best and only way to ensure your client's safety is to observe every precaution and take special care not to use excessive heat during the actual thermal service.

It is important to know that if you apply too much heat or do not understand the tools you are using, you could damage your client's hair with thermal heat services. Your clients are seeking you out for healthy hair choices, so it is important for you to do everything you can to avoid damaging their hair. Be aware that many clients receiving your services will have a history of chemically treated hair, and some will have a history

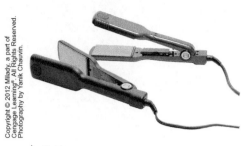

▲ Flat iron.

of thermal straightening of the hair. While clients are in transition to going "totally natural," the hair follicles are under an extreme amount of stress. Each strand has two textures: natural and chemical. At the point where these two textures meet, the shafts are weak and may snap off during the comb-out and sectioning. Be very gentle with hair in transition. In most cases, the client has experienced some form of hair damage or scalp irritation.

Flat Irons

Flat irons have two hot plates, ranging in size from ½ inch to 3 inches (1.3 cm to 7.5 cm) across. Flat irons with straight edges are used to create smooth, straight styles, even on very curly hair. Flat irons with beveled edges can be manipulated to bend or cup the ends. The edge nearest the stylist is called the inner edge; the one farthest from the stylist is called the outer edge. Modern technology is constantly improving electric curling and flat irons by adding more heat settings for better control, constant, even heat on high settings, ergonomic grips, and lightweight designs for ease of handling.

Testing Thermal Irons

After heating the iron or flat iron to the desired temperature, test it on a piece of tissue paper or a white cloth. Clamp the heated iron over this material and hold for five seconds. If it scorches or turns brown, the iron is too hot! Let it cool a bit before using. An overly hot iron can scorch the hair and might even discolor white hair. Remember that fine, lightened, or badly damaged hair withstands less heat than normal hair.

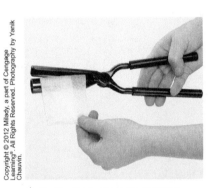

▲ Testing the heat of a thermal iron.

Care of Thermal Irons

Before cleaning a thermal iron, be sure to check the manufacturer's directions for care and cleaning. One way to remove dirt, oils, and product residue is to dampen a towel or rag and wipe down the barrel or plate of the iron with a soapy solution containing a few drops of ammonia. If you are using a nonelectrical thermal iron, immerse the barrel or plate in this solution. Do not clean your iron when it is turned on or when it is still cooling from a previous styling service.

Comb Used with Thermal Irons

The comb should be about 7 inches (17.5 cm) long, should be made of hard rubber or another nonflammable substance, and should have teeth to firmly hold the hair. Hold the comb between the thumb and all four fingers of the nondominant hand. For better control, rest the index finger on the backbone of the comb and rest one end of the comb against the outer edge of the palm. This position ensures a strong hold and a firm movement.

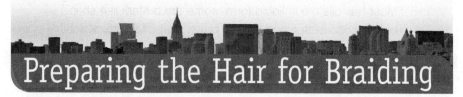

Preparing the Hair for Braiding

Preparing the hair for braiding means that you have thoroughly cleaned the hair and scalp. Hair should be dry, softened, and free of snarls, tangles, or knots.

- Before you begin braiding the client's hair, look for bald, thinning, or damaged hair areas. These problem areas will affect the style of the braiding design. Texture, length, and hair condition will determine the style design around the problem areas.

- Before you proceed with any braiding service, examine the scalp for scratches, abrasions, sores, irritations, birthmarks, or moles.

- The crown is your canvas. Be certain that the natural hair and the client's scalp condition can support the braiding style that you choose.

Hair Oil Preparation

Preparing the scalp for braiding also involves selecting a natural hair care product that will help soften the hair as well as moisten the scalp. The preparation should provide a light coat of moisture to the strands that will aid the braiding process. Natural hair oils have been part of the hair-grooming process since the ancient Khamit people used them in Egypt.

The scalp also produces its own natural oil, called sebum. Sebum is produced by the sebaceous glands that are connected to the hair follicle. Sebum travels along the outside of the hair shaft, acting as a lubricant and natural emollient that seals in moisture. However, with textured hair, the spiral structure of the hair shaft makes it difficult for the sebum to travel along the shaft. This is why in many cases, the scalp may be oily, but the hair remains dry.

The cellular structure of textured hair is different from that of other hair types. In the spiral pattern, the outer, shingled layers of cells that protect the hair cuticle lie closer together, making the hair look drier than other hair types. The hair can become fragile in cases where the scalp has fewer sebaceous glands and produces less oil or sebum.

Replacing the sebum with natural oils from vegetables, seeds, plants, and flowers can restore moisture and protect the hair. These oils add a thin lubricant for braiding, making both the client's natural hair and extension (if one is used) more pliable and softer on the braider's fingertips.

Heavy synthetic oils such as lanolin, petroleum, and mineral oils should be avoided because of their ability to attract dust and dirt (see Chapter 8). Synthetic oils do not absorb into the scalp and often leave a coat of residue, which ultimately creates blockage at the follicle base. This blockage eventually hinders the growth process.

Did you know?

Hair can become fragile in cases where the scalp has fewer sebaceous glands and produces less oil or sebum.

When removing braids:

- Pull clumped residue apart by hand, using your fingers to loosen the wax.

- Further removal requires the use of a wide-toothed comb.

- Lightly spray affected area with a rinse solution of water and cream to soften buildup.

- Always start at the ends of the hair, holding at the base so that the client is completely comfortable and hair is not overly stressed.

Most hair oils are in liquid form, some are butters like shea butter, coco butter, and mango butter that offer a thick rich nourishing emollient without a waxy deposit. These butters are great moisturizers and humectants. They are light to the touch and absorbed quickly into the hair and skin, giving the hair a rich moisturizing sheen.

Pomades are scented hair oils that have a cream or wax base. Be careful when using pomades with heavy wax bases. When selecting pomades, a stylist should look for natural ingredients that will stimulate hair growth and lubricate hair. Pomades should not be greasy, sticky, or pasty. Heavy pomades will block pores and cause wax buildup in the braids. Clots of wax buildup at the base of the braid are a major problem when removing braided styles. Wax from the heavy grease or pomade that is left in the hair collects dust and dirt from the environment. It then can become impacted or hardened between the new growth and hair extension. When combing out this wax residue, be careful to avoid breakage. ✓ **LO6**

Myth 13: Braids Must Be Tight in Order to Last

Tight braids pull out the hair. Too much tension on the hair with or without extensions can cause serious damage to the hair follicle. In many cases, prolonged tension will create permanent hair loss, damage, thinning, and balding scars. In some extreme cases, traction alopecia will occur, removing patches of hair pulled out as well as leaving sensitive areas of the scalp tender and scared.

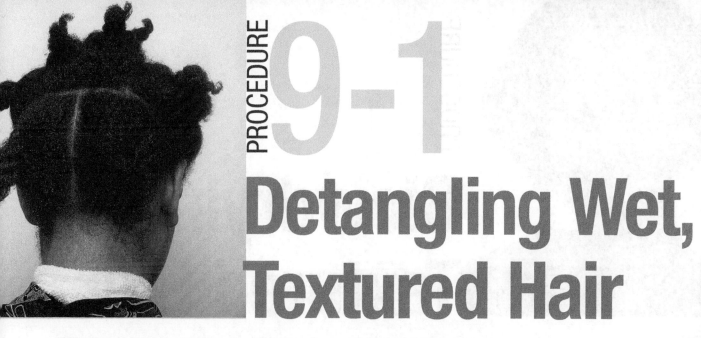

PROCEDURE

9-1

Detangling Wet, Textured Hair

Detangling wet, textured hair can be made much easier by following these steps.

1 Start at the nape of the neck. Using a tail comb with large rounded teeth, part the crown of the head from ear to ear. Use butterfly clips to separate and hold the front section away from the back section.

2 Part the back of the head into four to six sections. For thick textured hair, make more sections to allow for ease and control. For thinner hair, use fewer sections. The front half of the head can be parted in three sections or more, because some clients' hair is less dense in the front. Separate sections with clips. Gently spray each section as you go along, using a solution of 4 parts water with 1 part cream rinse or oil.

3 Begin with the left section. There should be enough hair to hold in the palm of your hand. Too much hair in this section can cause you to lose control, which could result in hair breakage.

4 Holding the palm upward and close to the scalp, start combing with a wide-toothed comb at the ends of the hair first, working your way up to the base of the scalp. Work from the bottom up, because hair tangles at the ends.

5 The combing movement should be steady and rhythmic, but should not put tension on the scalp. It is better to use a picking motion to comb through the hair.

6 Once the hair is combed thoroughly, divide the section into two equal parts and twist it together to the end to separate and hold the combed section in place.

7 Repeat steps 4 through 6 for the other sections of the hair to finish the entire head.

8 Place the client under a hood dryer on medium heat for about five minutes to remove excess water.

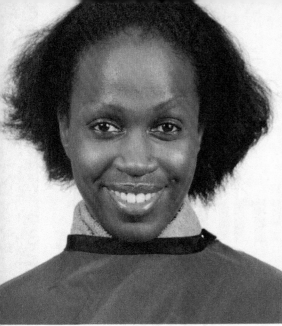

9-2

Blowdrying Textured Hair

1 After shampooing, conditioning, and properly sectioning the hair, place the client under the hood dryer for 5 to 10 minutes (depending on the density of the hair) to remove excess water.

2 Blowdrying creams and lotions protect the hair from direct heat and help control the manageability of textured hair. These creams or lotions can be applied before blowdrying each section, if combed through thoroughly, as well as afterward.

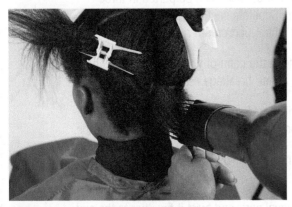

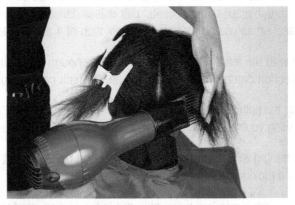

3 Open one of the combed sections. Use a pick nozzle attachment on the blowdryer and begin drying, using the comb-out motion.

4 Holding the hair down and away from the client's head, start the comb-out motion. Always point the pick nozzle away from the client. As the end stretches, move the blowdryer, heat blowing downward, away from the scalp. Blowdrying directly into the scalp could cause burns.

5 As the longer hair dries, some shorter lengths of hair may have curled closer to the scalp. To get closer to the scalp, reduce the blowdryer heat and speed. This technique allows the pick nozzle to reach shorter, more resistant textured hair and loosen the curl pattern. It also prevents the client from being burned by the heat of the blowdryer.

6 Check each section to be sure it is dry. If so, the hair is ready to be braided or styled.

Review Questions

1. Name three tools used in braiding and natural hairstyling, and give an example of how each tool is used in braiding and other natural styling techniques.

2. Why is it important for the natural hair care client to receive regular haircuts and trims?

3. What are some measures that need to be taken to safely comb and brush out textured hair?

4. Name a method used to straighten natural hair without the use of chemicals.

10 Natural Hair and Braid-Sculpting Techniques

Chapter Outline

- Why Study Natural Hair and Braid-Sculpting Techniques?

- Protective Transitional Styling versus the Big Chop

- Textured Styles and Braiding Terms

- Procedures: Textured Styling and Braid-Sculpting Techniques

- Final Reflections

Learning Objectives

After completing this chapter, you will be able to:

☑ **LO1** Identify the fundamental terms used in the industry.

☑ **LO2** Explain the general information about the benefits of transitional styling, protective styling, and the "big chop."

☑ **LO3** Perform a range of textured, transitional, and protective styles.

Key Terms

Page number indicates where in the chapter the term is used.

big chop
p. 226

demarcation line
p. 225

long-term transitioning
p. 225

protective styles
p. 224

transitional textures
p. 224

transitioning
p. 224

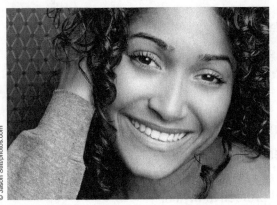

© Jason Stitt/photos.com

▲ Figure 10–1
Having a clear understanding of the techniques will help ensure a satisfied client.

The creative art form of natural hairstyling and braiding is unlimited. The techniques offered here are fundamental and can be improvised to allow self-expression. As demand increases for the natural hairstyles, **protective styles**, and transitional styling, the styles will become more diverse. More important, the stylist must be aware of the different styles and options that are available to the client. By completely understanding naturally textured hair, the variety of natural styles, and above all, the required hands-on experience and practice, you can be among the best in the industry **(Figure 10–1)**.

Why Study Natural Hair and Braid-Sculpting Techniques?

It is important for the natural stylist to study and thoroughly understand the importance of natural hair and braid-sculpting techniques because

- All stylists should be prepared to work with every hair type and be able to create hairstyles that the client wants.

- These styles are very popular, and customers are interested in wearing styles specific to their hair texture.

- Knowing these fundamental techniques will expand the styling options that you can give to your client no matter what the hair texture is.

protective styles extension styles that include braid extensions, twist extensions, weaves, and wig styles that can be worn while transitioning from a relaxer and are great for natural textured hair.

transitioning also known as "going natural." This process involves growing out chemically relaxed hair to natural hair. It is a conscious approach to stop relaxing or using harsh chemicals or extreme heat to reduce or modify the client's natural, virgin hair texture.

transitional textures occur when the hair has two textures on one strand. The hair is allowed to grow without chemically "retouching" the new growth. This is the first step toward growing out natural hair. The new growth or natural portion is strong and vital while the relaxed portion of the hair is weak, thin, and breaks easily.

Protective Transitional Styling versus the Big Chop

"Going natural" means many things for many people. There are several ways to achieve the ultimate goal of naturally healthy hair. **Transitioning** from chemically relaxed hair to natural is a conscious approach to stop relaxing or using harsh chemicals or extreme heat to reduce or modify the client's natural, virgin hair texture. The condition called **transitional textures** occurs when the hair has two textures on one strand. The hair is allowed to grow without chemically "retouching" the new growth. The new growth or natural portion is strong and vital while the relaxed portion of the hair is weak, thin, and breaks easily. This is the client's first step toward having natural hair.

Once the client is committed to discontinuing the process of chemically relaxing her hair, the transitional process begins **(Figure 10–2)**. During this phase, the hair fiber will have two distinctly different textures on one strand—the new growth at the root and the previously relaxed portion of the hair. It is important to note that the **demarcation line**, the point where the natural hair and the chemically treated hair meet, is extremely fragile. Excessive hair combing and style manipulation during transitioning will cause stress, breakage, and hair loss. To minimize hair loss, the hair must be treated, protected, and styled in various methods that nourish and reduce stress. You must use conditioning treatments that address the needs of naturally textured hair. Daily cleansing, combing, and styling must be altered, reduced, and in some cases prohibited. ✓ **LO1**

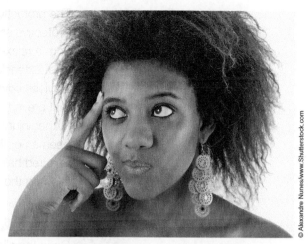

▲ Figure 10–2
The beginning of the transitional phase.

Transitional Hair: Brittle, Damaged, and Thinning

Going natural is a huge decision for most clients. Although they may want natural hair, the transitional phase can be perplexing. Going natural requires adapting to new hair regimes, new products, new hairstyles, and a different life. Going natural is more than just the decision to stop using chemicals for the client with textured hair. It is also an emotional and practical decision to allow the community where they live to see their vulnerability and their uniqueness. **Long-term transitioning** provides many clients the opportunity to try protective styles and to allow the hair to grow out of the relaxer without removing or cutting the fragile ends. This process allows the hair to grow over time. Natural sets and protective styles like rod sets, twist-outs, braid-outs, extensions, weaves, and wigs can aid the client who wants to have a long-term transition. Many clients opt to service their new growth by long-term transitioning because they want to retain the length of their hair.

demarcation line the point where the natural new growth of hair meets the old relaxed hair. This point of the hair is weak and can easily break and snap off.

long-term transitioning gives many clients the opportunity to try protective styles that allow the hair to grow out of the relaxer and avoid removing or cutting the fragile ends. This process allows the hair to grow over time. Natural sets and protective styles like rod sets, twist-outs, braid-outs, extensions, weaves, and wigs can aid the client who wants to try long-term transitioning.

Transitioning is a process; it is often referred to as a journey. This process gives clients, as well as family and friends, time to adjust and see the person who is transitioning from long, straight relaxed hair into a new short natural style **(Figure 10–3)**. The journey can be challenging for many clients, because some have not managed their own natural texture as an adult. They may remember only the pain and discomfort of their childhood experiences. As natural stylists, our job is to help clients get reacquainted with their hair. You must educate them by offering options, which includes a full range of texture-enhancing products and styling solutions that keep their hair healthy and manageable. Long-term transitioning may work for a few months, but the two different textures on one strand eventually become more fragile, get thinner, and require trimming or total removal. Long-term transitioning can take from six months to one year.

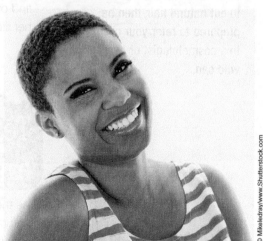

▲ Figure 10–3
Sometimes cutting the hair in the transitional phase is a good option.

The protective style is an effective option for the client who is in transition. Protective styles are extension styles that can be worn while transitioning from a relaxer and are great for the natural textured hair. Braid extensions, twist extensions, weaves, and wigs are all protective styles. These hair services cover, embellish, and safeguard the delicate weakened strands that are in transition. Protective styling safeguards the two textures from further injury or breakage by manipulation. Protective styling has always been an option to enhance and preserve the wholeness of naturally textured hair. Natural hair can also benefit from protective styling by allowing the natural tresses to rest from daily styling.

Short Afro After the "Big Chop"

Once the client has decided to go natural, she may not want the long-term effects of transitioning or protecting the hair with extensions. Some clients opt to make an appointment to totally remove or cut the relaxed portion of the hair. This is referred to as the **big chop**. The results of the big chop are immediate and dramatic. Most clients find it is refreshing, uplifting, and totally gorgeous. For others it is traumatic, intimidating, and unattractive. It is your responsibility to help the client embrace this new natural style.

After the relaxed hair is removed, the natural texture will no longer look elongated or have much length. The coil or curl pattern will be more pronounced, and the hair length will reduce or shrink. The shrinkage for natural hair depends on the coil configuration and hair density. Some clients feel comfortable with short, textured hair, and others have more difficulty. Their facial features, head size, and head shape will be more pronounced. There is no longer any hair to hide behind after the big chop, nor any hair to camouflage perceived imperfections. A consultation is highly recommended and should be required before the big chop. Talk to the client before any cutting service is performed. If your scope of license does not allow you to complete the cutting service, refer your client to a trusted professional who can. It is extremely important to listen to the client's doubts, fears, and concerns about wearing a short natural Afro. Ask the client questions to find out how the client feels about having a short Afro—what it means for her lifestyle and for her self-image. ☑ **LO2**

big chop The total removal or cutting off of the relaxed portion of all hair strands leaves naturally curly hair as a teeny weeny Afro (TWA). The results of the big chop are immediate and dramatic.

CAUTION

In several states your natural hair care and braiding license does not permit you to perform a haircut on natural hair. Be guided by your instructor concerning your state mandatory requirements regarding haircutting. If your state does not allow you to cut natural hair, then be prepared to refer your client to a cosmetologist or barber who can.

Textured Styles and Braiding Terms

As the natural hairstyling industry becomes more popular, innovative natural stylists will create many beautiful styling options. The names may vary from state to state; however, it is necessary to know the featured styles. The following descriptions provide you with the basic knowledge of the most popular natural, protective, or transitional styles and techniques.

Afros

The Afro can be achieved on long or short wavy, curly, coiled, or highly textured (kinky) hair. Hair that is cut and textured can vary in its final shape. The Afro-twist extensions style is achieved when human hair or synthetic hair fibers are anchored with a braid-and-twist combination. Gel is used to seal the twist and enhance texture. The Afro weave style is achieved by attaching textured hair on a weft to a designated cornrow base. The wefted hair extension is sewn with a cotton thread.

Braids and Cornrows

Braids can be formed as single, box, and individual braids. These names are interchangeable for most braid stylists across the country. These techniques are basic free-hanging braids with or without extensions. The hair is divided into three equal sections that are intertwined or weaved into one single braid. Casamas braids are extended braids that are large, single braids with a tight stitch; they are tapered and/or curved at the ends. Cornrow and canerow braids are underhand, three-strand braids interwoven to lie flat on the scalp. They can be designed and sculpted into varying patterns with or without extensions.

Coil Styles

Coils or comb twists are small sections of natural hair that are gelled and spiraled with fingers or a comb to create individual formations of tight, cylindrical coils. The Nubian coils technique is styled on naturally curly or textured hair. Hair is curled into a cylindrical shape with a comb or hands.

Locked Styles

Locs, also called dreadlocks, are natural textured hair that is intertwined, meshed, and interlaced to form a solid cylinder and separate network of hair. Locs can be started at various sizes: extra small, small, medium, or large. Nu-locs is a technique that is done with yarn fiber, giving the extension a matte finish to look like locs. A single-braid technique is used.

Textured Sets and Styles

For the Bantu knot-out style, the hair is double-strand twisted or coil twisted and wrapped around itself to make a knot. Knots are secured by bobby pins or elastic bands. Knots can be opened and released to create wavy and fuller loose curls. The braid-out set involves braiding the hair when either wet or dry and then opening the braid to create a crimped texture-on-texture effect with added volume. The flat twist involves a parted row of hair that is first divided into two sections and then twisted and interwoven to lie flat on the scalp. It can be made in varying patterns with or without extensions. Spiral rod sets can be done with rods or flexi-rods or curl reformers of all sizes. Hair is wrapped around a vertical rod, going up the rod in a spiral movement. Hair must completely dry, or the style will appear frizzy.

Twist Styles

Double-strand twist styles start with wet, gelled, or dry hair. The stylist divides hair into two sections and then overlaps them to create a twisted rope effect (dry) or textured effect (wet). A twist set is a two-part set that can be done on natural hair, transitional hair, twists extensions, weaves, wigs, and locs. Hair is double-strand twisted and then set on rods. Rods can be placed only at the end of the hair or loc. For a full set, rods can also be placed vertically all the way to the base of the hair. Twist curls on textured hair are achieved by using a double-twist technique. The twisting technique is done on wet hair to define the textured curls and waves. The "twist-out" involves unraveling the twist to add fullness and a crimped effect. The twist-out's double-strand twists can be made in any size and length. Hair is wet, and gel or crème is applied to set the textured hair. After hair is dried, twists are opened to provide texture and volume.

Myth 14: Transitioning Means the Client Grows Out Her Relaxed Hair Over an Extended Period before Cutting Off All Her Hair to Get an All Natural Style; Also Known as the Big Chop

The big chop—cutting all the relaxed hair—while the client is in transition is always an option, but it is not necessary. If the client is not ready to deal with a short Afro, then offer her time to adjust and allow the hair to gain some length with transitional styles or protective styles (these terms are often used interchangeably). Eventually, the relaxed hair must be removed by cutting before there is extreme breakage. Protective styling is a style that protects the hair from style manipulation and allows the hair to rest while transitioning to the new style.

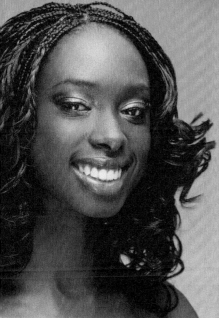

10-1

Single Box Braids

This classic single-braid style is timeless and regal. Box braids can be set crimped, spiraled, or twisted to create soft movement. As a protective style, human hair extensions are incorporated for body and length. This style is versatile and liberating by reducing style manipulation for clients that are in transition.

Tools

- 6 oz. loose human hair
- 5 butterfly clips
- wide-toothed comb
- tail comb
- long duckbill clips
- shears
- spray bottle with detangling and moisturizing solution
- spray bottle with setting lotion
- steamer
- blowdryer with nozzle comb attachment
- hood dryer

Hair Type

- Texture—coily, fine, very dense
- Coil pattern—tight spiral, wiry bends
- Hair condition—very dry, fragile, needs added moisture

Hair Prep

- To cleanse the hair, use a sulfate- and surfactant-free moisturizing shampoo.
- Treat with humectants and moisturizing conditioner with steamer for 20 minutes.
- Spray leave-in conditioner with protein to strengthen hair, or apply cream leave-in conditioner with natural butters.

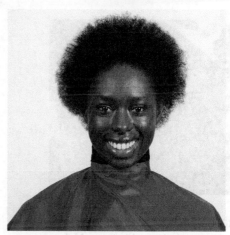

Procedure

1 After hair prep and steam treatment, detangle with large-toothed comb and divide into five manageable sections.

2 Blowdry with nozzle comb.

3 Prepare hair fiber for easy distribution.

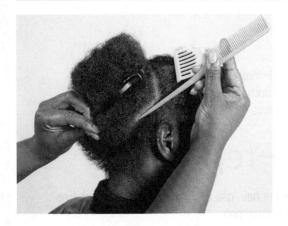

4 Starting at the side crown and going to the nape, create a ¼-inch (0.6-cm) diagonal parting with ¼-inch subsections.

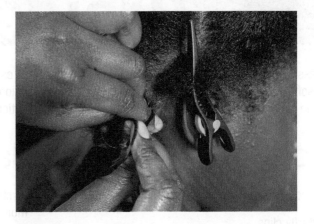

5 Prepare hair for braid: Divide base hair into three equal parts, placing three interlocked strands of the hair fiber; one strand in the middle as well as on the outside strands.

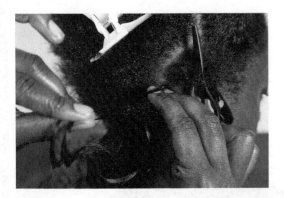

6 When applying hair fiber to natural hair, introduce equal amounts to avoid stress. Make one rotation and split hair fiber to cover the third hair strand. Each of the three hair strands should have a hair fiber to extend its length. Alternate center hair strand to the outside strand to complete a rotation. Continue to braid down ½ inch (1.2 cm) past the length of the natural hair. Complete that section.

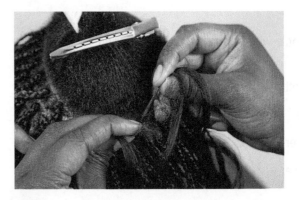

7 Part the next horizontal row, and create a braid that is ¼ inch (0.6 cm) with ¼-inch subsections in a bricklaying formation. Using the same braiding technique, continue to work up and around the back of the head.

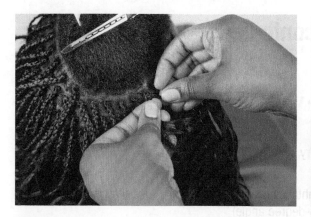

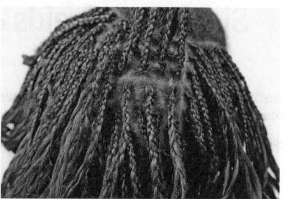

8 Every braid created will need to hang directly over the existing partings of the row below, in a bricklaying fashion. This technique creates fullness and shows less of the scalp.

9 Complete entire back section with the bricklaying technique.

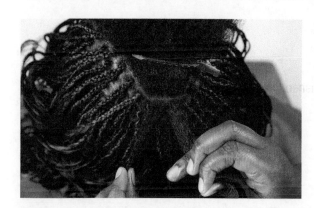

10 Start the front by parting into three sections; clip them for control.

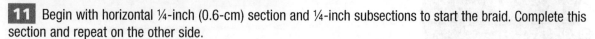

11 Begin with horizontal ¼-inch (0.6-cm) section and ¼-inch subsections to start the braid. Complete this section and repeat on the other side.

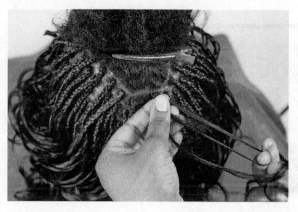

12 At crown, use bricklaying in smaller subsections to diminish partings and to create fullness. Repeat until entire head is completely braided.

13 Spray braided base with setting lotion. While the braid is wet, use a two-strand twist to create a texture-on-texture finish.

14 Place client under hood dryer. When braids are completely dry, untwist them.

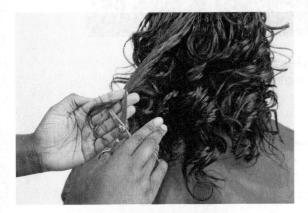

15 Lightly oil scalp, trim, and style (use a scissor cut at 45-degree angle)

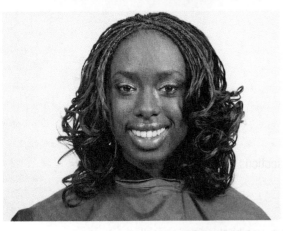

16 Finished look.

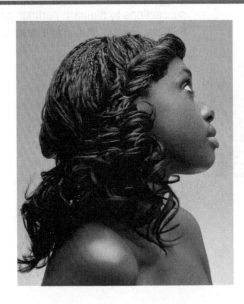

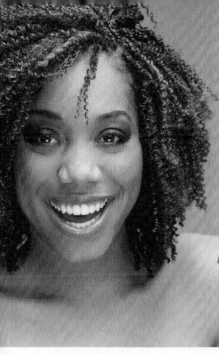

Copyright © 2014 Milady, a part of Cengage Learning. Photography by Visual Recollection

10-2
Afro-Twist Extension

The client with Afro-twist extensions will certainly be noticed. This show-stopping hairstyle is an excellent protective style to embellish the client's natural hair texture. For those in transition, this braid-twist combination allows the hair to grow without damage or stress.

Tools

- 5 oz. Afro kinky custom blend human hair
- 5 butterfly clips
- wide-toothed comb
- tail comb
- long duckbill clips
- shears
- spray bottle with detangle/moisturizer solution
- gel or curling cream
- steamer
- blowdryer with nozzle comb attachment
- hood dryer

Hair Type

- Texture—soft, highly textured, curls; fine, not very dense
- Curl pattern—small loops, curly ends
- Hair condition—dry, dull

Hair Prep

- To cleanse, use a sulfate- and surfactant-free moisturizing shampoo.
- Treat with moisturizing conditioner.
- Spray leave-in conditioner with protein and vitamins to strengthen hair, or apply cream leave-in conditioner with natural butters.

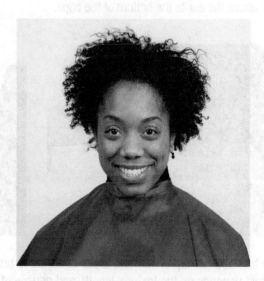

Procedure

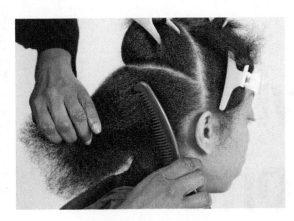

1 After hair prep and steam treatment, detangle with wide-toothed comb and divide into five manageable sections.

2 Blowdry with nozzle comb.

3 Prepare human hair fiber.

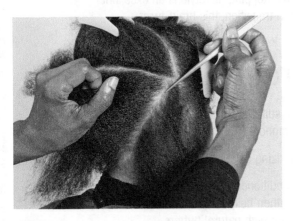

4 Begin at the ear, on the right side of the head. Part hair on a 45-degree angle into a ¼-inch (0.6-cm) section from above the ear to the bottom of the nape.

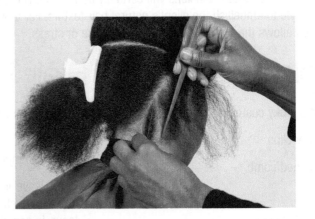

5 Create a diamond-shaped ¼-inch (0.6-cm) subsection.

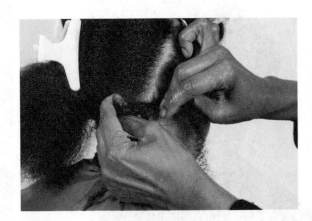

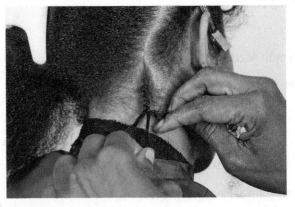

6 Place hair fiber on top of hair and braid. Continue to braid for five to seven rotations. The length of the extended braid depends on the texture, length, and density of the client's hair. If hair is in transition, increase the braid base and rotations.

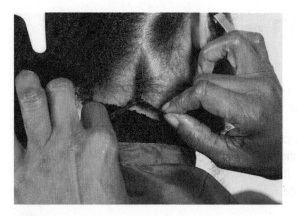 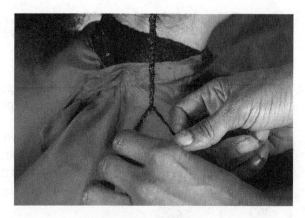

7 Holding all three strands of the braid, divide the center strand into 2 equal parts and braid into outside strands. In the same direction, apply one roll to the two strands, incorporating the natural hair into the twist extension.

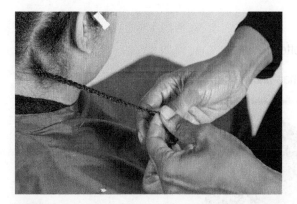 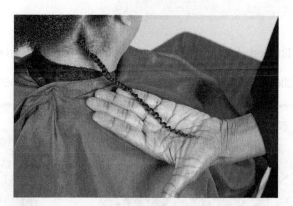

8 Apply gel to two equal sections and create the twist with an overlapping motion, strand over strand. Repeat the overlapping motion down the entire unit.

9 Apply gel to seal ends. Continue until section is complete.

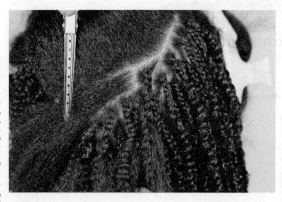 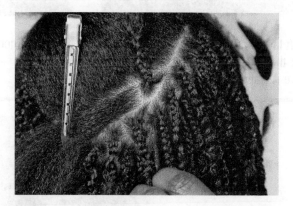

10 On the right side of the back section, create a 45-degree diagonal ¼-inch (0.6-cm) section with ¼-inch subsection. Continue to add extensions with the braid-twist-gel combination. Part the back triangular center section on the same 45-degree angle.

11 Continue bricklaying the subsection until entire back is complete.

12 Front, side, and crown sections are parted on the same angle. Front sections and subsections may be smaller and closer together to create fullness and to diminish parts.

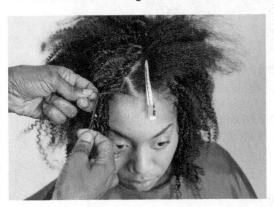

13 Crown sections and subsections are small and in bricklaying style. Anchor braid-twist in the direction of the finished style. Continue until entire head is complete.

14 Spray finished style with leave-in moisturizing conditioner to soften hair.

15 Place client under preheated hood dryer for 30 minutes. When hair is dry, open twists for fullness.

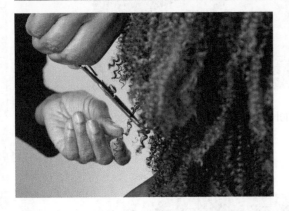

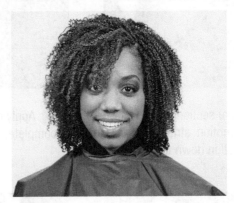

16 Cut soft layers and shape textured hair by cutting under the curl. Gently pull curl out and cut the curl where it stands.

17 Add nonalcoholic holding spritz. Finished style.

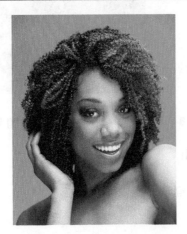

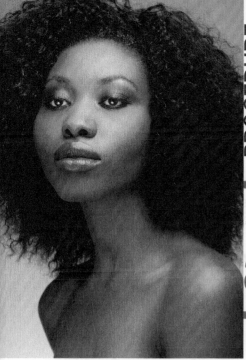

10-3

The Afro Weave and the Mixed Texture Afro Weave

Afros are back and hotter than ever! They are fun, versatile, and can be styled in any color, length, or shape. The Afro weave adds a new dimension to textured hairstyling. This weave can be created with synthetic hair, human hair, or blends of yak and human hair. The look is as contemporary today as it was in the 1960s. Weaving in hair can protect natural hair, transitional hair, and hair that has been chemically damaged. It covers balding or thinning spots, allowing the natural hair to regenerate and grow.

The traditional Afro weave has a new approach with two alternating hair textures to create a full, realistic, and individualized style. The kinky crown is great as a protective style for natural styles and for those in transition. It gives total coverage while hair grows and stays healthy.

Tools

- 8 oz. wefted human hair fiber
- 1 oz. synthetic hair
- 4 butterfly clips
- wide-toothed comb
- tail comb
- long duckbill clips
- shears
- spray bottle with detangling and moisturizing solution
- curved needle and cotton thread
- steamer
- blowdryer with nozzle comb attachment
- hood dryer

Hair Prep

- To cleanse, use a sulfate- and surfactant-free moisturizing shampoo.
- Treat with moisturizing conditioner.
- Spray leave-in conditioner with protein to strengthen hair, or apply cream leave-in conditioner with natural butters.

Hair Type

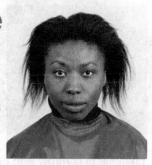

- Texture—highly textured, fine, dense
- Curl pattern—small loops and spirals, coiled ends
- Hair condition—dry, dull

The Afro Weave and the Mixed Texture Afro Weave continued

Procedure

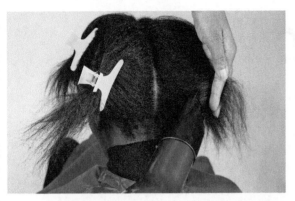

1 After hair prep and steam treatment, detangle with wide-toothed comb. Divide into four manageable sections and blowdry with nozzle comb.

2 Prepare human hair on tray.

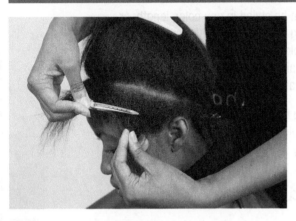

3 Following the contours of the hairline, leave out a ½-inch (1.3-cm) section of hair around the nape of neck and perimeter of hair line from ear to ear. Use a clip to secure hair left out around the perimeter.

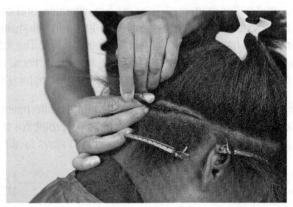

4 Starting at the nape, above the ear, create a horizontal ¼-inch (0.6-cm) wide section. Add a small amount of synthetic hair to the natural hair, and cornrow across back of head.

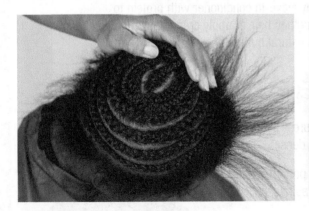

5 Continue to cornrow with the hair in a circular pattern until all the natural hair is braided. Extend cornrow past the scalp, and braid behind the length of natural hair.

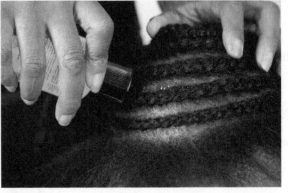

6 Add oil to the scalp.

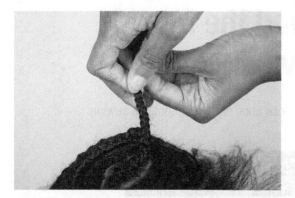

7 Extend cornrow on scalp, and braid it after the length of natural hair.

8 Secure all braided ends with needle and cotton thread. Tuck the ends down into cornrow; sew braided ends to base of cornrow. Cut thread and any excess hair.

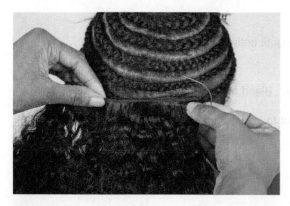

9 Braid and sew attaching method: Starting at the back, place human hair weft (track) on top of the length of cornrow.

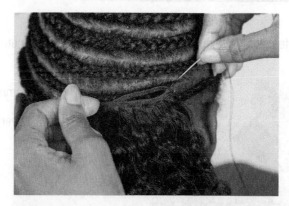

10 Gently push double-threaded needle through the base or track, also known as the braided cornrow, and connect it to the weft of human hair.

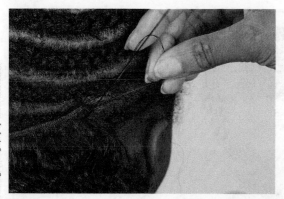

11 Pull the thread through the hair, creating a loop, and then pass the needle through loop a second time to secure the stitch. Make sure the stitch is flat and secure, but not tight.

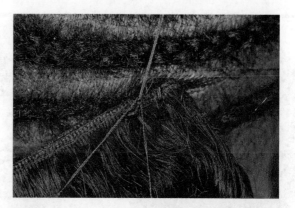

12 End sewing by looping thread several times or knotting.

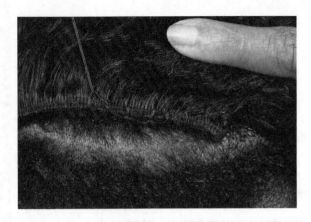

13 Cut all loose ends of thread. Continue sewing.

CAUTION

Excessive tension from this sewing process can cause breakage—or worse, traction alopecia.

14 Alternate colors or textures as desired. Continue sewing method until entire head is complete.

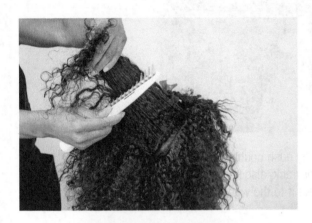

15 Comb out. Blend hair left out at perimeter.

16 Layer cut to desired length and shape.

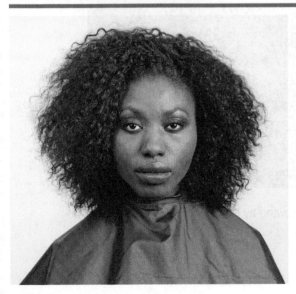

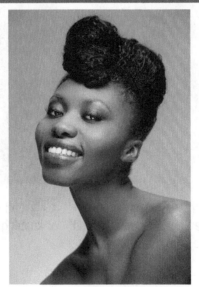

17 Finished style.

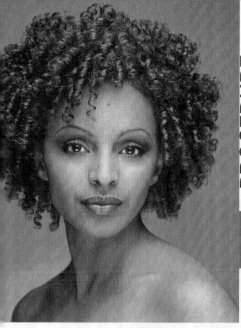

PROCEDURE
10-4
Flexi-Rod Set

Natural hair has its own inherent texture and quality. With the following sets, you can change, embellish, and elongate those qualities. Texture-on-texture sets are perfect for natural and transitional hair. These sets are low maintenance and require low manipulation. Depending on the hair type, they can be worn for up to four weeks.

Tools

- wide-toothed comb

- tail comb

- long duckbill clips

- spray bottle with detangling and moisturizing solution

- setting lotion

- steamer

- rods

- hood dryer

Hair Type

- Texture—soft curls, not very dense

- Curl pattern—medium spirals, curly ends

- Hair condition—dry, dull

Hair Prep

- To cleanse, use a sulfate- and surfactant-free moisturizing shampoo.

- Treat with deep moisturizing conditioner.

- Spray on leave-in conditioner with protein to strengthen hair.

- Steam scalp with steamer.

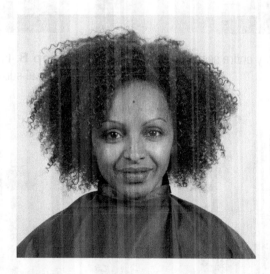

Procedure

1 Detangle hair with wide-toothed comb.

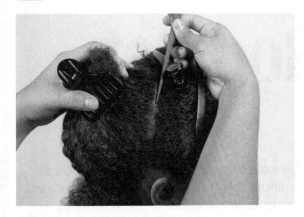

2 Divide hair from ear to ear, and divide front from back.

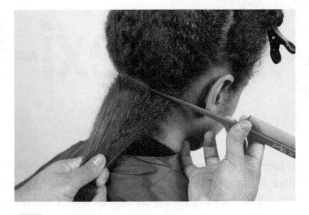

3 At the nape, part hair in a 1-inch (2.5-cm) horizontal section.

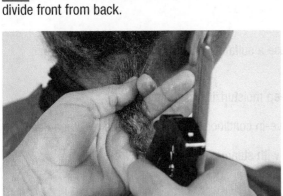

4 **Step A.** Spray entire section with setting solution.

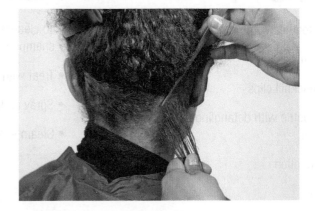

Step B. In this section, make ½-inch (1.3-cm) vertical subsections.

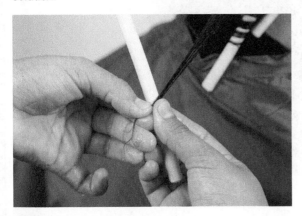

5 Wrap ends of hair around the bottom of the rod.

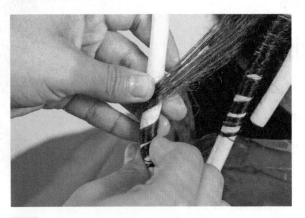

6 Move up the rod by making tight spirals; spiral hair up with each turn of the rod.

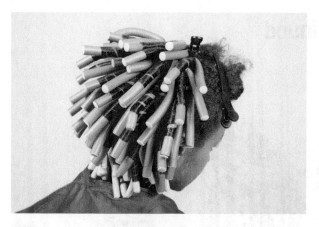

7 Continue throughout back of head, bricklaying as you repeat the spiraling method.

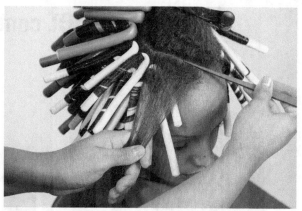

8 Repeat the same spiral method in front and crown sections. Part crown in the desired direction.

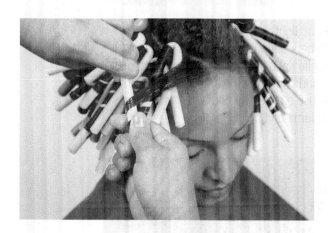

9 Directional subsections give finished style movement and dimension.

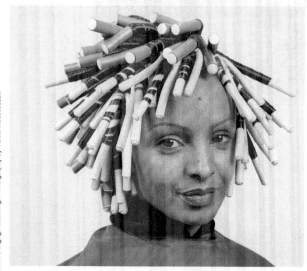

10 Set is complete. Saturate hair with setting solution. Place client under hood dryer. Hair must be completely dry.

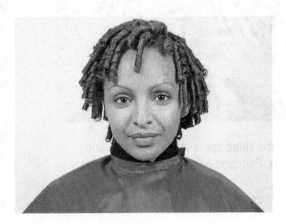

11 Once hair is dry, unwind rods, keeping each spiral in place.

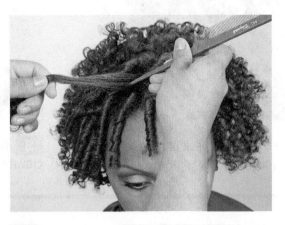

12 Place light natural oil or serum on the tips of fingers and, using the fingertips, apply serum while splitting open the spiral curls. After all curls have been opened to the desired fullness, use a small tail comb or lifting comb to add volume and height.

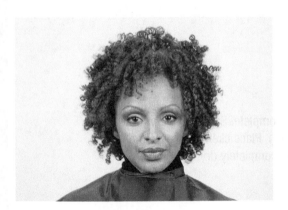

13 Finished style.

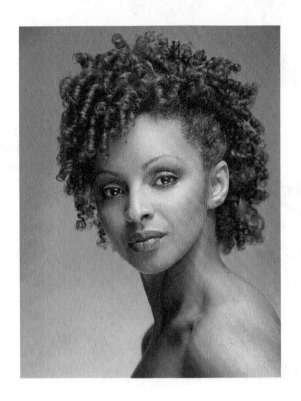

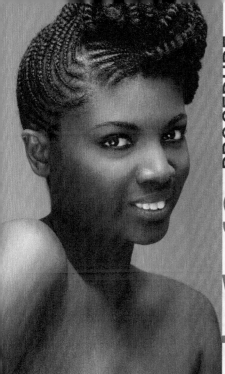

10-5

Sculpted Cornrows with Feed-in Technique

There are many techniques for starting the traditional on-the-base braid known as the cornrow. The cornrow is a three-strand, on-the-scalp braid created by using an underhand "pickup" technique. According to master braid designer Anu Prestonia, co-owner of Khamit Kinks in New York and celebrity master braid designer, cornrows are the foundation of all braiding styles. (Her clients include such notables as Stevie Wonder and Angela Basset.) "If you excel at the art of cornrows, all other braiding techniques are at your disposal," says Prestonia.

To cornrow like a professional, you must practice and have patience. A skilled braider takes time every day to practice cornrows. Cornrowing is the repetition of the entire woven patterns; the sequence of weave patterns may vary and will determine the style. However, the series of revolutions are created by a simple, repetitive pickup motion. Practicing on a mannequin will help you develop speed, accuracy, and dexterity. Braid services can vary in time from two hours for a large braid to two days for a micro braid.

After mastering the basic cornrow technique, you can approach other braid styles with confidence. Cornrows are skillfully designed by sculpting the parted sections. Sculpting is more than just vertical or horizontal partings. When sculpting the braid, you must first visualize the finished look. This will allow you to create smooth and consistent curved partings that follow the contour of the head. The curve partings are a part of the design, so they must be neat and even. The more creative you are in designing the partings, the more beautiful the finished sculpted look will be. This contouring or sculpting is especially beautiful on small to medium-sized cornrows.

Tools

- 5 butterfly clips
- 8 oz. synthetic hair
- wide-toothed comb
- tail comb
- long duckbill clips

- hairpins
- spray bottle with detangling and moisturizing solution
- shears
- waxy gel
- blowdryer with nozzle comb attachment

Hair Prep

- To cleanse, use a sulfate- and surfactant-free moisturizing shampoo.

- Treat with deep moisturizing conditioner.

- Spray leave-in conditioner with protein to strengthen hair.

Hair Type

- Texture—coily to highly textured, very dense

- Curl pattern—medium coils, tight coiled ends

- Hair condition—healthy but dry and lacks sheen

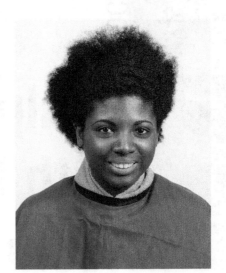

Procedure

1 Detangle client's hair. Blowdry with nozzle comb attachment to elongate.

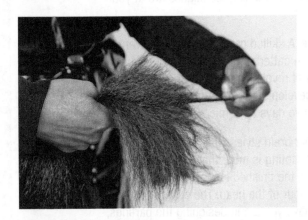

2 Part synthetic hair in half. Stretch hair to taper.

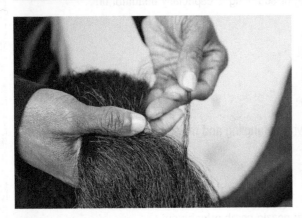

3 Smooth hair.

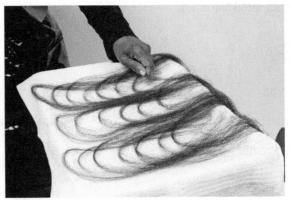

4 Separate and prepare extension hair.

5 Starting at the nape, part hair in a forward direction, ending above the left ear.

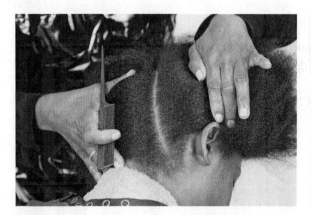 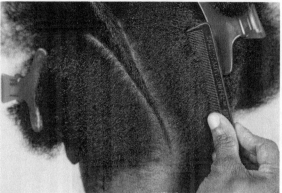

6 Part hair with clean contoured parts to create a sculpted movement.

7 Partings are ¼ inch (0.6 cm) or smaller, depending on the density and length of hair.

---

8 At the nape, start cornrow with natural hair. Pick up and divide into three equal strands.

9 Begin cornrow by moving outside-right strand under the center strand to become the new center strand.

10 Now, move the outside-left strand under center to become the new center. With each crossing under or rotation, pick up hair strands from scalp base.

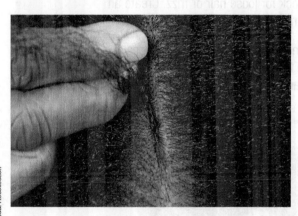

11 Pick up hair strands from directly under your finger. Passing the strand under the center with each rotation creates the underhand cornrow braid. Hydrate hair as needed.

12 Do not overdirect hair. Overdirected hair adds tension to the scalp, creates stress on the hair and scalp, and promotes breakage.

13 After four to eight rotations, introduce hair fiber by placing the extensions on the inside strand and leaving the outside strand of the extension to be picked up at the next rotation.

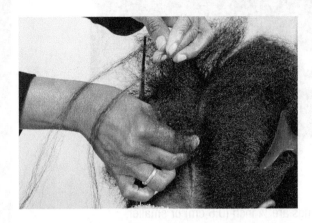

14 Continue to feed the extension into the cornrow until the desired width and length are achieved.

15 Contour and sculpt cornrows over to left side of crown. Continue to create asymmetrical cornrow until crown is reached.

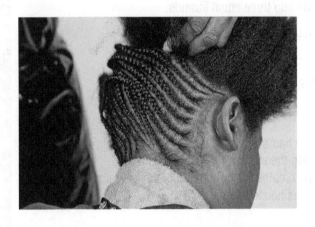

16 Proceed to braid or two strand twist excess extension to ends.

17 With a scissor, groom each braid. Move up braid slowly. Avoid cutting into braid.

18 Check for loose hair or frizz. Create an asymmetrical stuffed bun with extensions.

19 If more height is desired, add pieces of extension fiber to fill in bun. Apply natural botanical oils to scalp, and use waxy gel to keep all hair in place.

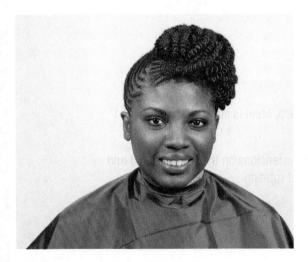

20 Finished style.

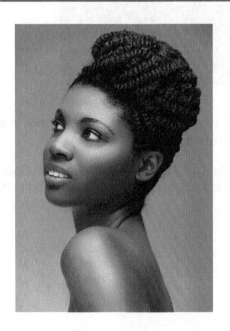

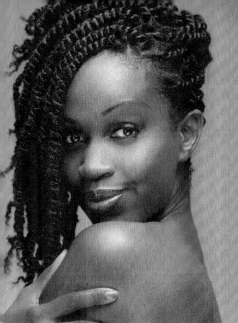

PROCEDURE

10-6
Large Twist Extensions

This twisted style provides a soft, romantic silhouette that adds length and volume with synthetic fiber. It's great as a protective style for natural hair and excellent as a transitional style.

Tools

- 5 butterfly clips
- wide-toothed comb
- tail comb
- long clips
- spray bottle with detangling and moisturizing solution
- shears
- steamer
- blowdryer with nozzle comb attachment
- moisturizing cream

Hair Prep

- To cleanse, use a sulfate- and surfactant-free moisturizing shampoo.
- Treat with deep moisturizing conditioner.
- Spray on leave-in conditioner with protein to strengthen hair.

Hair Type

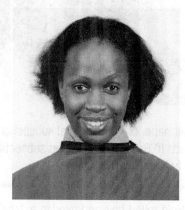

- Texture—highly textured, very dense
- Curl pattern—tight coils
- Hair condition—healthy but dry; lacks sheen

Procedure

1 After hair prep and steam treatment, detangle with wide-toothed comb.

2 Apply moisturizing cream to wet hair.

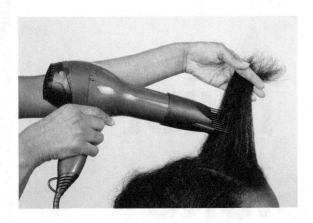

3 Blowdry hair and divide into five manageable sections.

4 Prepare hair fiber for easy distribution.

5 Starting at the nape, make a diagonal 45-degree part that goes from the top of the ear to the bottom of the nape.

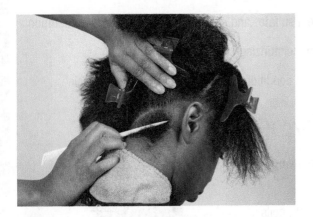

6 At nape, create diagonal subsections. Part hair in ¼-inch (0.6-cm) sections and subsections to create fullness.

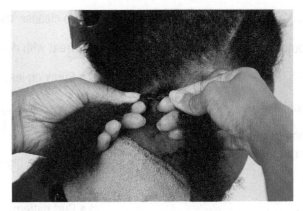

7 Divide the subsection into two equal parts. Lay extension flat on the base, and anchor the twist by rolling the extension onto the base.

8 Hold rolled hair and overlap extension between thumb and first two fingers.

9 The roll-overlap-roll movement anchors the twist and blends the natural hair into the extension.

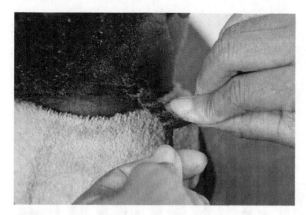

10 Continue down the twist with overlapping movement.

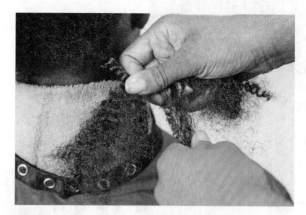

11 To lengthen twists, add equal amounts of extension to twist. Place extension fiber on top of two strands, pushing the extension up as you roll.

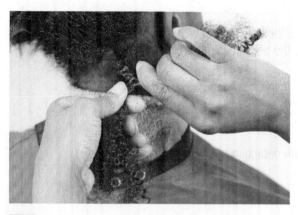

12 Repeat the roll-overlap-roll sequence for several revolutions.

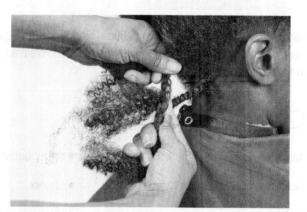

13 Next return to the basic twist movement, which has less tension and gives the twist a fuller finish.

14 Continue until the entire head is complete. Use scissors to groom and trim twists.

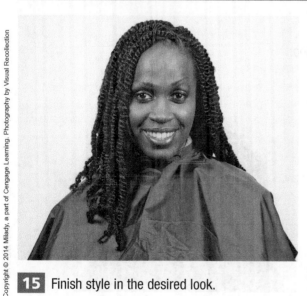

15 Finish style in the desired look.

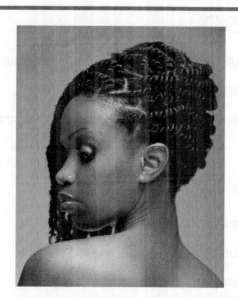

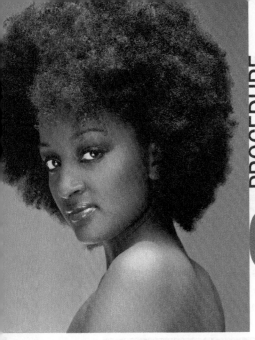

10-7

Crochet Weave

The goddess weave is current and distinctive. This full-head weave is ideal for clients wishing to protect their natural hair by giving it a rest from styling manipulation. Weaves are the perfect solution, while making the transition from a relaxer.

Tools

- 8 oz. packs of textured synthetic hair
- latch-hook needle and cotton thread
- 5 butterfly clips
- wide-toothed comb
- tail comb
- long clips

- spray bottle with detangling and moisturizing solution
- shears
- thinning shears
- blowdryer with nozzle comb attachment
- light herbal oil

Hair Prep

- To cleanse, use a sulfate- and surfactant-free moisturizing shampoo.
- Treat with deep moisturizing conditioner.
- Spray on leave-in conditioner with protein to strengthen hair, and apply cream-based leave-in conditioner with natural butters.

Hair Type

- Texture—hair in transition, fragile, spit ends
- Curl pattern—medium tight coils
- Hair condition—healthy new growth, relaxed ends dry; trimming required

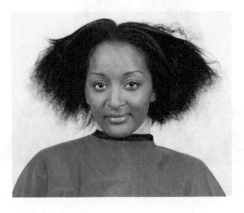

Procedure

1 Detangle and blowdry client's hair with nozzle comb to elongate hair.

2 Prepare extension hair by cutting to the desired length.

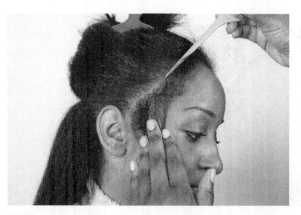

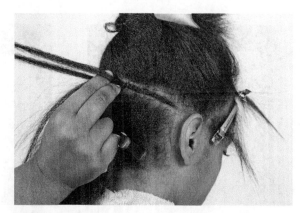

3 Following the contours of the hairline, leave out a ½-inch (0.3-cm) section of hair around perimeter from ear to ear. Use a clip to secure hair left out around the perimeter.

4 Starting at the nape, above the ear, create a horizontal ¼-inch (0.6-cm) wide section. Add a small amount of synthetic hair to natural hair, and cornrow across back of head.

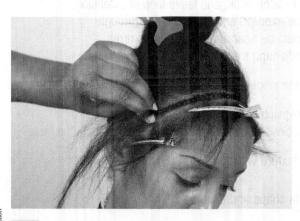

CAUTION

Be careful not to overextend or elongate the hair at a part. Pick up hair directly from under your finger. Failure to do so could cause breakage.

5 Extend cornrow past scalp, and braid behind for the length of natural hair.

---

6 Continue to cornrow with synthetic hair in a zigzag pattern until all the natural hair is braided.

7 Secure all braided ends with needle and cotton thread. Tuck the ends down to cornrow; then sew braided ends to base of cornrow.

8 Cut any excess hair.

Latch-Hook Method

9 Insert the latch hook into the middle of cornrow until entire latch is seen from the other side.

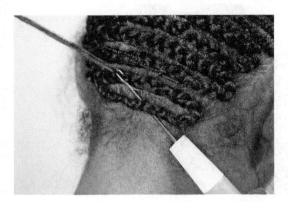

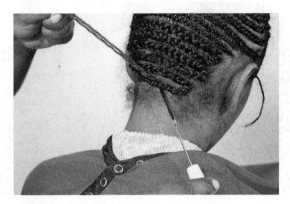

10 Place small amount of hair inside latch hook.

11 Pull latch hook through until a loop of the extension is formed.

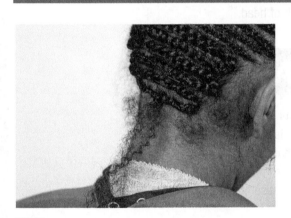

12 Remove latch hook, and leave loop of extension open. Pull two exposed ends of extension through loop. Loop must be near and secure on cornrow. Extension ends hang freely.

13 Continue looping movement throughout the entire head.

14 For a highlighted appearance, place lighter textured synthetic hair close to hairline, crown, and sides to frame the face.

15 Open texture with fingers, and lift with small pick.

16 Use thinning shears to remove bulk. Cut with scissors to create shape and contour.

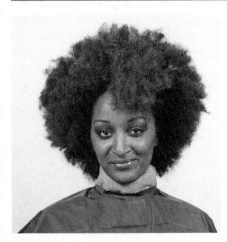

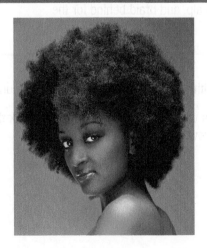

17 Style for desired finished look.

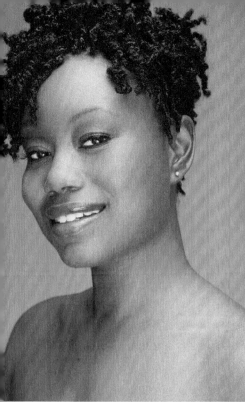

10-8

Coils and Twist Extensions

This exotic tribal style has a fresh, urban feel. This combination style is great for clients who want to protect their natural hair or for transitional clients, where knots on the relaxed ends may be stressful.

Tools

- 2 oz. Afro kinky bulk hair
- 5 butterfly clips
- wide-toothed comb
- tail comb
- long duckbill clips
- hairpins and bobby pins

- spray bottle with detangling and moisturizing solution
- shears
- holding gel and stretching cream
- blowdryer with nozzle comb attachment
- hood dryer

Hair Prep

- To cleanse, use a sulfate- and surfactant-free moisturizing shampoo.
- Pretreat hair with deep moisturizing conditioner and botanical oil treatment.
- Spray on leave-in conditioner with protein to strengthen hair, and apply cream-based leave-in conditioner with natural butters.

Copyright © 2014 Milady, a part of Cengage Learning. Photography by Visual Recollection

Natural Hair and Braid-Sculpting Techniques   Chapter 10   **255**

Coils and Twist Extensions continued

Hair Type

- Texture—coily, highly textured, dense

- Curl Pattern—small coils; fine; tight coiled ends

- Hair condition—healthy but dry; lacks sheen

Procedure

1 Detangle and blowdry with nozzle comb to elongate hair.

2 Clip hair into three distinct sections.

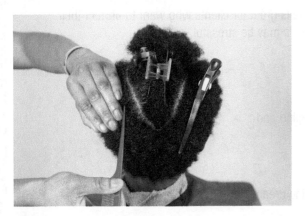

3 Part crown section into V shape. The point of the section starts at the back of crown.

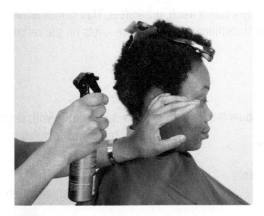

4 Spray on setting lotion with gloss.

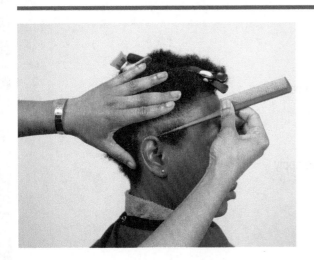

5 Part from hairline to top of the ear, starting above the ear using a ½-inch (1.3-cm) section and parting diagonally from ear to nape. Coils will lie from front to back.

6 Apply waxy gel to subsection; comb gel through for even distribution.

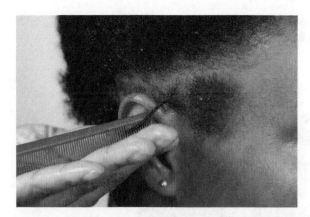

7 Roll and twist hair into a solid cylinder with comb.

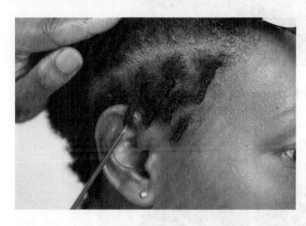

8 Continue parting from the hairline to nape, diagonally coiling in ⅛-inch (3.5-mm) subsections in vertical bricklaying technique.

Optional: Either counterclockwise or clockwise twisting is acceptable.

9 Trim extension and twist hair in direction of desired coil.

10 Continue until you reach the other side of the nape. Rehydrate hair as needed. Begin on opposite side at the nape, diagonally coiling hair into ⅛-inch (3.5-mm) vertical bricklaying sections and connecting left side to complete the V shape.

11 Add twist extension with synthetic hair (refer to braid-twist procedure).

12 Braid the front in the desired direction with ⅛-inch (3.5-mm) diagonal bricklaying parting.

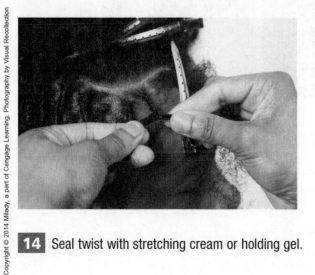

13 After four or five braid rotations, split middle and divide into two equal parts and twist.

14 Seal twist with stretching cream or holding gel.

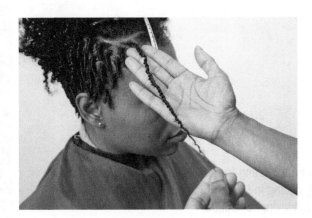

15 Twist down length of hair.

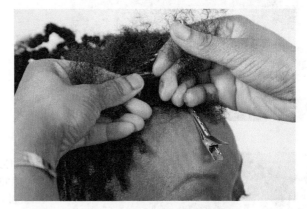

16 Continue until crown is complete.

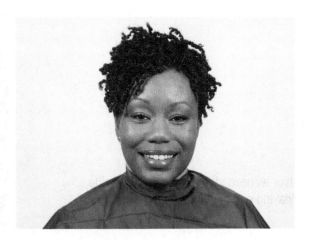

17 Finished style.

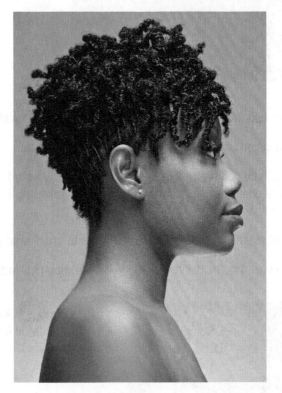

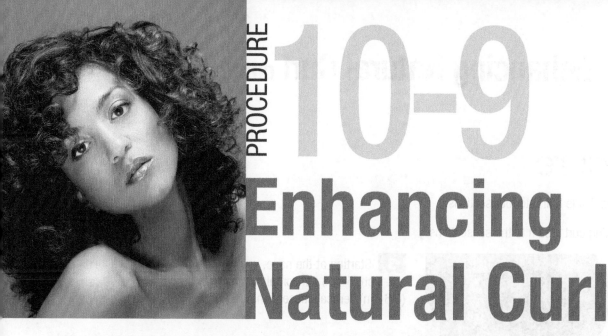

PROCEDURE 10-9

Enhancing Natural Curl

This natural style has cascading ringlets that can range from easy day styling to elegant evening chic. These crisp spiral curls add fullness and dimension to layered cuts. To keep the winding curls crisp and free from frizz, select products that offer to redefine texture, smooth and hydrate the hair, and reduce frizz.

Tools

- natural-curl–enhancing products
- setting spray
- hydrating curl cream
- 5 butterfly clips
- tail comb
- lifting comb
- long duckbill clips
- bobby pins
- hood dryer

Hair Prep

- To cleanse, use a sulfate- and surfactant-free moisturizing shampoo.
- Treat with moisturizing/detangling/curl-enhancing conditioner.
- Spray on leave-in conditioner with protein to strengthen hair.

Hair Type

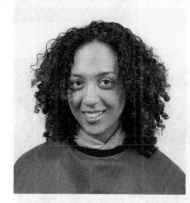

- Texture—curly, dense
- Curl pattern—large corkscrew, spiraled ringlets
- Hair condition—healthy, shoulder length, lacks sheen

Copyright © 2014 Milady, a part of Cengage Learning. Photography by Visual Recollection

Natural Hair and Braid-Sculpting Techniques   Chapter 10   **259**

Procedure

1 Detangle and divide hair into four sections.

2 Apply hydrating curl cream to the subsections.

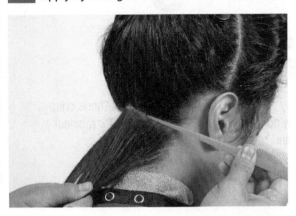

3 Starting at the nape, you will begin to take a 2-inch (5-cm) horizontal section with ¼-inch (0.6-cm) vertical subsections.

4 After curl cream has been distributed, create a finger curl.

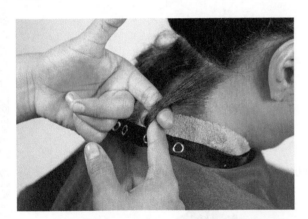

5 Begin to whirl or wrap strands around finger. Continue to roll up the shaft with each rotation, forming a barrel ½ inch (1.3 cm) from base; then pin curl to itself for closure.

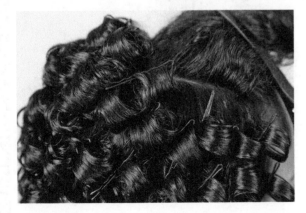

6 Continue to move up to the crown on both sides. Set the hair in the desired direction.

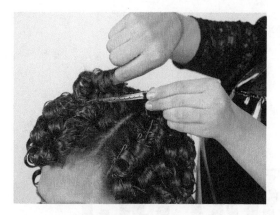

7 Spray with setting spray and add duckbill clips to add height. Place under a hood dryer.

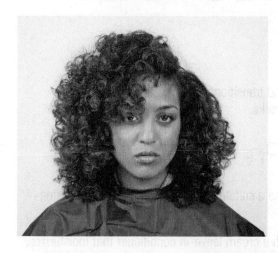

8 Finished style.

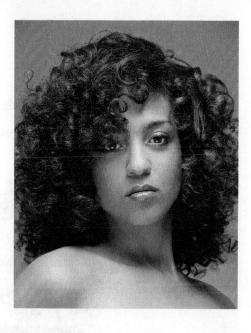

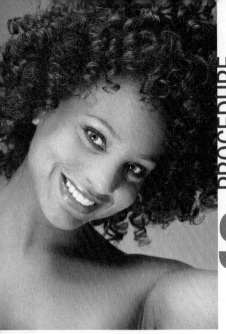

10-10
Spiral Rod Set

The prestige spirals curls are the new classic hairstyle for both natural and transitional clients. This impressive style can transform any texture into crisp, swirling tendrils that last for weeks.

Tools

- natural-curl–enhancing products
- large orange perm rods
- 5 butterfly clips
- wide-toothed comb
- tail comb or lifting comb
- long duckbill clips
- setting lotion
- end wraps
- blowdryer with nozzle comb attachment
- hood dryer

Hair Prep

- To cleanse, use a sulfate- and surfactant-free moisturizing shampoo.
- Treat hair with a cream leave-in conditioner that moisturizes, detangles, and enhances curl.

Hair Type

- Texture—curly
- Curl pattern—spiraled ringlets, front straighter and finer
- Hair condition—dry, lacks sheen

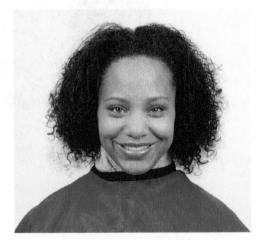

Procedure

1 Detangle hair and divide into five sections. Clip for control.

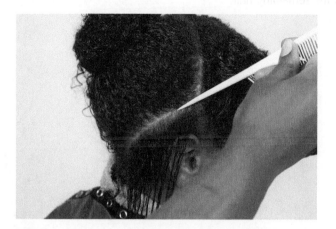

2 Starting at the nape, on a 45-degree angle, make a ½-inch (1.3-cm) diagonal part with ¼-inch (0.6-cm) subsection.

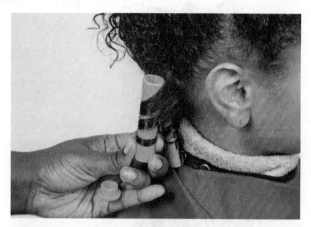

3 At the base of subsection, place setting lotion on strands and begin to whirl or wrap strands around the rod, moving down the shaft with each rotation.

4 Continue to move up to crown on both sides, maintaining ¼-inch (0.6-cm) subsections.

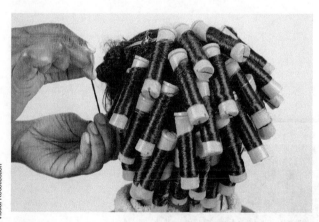

5 Continue parting into ¼-inch (0.6-cm) subsections.

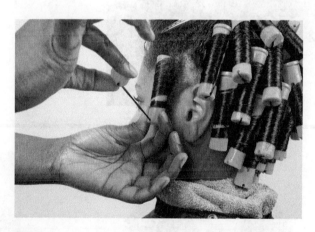

6 Inside 1-inch (2.5-cm) front sections, continue ¼-inch (0.6-cm) subsection vertical parting until you reach crown.

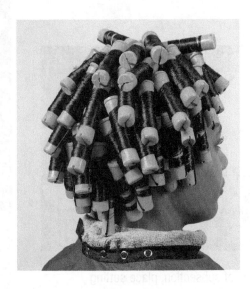

7 Complete the remaining hair.

8 Place under dryer. Allow curl enhancer to penetrate and set hair. When hair is completely dry, remove rods.

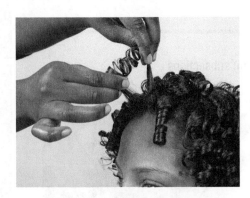

9 Separate curls to add fullness and height. When separating the curl, apply oil or serum to add shine, close cuticle, and decrease frizz.

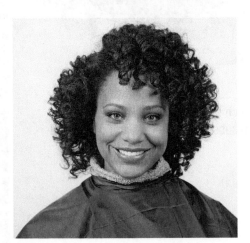

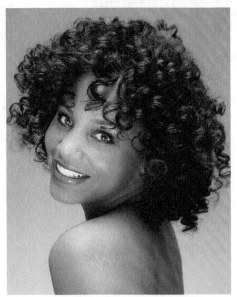

10 Style as desired. Finished look.

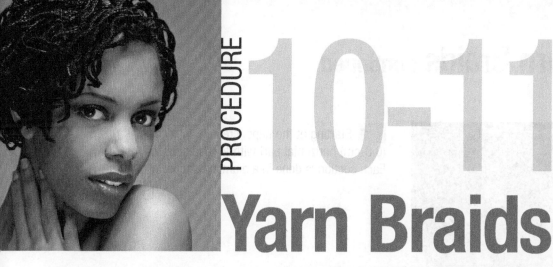

10-11
Yarn Braids

Yarn braids are single braids created with yarn as the extension. They are considered a loc alternative or loc extension. Clients enjoy the style because of its aesthetics and the benefit of the look of locs without the permanent commitment. This pixie style is excellent on short natural hair or short transitional hair.

Tools

- yarn: black or brown precut to desired length
- 4 butterfly clips
- wide-toothed comb
- tail comb
- long duckbill clips
- steamer
- shears

Hair Type

- Texture—relaxed/transitioning
- Curl Pattern—highly textured
- Hair Condition—very dry, brittle, lacks sheen

Hair Prep

- To cleanse, use a sulfate- or surfactant-free moisturizing shampoo.
- Treat with moisturizing/detangling/curl-enhancing conditioner.
- Spray on leave-in conditioner.
- Apply natural botanical oil.

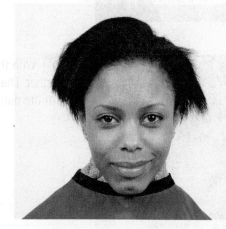

Procedure

1 Prepare hair for braid. After hair prep and steam treatment, detangle with wide-toothed comb and divide into five manageable sections.

2 Blowdry with nozzle comb attachment.

3 Prepare hair fiber for easy distribution. Precut yarn before braiding.

4 Cut yarn slightly longer than hair. This leaves room to finish ends.

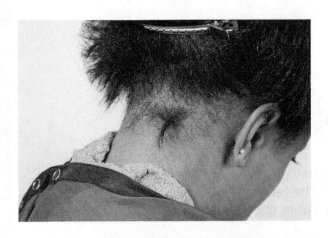

5 Starting at the nape, create a ¼-inch (0.6-cm) horizontal part with ¼-inch subsections. Each section is done in a diamond shape.

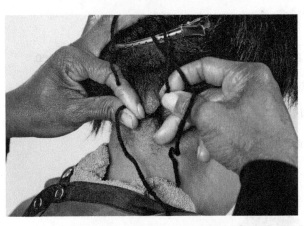

6 Pick up two pieces of yarn from precut pile. Hold yarn in the center, pick up parted-off section of hair, and create three sections (center, left, and right).

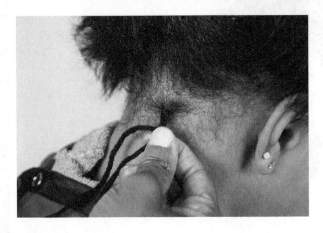

7 With the three sections, braid the yarn and hair together. The stitch of the braid must be very tight to form the natural curve.

8 Continue to braid to your desired length.

9 Remember that for a pixie, every other row should lie on top of another to create depth and layers (bricklaying technique).

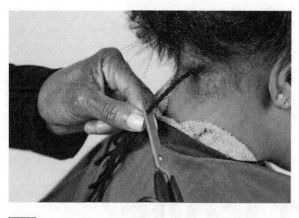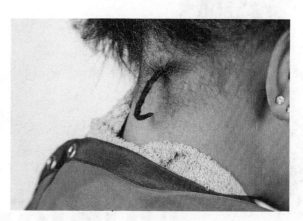

10 Cut to desired length and then finish ends.

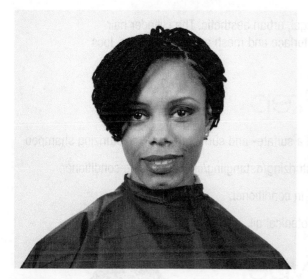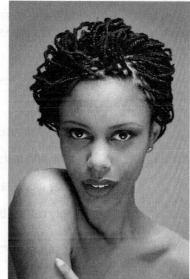

11 Finished style.

How to Finish the Ends of Yarn Braids

Yarn braids can be finished by knotting, melting with a heat source, or tying them off with a small rubber band.

CAUTION

When finishing the ends of yarn braids, use of an open flame is prohibited in hair salons in most states. Using an open flame will place you and your client at risk for a burn and burning acrylic yarn can also release toxic flumes. Check with your state regulatory board before using any type of open flame in the salon.

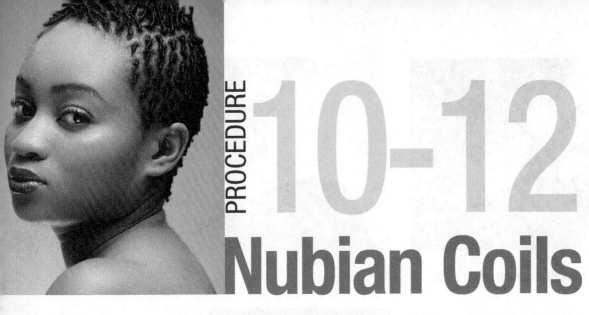

10-12
Nubian Coils

This tribal, natural hairstyle makes a beautiful statement with its regal, urban aesthetic. The cylinder hair formations catch the eye with swirling movement. As these coils interlace and mesh as separate units, locs are formed. Coils are a great way to transition into locs.

Tools

- holding gel
- sulfate- and surfactant-free moisturizing shampoo
- moisturizing/detangling/curl-enhancing conditioner
- leave-in conditioner
- natural botanical oil
- 4 butterfly clips
- wide-toothed comb
- barber's comb
- long duckbill clip
- hood dryer

Hair Prep

- To cleanse, use a sulfate- and surfactant-free moisturizing shampoo.
- Treat with moisturizing/detangling/curl-enhancing conditioner.
- Spray on leave-in conditioner.
- Apply natural botanical oil.

Hair Type

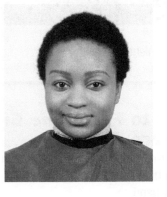

- Texture—wiry, highly textured
- Curl pattern—tight small, coils/zigzag
- Hair condition—very dry, brittle, lacks sheen

Procedure

1 Detangle and divide hair into two sections.

2 Clip for control.

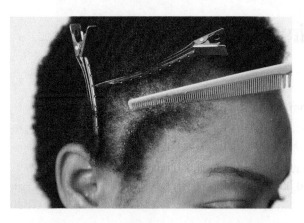

3 To create movement, start at the hairline and create a ¼-inch (0.6-cm) crescent shape part with smaller end of comb. Apply gel to tip.

4 Comb gel through strands of crescent subsection. At the base, start to rotate or roll-comb down the hair shaft to the end. Hair is curled toward the end, and the coil lies flat.

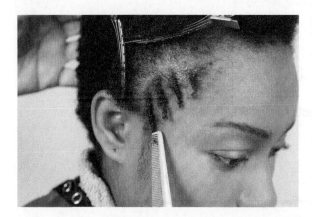

5 Place coils by using comb. Twirl subsection in direction coil will lay.

6 As you move up the head, start to create a sculpting movement that features the contour of the head.

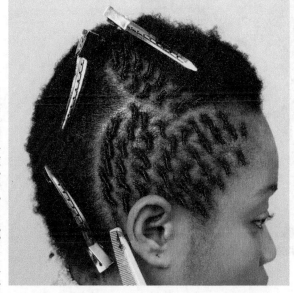

7 Movement can be in multiple directions with different channels for dimension.

8 Coiling movement on the front and sides is a continuation from the back section. Make sure to diminish any parts that divide the back from the front.

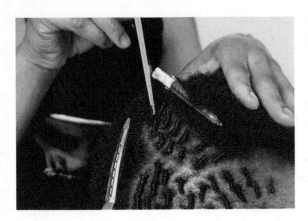

9 Style will have one continuous movement from front to back.

10 Continue coil movement at crown, keeping contours and directions of coil uniform.

11 While front coils are still damp, fine-tune. Create a soft bang.

12 Place client under hood dryer. Add oil for more sheen.

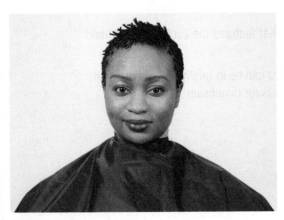

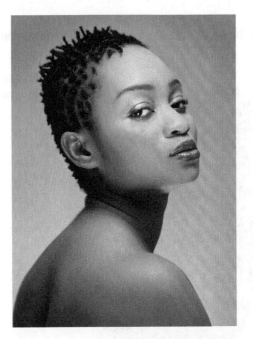

13 Finished style.
(Optional: Open coils for more fullness.)

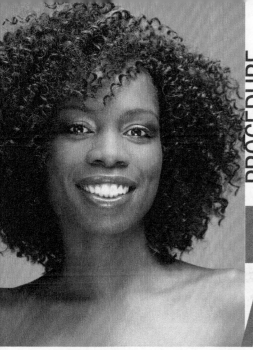

10-13

Making and Applying Wigs

Wigs are the new accessory. They are perfect as a fashion statement alternative or a temporary hairstyling option. They can reflect your client's mood or complement the suit she is wearing. Traditionally, wigs express social or religious status in African society. In our contemporary culture, wigs are beautifying—they embellish and conceal unhealthy hair. For clients who are in transition, a wig is a great way to contain and cover broken or damaged relaxed hair. Wigs are also a wonderful alternative for natural hair, because they protect healthy hair from excessive styling manipulation. Important note: Clients should understand that the hair requires daily moisturizing products and professional steam treatments to keep it nourished if they wear wigs to transition or to conceal their natural hair. Always explain to the client that excessive wig wearing can erode the fragile hairline and lead to traction alopecia. To prevent hair breakage or thinning, it is imperative that the clients place a wig net on the head before the wig, which protects the natural hair, avoids hairline erosion, and allows the scalp to breathe.

Tools

- 8 oz. of human hair—curly mixed with wavy
- wig net
- pins
- fabric glue
- wig head
- weaving thread and curved needles

- spray bottle with detangling solution
- scissors
- shears
- hairpins or bobby pins
- blowdryer with diffuser attachment

Hair Prep

- To cleanse, use a sulfate- and surfactant-free moisturizing shampoo.
- Treat with deep moisturizing conditioner steam treatment.
- Spray on leave-in conditioner with protein to strengthen hair.
- Apply cream-based leave-in conditioner with natural butters.

10-13 **Making and Applying Wigs** continued

Hair Type

- Length—4 to 5 in. (10 to 13 cm), extension hair—14 in. (35 cm)

- Texture—highly textured, tight, dry

- Curl pattern of extension hair—spiral, deep waves

- Condition of extension hair—Colored and chemically treated to create curl pattern

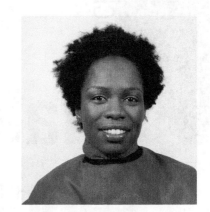

Procedure

1 Detangle and divide hair into four sections to blowdry.

2 Leave out ½ inch (1.3 cm) of hair around the hairline. Make ½-inch parts for cornrows.

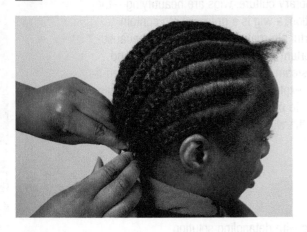

3 Cornrow hair without extensions, making six to eight sections from the front to the nape. Braid to the end and sew hair together at the nape.

4 Apply natural oil to scalp. Hair is now ready for wig.

Creating a Wig 101

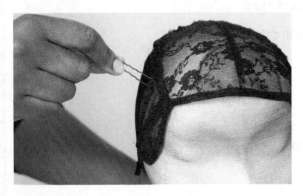

5 Place packaged wig net on wig head and secure with hair or wig pins.

6 Prepare hair: Open packages of hair and arrange in the order of desired color pattern.

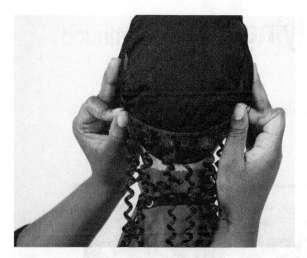

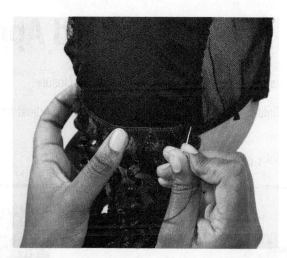

7 Starting at the back of the wig head, pin weft onto wig net to measure proper length.

8 Cut weft to desired length. Place weft facing down so that hair lies flat. Make sure weft is sewn on the correct side (stitching on wrong side reveals double folded hair, and shorter hairs are noticeable).

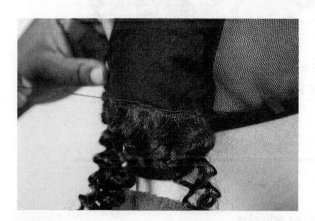

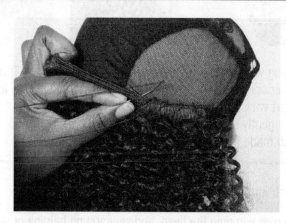

9 **Step A** Begin to sew by placing curved needle into folded section of weft on netting.

Step B Stitches are ¼ to ½ inch (0.6 cm to 1.3 cm) apart and are finished with a double loop.

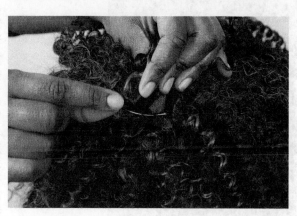

10 To create a closure: Take 6 inches (15 cm) of wefted hair and roll it onto itself.

11 Sew weft together and flatten with hands for closure.

12 Place finished wig on client's head for custom fit. Adjust back elastic hooks until cap is secure and comfortable.

13 Use bobby pins to secure sides while styling.

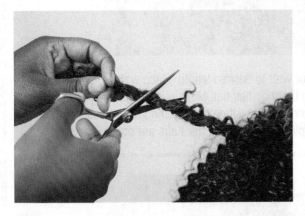

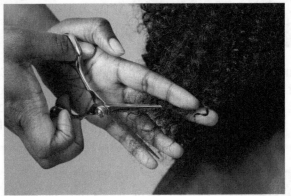

14 Thin wig with shears by gently rolling a small section of hair and inserting the shears and closing the blade part way, three times. Rack or comb out loose hair by gently removing excess hair with a paddle brush made for weaves.

15 Trim the wig hair as needed to create a shape suitable for your client.

16 Cut hair into layers.

17 Place new wig onto the head, and sew around hairline or secure with pins.

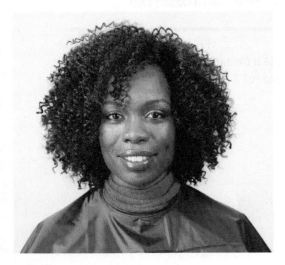

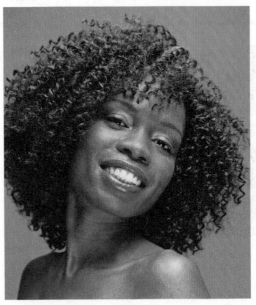

18 Finished look.

☑ LO3

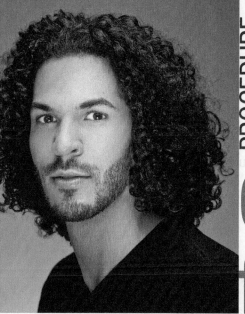

10-14
Curly Haircut for Men

Curls are not just for girls. Spiral, rich curls have become popular for men. Textured hair requires a good cut and quality products to maintain the curl and reduce frizz.

Tools

- curl enhancer and frizz control products
- blowdryer with nozzle comb attachment
- lift comb
- tail comb
- hairnet (optional)
- shears
- spray bottle

Hair Prep

- Shampoo with a mild conditioning shampoo or sulfate-free shampoo.
- Apply a light moisturizing conditioner.
- Spray on leave-in conditioner.

Hair Type

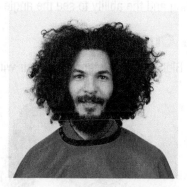

- Texture—small to large curls
- Length—shoulder length
- Curl pattern—varying spiral formations, frizz
- Condition—healthy but with split ends

Procedure

1 After shampoo, use a wide-toothed comb and draw conditioner through to ends.

2 Rinse out conditioner lightly, leaving some conditioner in hair.

3 Do not comb anymore. This will help reduce frizz and establish the natural curl pattern.

4 Blot-dry hair with cloth or paper towel.

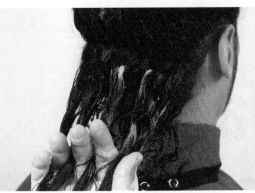

5 Apply silicone-free curl enhancer to hair: Taking 2-inch (5-cm) sections and with small amount of product on the fingertips, smoothly rack or "shingle" through hair. Be sure to apply enough product to the ends.

6 Repeat shingle movement, applying product throughout the head until entire head is complete. Scrunch hair by cupping hair in the palms of hands.

Cutting Curly Hair

- Cut curly hair dry. When wet, curly hair can be deceiving because of its elasticity; curly or wavy hair can appear to be longer when wet. When curly or wavy hair dries, it "shrinks" or springs back to its natural form and length.

- When cutting curly or wavy hair, never cut blunt or horizontal uniform lines for final cut. Cut hair vertically or diagonally under the curl to keep spiral movement.

- To cut curly or wavy hair, extend curl strands and cut underneath the "C" or "S" pattern of the texture. Do not cut midway through curl; this will make the strand stick out or have a hook effect. Make medium to long, tapered layers; this technique creates fullness without making hair look round. One length gives the hairstyle a heavy look.

- Please note: Cut coily, highly textured, wiry hair by elongating the texture using a blowdryer with a nozzle comb attachment first. This helps extend the ends, unravel the tight strands, and allows for even, smooth hair texture for cutting and the ability to see the angle adjustment made during the cut.

The Curly Cut

7 Blot-dry hair. Detangle wet hair with fingers—this allows curls to form and separate.

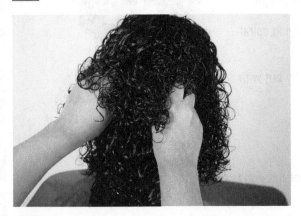

8 **Step A** Rack or shingle leave-in conditioner through to ends.

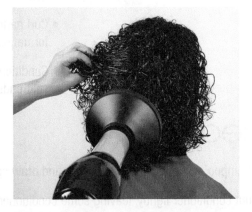

Step B Diffuse on medium heat and scrunch until dry to minimize frizz and define curls. Section hair into a U-shaped parting extending from eyebrow to eyebrow and the crown into a right and left section. Cut the perimeter at zero degrees using ½-inch subsections. When complete, re-section into three.

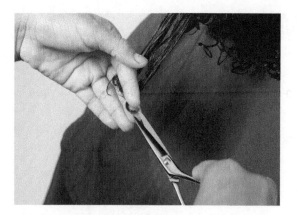

9 Starting at the back and holding the scissors at a 45-degree angle, gently extend single curls and cut ¼ inch (0.6 cm) of hair. Working your way around the head taking vertical subsections, cut hair at 45 degree layers.

10 Gently move hair from the base by lifting strands to see where it falls as well to check cutting lines and layers.

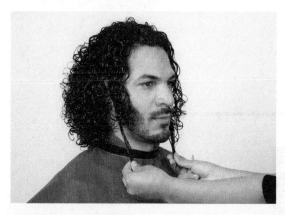

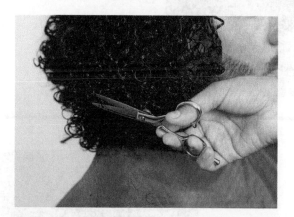

11 Gently pull curls out to see length and move over to the next curly section. If the client wants a tapered curl, cut curls diagonally, not straight across.

12 Continue to cut ¼ inch (0.6 cm) of hair on the diagonal, lifting and moving curls to check length.

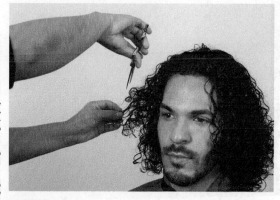

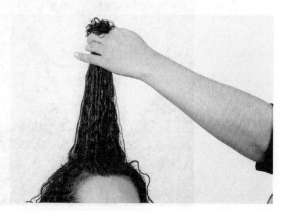

13 To add more layers, hold curl out around crown and see where hair falls in the same line to the previous curl.

14 Use that curl as a guide and cut desired length. The crown will be cut at 90 degrees. Do not cut crown sections too short. Keep layers around eyes and chin to create volume around face.

15 Open curls more to fine-tune cut and make hair fuller. Look for a consistent and even silhouette to frame the face.

16 Have client shake head to see if any curls fall out of place. Check and correct.

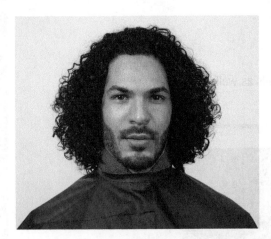

17 Finished style.

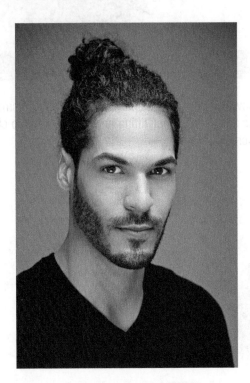

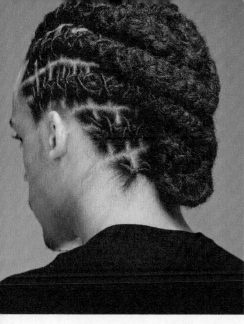

PROCEDURE

10-15

Loc Groom and Style for Men

Locked hair is the ultimate natural hair statement. If coily or highly textured hair is left to take its own natural course, the hair will interlace and mesh together to form a loc. These "organic" locs would not have a separated, groomed, or manicured finished appearance. Cultivated locs are interspaced, and they have symmetry and balance. Symmetry is not easy to accomplish with textured hair. Although the hair is programmed genetically to curl, twirl, and turn, no two coils are exactly alike. It is the loctician or natural stylist's responsibility to develop a system that promotes symmetry into the textured hair. There are several ways to groom locs. The comb technique is an effective system for loc grooming.

Tools

- tapered barber's comb—#55
- French pins or hairpins
- water-soluble gel
- steamer
- natural herbal oil
- 5 butterfly clips
- box of small double-pronged roller clips

Hair Type

- Texture—wavy, coily
- Length—below shoulder
- Curl pattern—varying spiral formations
- Condition—dry, requires deep moisture treatment with steam

Hair Prep

- Shampoo—sulfate-free shampoo.
- Conditioner—natural oil and light moisturizing conditioner with steamer.
- Herbal rinse—use botanicals that soothe the scalp.

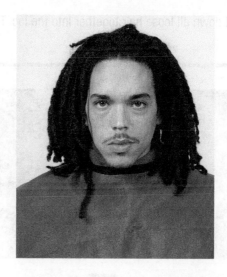

Procedure

1 After prep, towel-dry locs.

2 Apply oil to scalp and length of loc to seal in moisture.

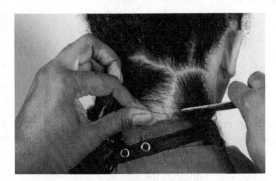

3 Starting at the base, use larger end of barber's comb to square off loc.

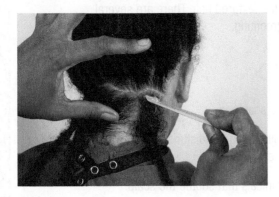

4 Apply gel to comb. Place small amount of gel at new growth base.

5 With comb and gel, pull down all loose hair together into the loc. This will compact the loose hair and help build the loc base.

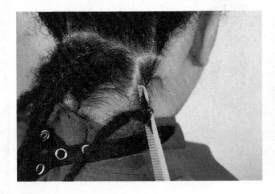

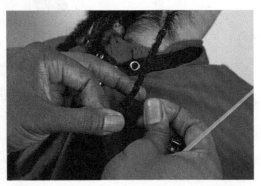

6 Rotate twice.

7 Remove comb. Wrap hair using index and thumb; then use your palm to roll down the loc.

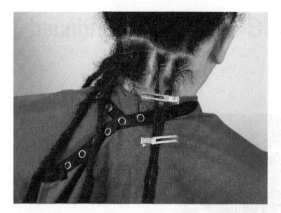

8 Clip sections as you complete each one.

CAUTION

The texture and amount of regrowth will determine if you should use your palm or fingers to smooth the loc. Using your fingers on shorter locs will make the locs neat and tight. Palm rolling with the palms of your hands are reserved for locs that are 4 inches (10 cm) or longer.

9 Place client under hooded dryer to reduce moisture and set locs in place with heat—locs are still damp.

Styling Locs

10 Starting above the ear, take 2-inch (5-cm) sections of loc, place outside loc, and wrap with inside loc for a inverted braid.

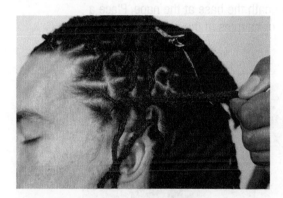

11 Continue picking up additional locs as you cross down the contour of the head to the occipital bone.

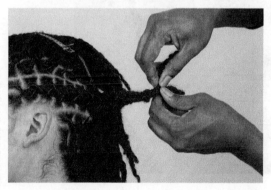

12 At the occipital lobe, split hair into three sections and braid to the end of the hair.

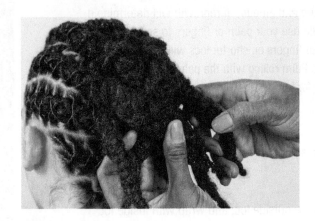

13 Starting at the crown, create a fishtail braid, crossing the outside and the inside sections over each other.

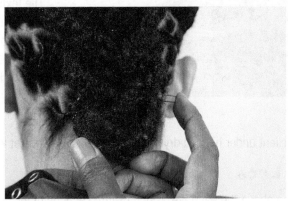

14 Continue moving down the head and then tuck ends underneath the base at the nape. Place a few French pins or hairpins in the hair to secure the tuck.

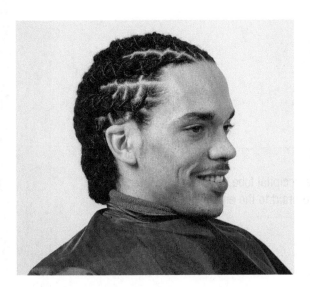

15 Finished style.

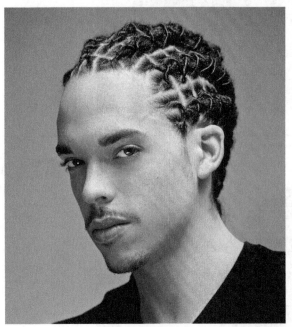

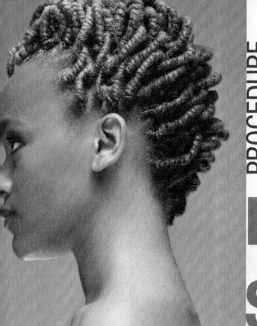

PROCEDURE

10-16

Loc Groom and Style for Women

Locked hair worn neat and groomed, whether conservatively or stylized, is a major commitment for most women. When locs are grown to a desired length, it is one of the most beautiful styles for showcasing a woman's crown and glory. Natural coily and highly textured hair can be unmanageable at times. Locs are ideal for these textures and allow clients to have more flexibility and versatility. Locking and grooming the hair give the client a long-lasting, fuss-free style that can be additionally stylized with curls, crimps, and updo styles.

Tools

- tapered barber's comb
- #55 pipe cleaners
- water-soluble gel
- steamer
- natural herbal oil
- 5 butterfly clips
- box of small double-pronged roller clips

Hair Type

- Texture—coily
- Length—mid-back length
- Curl pattern—varying spiral formations
- Condition—color-treated, dry, and requires deep moisture treatment

Hair Prep

- Shampoo—sulfate-free shampoo.
- Conditioner—natural oil and light moisturizing conditioner with steamer.
- Herbal rinse—use botanicals that soothe the scalp.

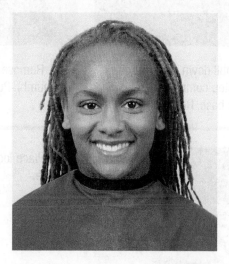

Procedure

1 After prep, towel-dry locs.

2 Apply oil to scalp and loc length to seal in moisture.

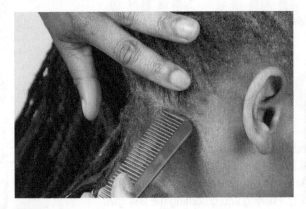

3 Starting at the base, use larger end of barber's comb to square off loc, creating a cleaner part.

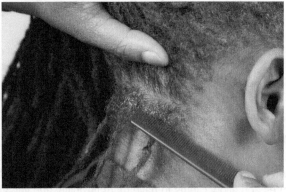

4 With the smaller end of comb, apply gel to comb. Place small amount of gel at new growth base.

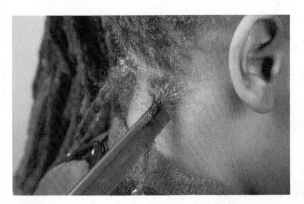

5 With comb and gel, pull down all loose hair together into the loc. This step compacts the loose hair and helps build the loc base. Rotate once.

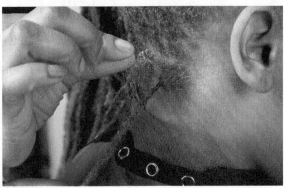

6 Remove comb using two fingers (index finger and thumb). Push loose hair.

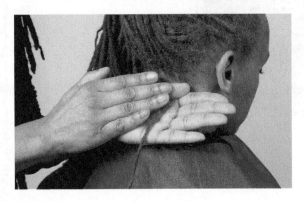

7 Place loc between palms. Rotate once or twice.

8 Smooth any remaining hair; gently press and rotate loc in palm with a back-and-forth motion.

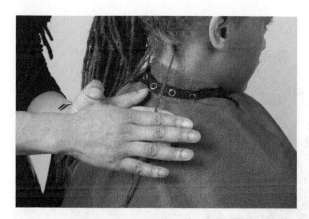

9 Move down loc to help smooth loose ends within the loc.

CAUTION

Avoid overtwisting. Base should remain flat and not crimped. Too much twisting thins out and damages hair.

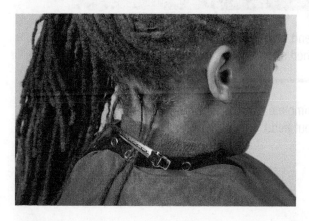

10 Clip sections as you complete.

11 Place client under hooded dryer. To reduce moisture, locs are still damp.

12 Apply pipe cleaners, one per loc. In a spiral motion, wrap pipe cleaners around loc.

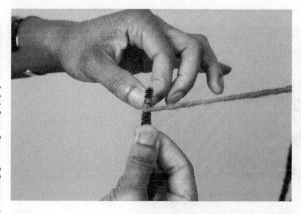
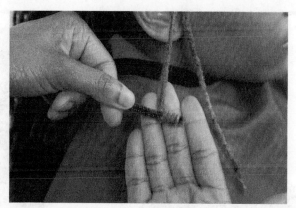

13 Depending on the length and density of the hair, one or two locs on each are needed.

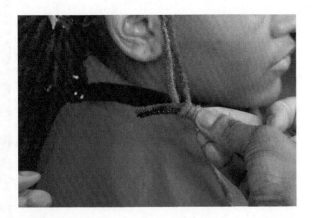

14 Trim or bend the excess pipe cleaner to complete wrapped loc.

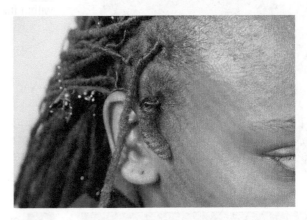

15 Bend wrapped locs in the direction you wish the finished style to flow.

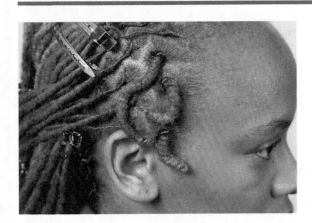

16 Complete the locs wrapped with pipe cleaners throughout head.

17 Place client under hooded dryer until locs are completely dry. Remove pipe cleaners and style.

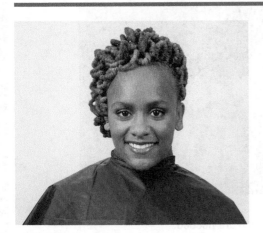

18 Finished style.

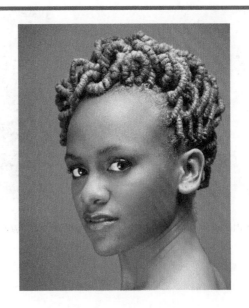

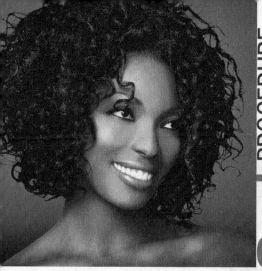

10-17
Transitional Haircut on Extensions

Being able to service style a client with extensions will broaden your abilities and client base. You should know how to give them a cut and style for the look they desire.

Tools

- curl enhancer/frizz-control products
- blowdryer with nozzle comb attachment
- lift comb
- tail comb
- hairnet (optional)
- shears
- spray bottle

Hair Prep

- Shampoo—mild conditioning shampoo or sulfate-free shampoo.
- Conditioner—light moisturizing conditioner.
- Leave-in conditioner.

Hair Type

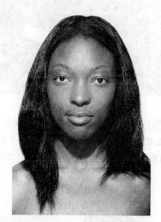

- Texture—small to large curls
- Length—shoulder length
- Curl pattern—varying spiral formations, frizz
- Condition—healthy but with split ends

Procedure

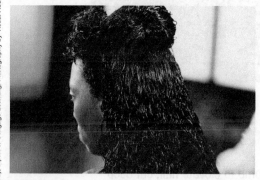

1 Isolate the top section in a horseshoe pattern, parting from temple to temple, just below the crown. To avoid pulling, use a wide-toothed comb when working with hair extensions.

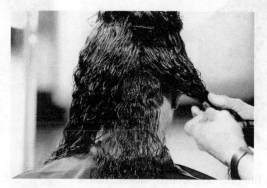

2 Section off the center back of the head by dividing into two sections.

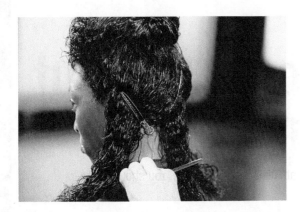

3 At the nape of neck, take a small diagonal section approximately 1 ½ inches (4 cm) in width.

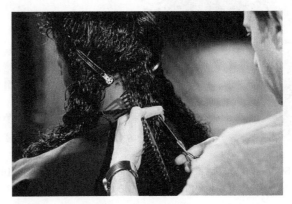

4 Elevate hair using one-finger elevation. Point-cut the guideline.

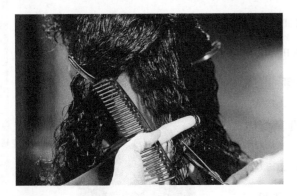

5 Mirroring your previous section, slightly increase elevation as you move up the head. Point-cut, working with very little tension on the hair.

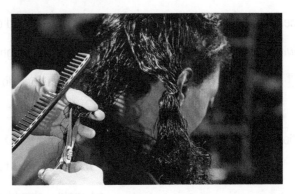

6 Take a small diagonal section to the top of the ear. The head is tilted slightly downward. Increase the elevation slightly higher than the previous. After finishing the haircut, check its balance and length.

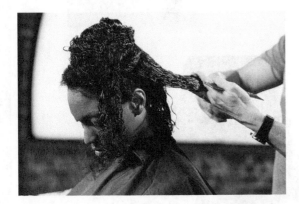

7 Mirroring the previous section, elevate hair to 45 degrees. Overdirect the hair above the back of the ear. Continue point cutting. Direct the hair at the sides to the back of the head and straight out from the temporal bone to increase side length.

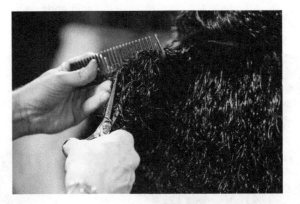

8 Using your comb to elevate hair, cut deep V's approximately 1 ½ inches (4 cm) into perimeter length, still elevating at 45 degrees.

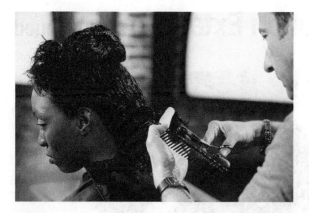

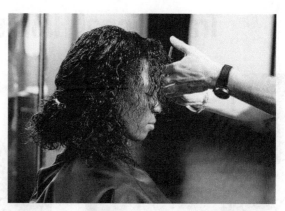

9 Drop the last subsection down (excluding the horseshoe-shaped section). Using very loose tension, point cut into the guideline length. Once the subsection is finished, check for balance.

10 Let the remaining horseshoe-shaped section drop down. Arrange the hair to the side that the client is going to wear it.

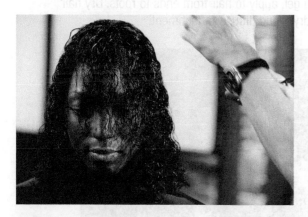

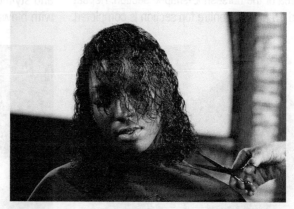

11 Using forward graduation, take about a 1- to 3-inch (1.3- to 8-cm) section from ear to ear. The size of the section depends on the thickness of the hair. Use wider sections for thicker hair. Take diagonal sections from the side parting.

12 Comb hair to the natural fall. Cut freehand to frame the face. Round off the corners.

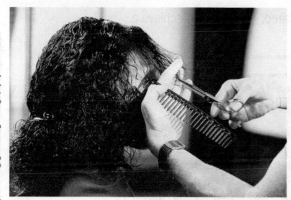

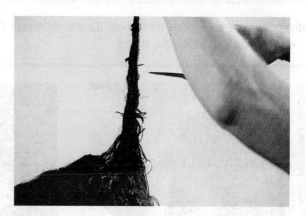

13 Using light tension, comb the hair down to frame the face around the fringe area.

14 Picking up a triangular section on top of the right crown area, twist the hair. Hold it straight up at 90 degrees. Cut random pieces of hair throughout the interior length of hair. Repeat step 14 on the top of the left crown area.

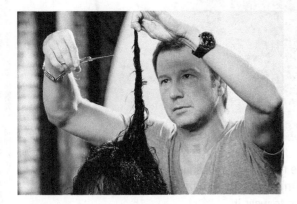

15 Take a third triangular section on the left front remaining area of the horseshoe-shaped section. Repeat steps 14 and 15 until the entire top section is completed.

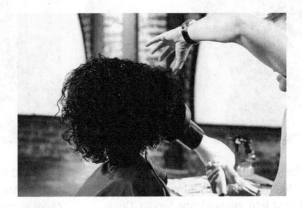

16 Using a mixture of smoothing balm, shine serum, and styling gel, apply to hair from ends to roots. Dry hair with blowdryer and diffuser attachment.

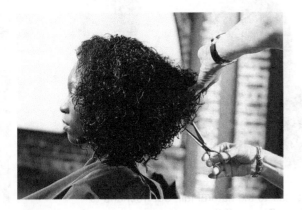

17 Randomly point-cut ends to emphasize the shape. Maintain disconnection.

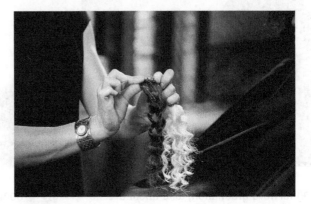

18 Prepare hair extensions in the desired color. Extensions should be 1 ½ inches (4 cm) in width. Sew a bobby pin or hair clip onto the extension.

19 Strategically place extensions throughout the hair wherever desired. The goal is to achieve a well-balanced look and emphasize the shape.

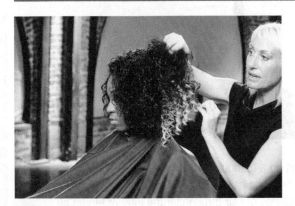

20 Finished style.

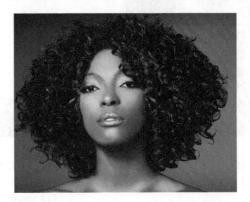

☑ **LO3**

Final Reflections

Healthy wavy, curly, coily, and highly textured hair has become the new aesthetic for textured hairstyling. The African American and the multi-textured hair markets are being fueled by the increasing demand for conditioning products for naturally textured hair. The largest segment of the natural hair care industry appears to be women who are in transition. They are looking for products and styles that minimize breakage, maximize growth, stop split ends, prevent dryness, and make the hair manageable. They also prefer products that are chemically free of harsh sulfates, parabens, propylene glycols, silicones, and petroleum. Women are looking for earth-friendly products and services that offer them the nurturing benefits of botanicals, natural oils, and butters to keep their hair healthy. As natural stylists, you can consult, guide, and service clients who are seeking transitional services to help them through these challenging times. After the client makes the transition and is totally natural, the natural stylist can offer a variety of products and services that embellish and maintain the varying textures.

Most of the clients who seek your services have used chemical relaxers since puberty. They have no idea what their natural hair texture looks like or how to address the needs of their hair type **(Figure 10–4)**. They search the Internet for Websites and blogs to get information and share hair and product experiences. Some information shared by consumers who are in transition provides only the essential elements for the individual "going natural." Therefore, the information communicated by the consumer-based market is often elementary or in some cases misleading. As a specialist, it is your responsibility to re-educate clients about their particular hair needs. The natural stylist must be proficient in several techniques and must be knowledgeable about various products to consult with clients and provide excellent services. Social media like YouTube, do-it-yourself bloggers, chat rooms, and product manufacturer's Websites all give this fast-growing industry a high profile.

It is a wonderful time to be a specialist in the field of natural hair! You should try new products to enhance your services. Make your own custom cocktails of conditioners and treatments that address your clients' needs. Learn the varying techniques that are offered to you in this text; never stop exploring the most current fashion-forward style combinations that will define your signature style and set you apart from other stylists. The natural hair industry is now a community, and it is growing. It is a culture with values and principles. It is a lifestyle that provides emotional, psychological, and physiological rewards, and the industry is earth and animal conscious. The natural hair care industry is here to stay—it is not a fad, but a financially rewarding endeavor that will take you on the journey to success and well-being. Enjoy your journey!

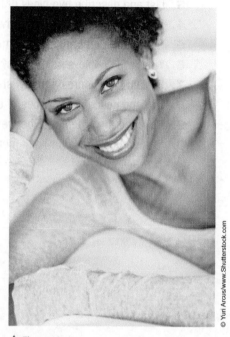
▲ Figure 10–4
The client journey.

Review Questions

1. Explain the general benefits of transitional styling, protective styling, and the big chop.
2. List and describe the different types of Afro styles.
3. List and describe two types of braids.
4. Describe how to create cornrows.
5. Name three other types of textured sets and styles.
6. What are double-strand twists?
7. Explain how to create the twist-out style.
8. List and describe two types of coil styles.
9. Describe the differences between locs and nu-locs.
10. Explain how the latch-hook method is used to create crochet weaves.

Glossary/Index

bacteria (*Continued*)

growth of, 32

infection, 32–33

nonpathogenic, 31

pathogenic, 31

Baker, Annabelle, 11

balance, 60, 63

baldness. *See* alopecia

balsam, 176, 178

*Baltimore Afro-America*n, 10

Bantu knots (Nubian knots or a knot out), created by twisting and twirling a geometric section of hair around its base. These knots can be worn as a style or as a way of setting the hair. When the knots are worn as a style, geometric designs can be parted into the head to separate each section, 5, 209, 227

Barker, Elizabeth Cardozo, 11

base oils, 195–196

basil, 176, 178

beauty, 78, 127. *See also* green beauty

established standards of, 11, 21

integrated, 19

natural, 11

paradigm shift in, 205

redefining concept of, 80–81

beauty industry

African American, 6–9, 13–14

white, 9, 13–14

beauty wellness, a holistic approach to natural hair services that views the client's beauty and health as being equally important, 72

bee balm. *See* bergamot

beeswax, 176, 178–179

behavior, 60, 69, 70. *See also* code of conduct

bergamot, 176, 179

big chop, the total removal or cutting off of the relaxed portion of all hair strands leaves naturally curly hair as a teeny weeny Afro (TWA). The results of the big chop are immediate and dramatic, 226, 228

binary fission, the division of bacteria cells into two new cells called daughter cells, 32

black power movement, 12

black seed oil, 128, 176, 179

bleach, a chemical (typically a solution of sodium hypochlorite or hydrogen peroxide) used to whiten or sterilize materials, 45

blood, fluid that supplies the body with oxygen and nutrients to the cells and tissues; circulates from the heart through the blood vessels to nourish the entire body. It also removes carbon dioxide toxins and waste from the cells, 141

bloodborne pathogens, 35–37, 44, 49–50

blowdrying, 211, 213, 220

body language, 69, 70

body systems (systems), groups of body organs acting together to perform one or more functions, 136–144

booking, 63

botanical, term relating to plants, 3, 171

colors and herbal rinses, 192–193

Bottner, Irving, 13

braid designer, one who is proficient and highly skilled in the art form of braiding; has more than just the technical skills and can incorporate skills into advanced techniques, such as creating and developing new styles. A braid designer is well-versed in client/stylist holistic relations and interpersonal communication satisfaction, 18

braid sediment, debris that accumulates on the hair and scalp over time; sediment from oils, creams, dirt, and debris resulting from improper cleansing and care, 157

braid stylist, one who has been trained and has adequate technical skills for braiding styles. The braid stylist is knowledgeable in hair loss, scalp disorders, health/cleaning and disinfection, proper hair tension, and interpersonal skills; he or she understands the holistic relationship between the client and the stylist, 15–16, 18

braid technician, an entry-level position—an assistant or apprentice in the specialty of braiding. The braid technician is in the process of acquiring technical skills and perfecting various braiding techniques, 18

braided style, 3, 20, 72. *See also specific braids*

beaded, 5, 14

combing out, 156–157

cream rinses and, 191

damage and, 157–158

preparing for, 217–218

removal of, 160–161, 197

restorative aspect of, 14–15

shampooing, 156–159, 198–200

single box braids, 229–232

terms, 226–228

traction alopecia and, 125–127

types of, 14–15

braid-out, the technique of using a single braid as a set to enhance, elongate, or define a client's texture. Hair is braided wet or dry and then opened to enhance original texture, 206, 225, 226, 227

brain, 140

Brandeis University, 12

breakage, 119

from relaxers, 118

breathing, 63, 143

Breedlove, Sarah. *See* Madame C. J. Walker

Brooklyn Museum, 4

Bundles, A'Lelia, 8

burdock root, 176, 179

Burkes, Hiddekel, 16

calcium hydroxide (Ca(OH)$_2$ no-lye), a non pre-formulated straightener, and inorganic compound with the chemical formula combining a cream containing calcium hydroxide (slaked lime) with an "activating solution" of guanidine carbonate, 115

calendula, 176, 179

California curls, 118

calmness, 63, 68, 184, 185, 186

canities (congenital and acquired), technical term for gray hair; results from the loss of the hair's natural melanin pigment, 115–116

carbon dioxide (CO$_2$), a colorless, odorless gas produced by burning carbon and organic compounds and by respiration. It is naturally present in air (about 0.03%) and is absorbed by plants in photosynthesis, 141

cardiac muscle, involuntary muscle that forms the heart. This type of muscle is not found in any other part of the body, 139

career opportunities, 3

carrot oil, 176, 180

castor oil, 122, 176, 180, 196

catagen phase, the transition or resting stage of hair development. During this phase, after years of growing, the hair cells stop reproducing. The hair begins to lose moisture and separates from the papilla. It is the signal of the end of the growth phase. This phase lasts from one to two weeks, 94

cationics, detergents or surfactants made of quaternary ammonium compounds, or quats, 165

CDC. *See* Centers for Disease Control and Prevention

cell enzymes, substances that help to produce amino acids, 150

cells, basic units of all living things from bacteria to plants to animals, including human beings, 136

Centers for Disease Control and Prevention (CDC), 42, 49

central nervous system (CNS), body system made up of the brain, spinal cord, spinal nerves, and cranial nerves. The CNS controls the mental activities; the five senses of seeing, hearing, feeling, smelling, and tasting; and all body movement and facial expression, 140

chamomile, 122, 176, 180

chemicals, 3, 16–17, 27, 87. *See also specific chemicals*
    causing damage, 116–119, 185
    in hair products, 174–175
    for straightening, 115, 117

children, 118

cilia, slender, hairlike extensions used by bacilli and spirilla for locomotion (moving about), 32

circulatory system, body system related to maintenance of good health. The cardiovascular or vascular system controls the steady circulation of the blood through the body by means of the heart and the blood vessels. It is made up of the heart, arteries, veins, and capillaries, 141

civil rights movement, 11–12

Civil War, 7

cleaning, a mechanical process (scrubbing) using soap and water or detergent and water to remove all visible dirt, debris, and many disease-causing germs. Cleaning also removes invisible debris that interferes with disinfection. Cleaning is what natural stylists are required to do before disinfecting, 3, 26, 30
    guidelines, 50–53
    logbook, 47
    routine, 40
    surfaces, 30, 47, 48
    tools, 30, 37, 41–42
    towels, linens, capes, 48

client
    with alopecia, 127–128
    with hair loss, 114–115
    history, 171
    natural hair stylist relationship with, 68–69, 72–73
    preparing, 71
    total well-being of, 72–73
    trust, 68–69

client consultation form, a questionnaire used to gather pertinent information about the client, 84

clover, 128

CNS. *See* central nervous system

cocci, round-shaped organisms that appear singly or in groups. The three types are staphylococci, streptococci, and diplococci, 32

cocoa butter, 176, 180

coconut oil, 176, 180–181, 187, 196

code of conduct, 65, 71, 73

COHNS elements, the major elements that make up human hair, carbon, oxygen, hydrogen, nitrogen, and sulfur, 97

coils, 5, 102, 107, 108, 227. *See also specific coils*
    creating, with extensions, 255–258
    shampooing, 156–159, 198–200
    short, 208
    thick and long, 208
    tight, 207

cold water conditioning, practice of rinsing the conditioner out of the hair using cool to cold water instead of hot water, 173

collagen, 147, 150, 189, 196

coltsfoot, 121, 176, 181

comb twists, 208

combing, 213
    finger, 206, 209
    out braided style, 156–157
    out locks, 196, 210

combs, 7, 9. *See also* hairstyling tools

comfrey, 176, 181

communication, 66
    effective, 77
    Internet, 17, 20
    skills, 59, 65, 69, 87
    styles, 70–71, 73

conditioning, 291. *See also specific rinses*
    instant, 193
    leave-in, 191–192, 215
    protein, 193–194
    types of, rinses, 190–196

connective tissue, 136

consultation, 72
    basics, 83–88
    beginning, 77–80
    client, form, 84
    questions, 85–86

contagious disease (communicable disease), disease that is spread from one person to another person. Some of the most contagious diseases are the common cold, ringworm, conjunctivitis (pinkeye), viral infections, and natural nail or toe and foot infections, 32, 33, 34

contamination, 34

cornrows, 14, 227, 238
    sculpted, with feed-in technique, 245–248

Cornrows and Company Salon, 15

cortex, the thickest and innermost layer of the shaft composed of elongated cells. This layer contains melanin and is responsible for the hair's elasticity, 95, 96

cosmetics, 3, 145

cosmetology, the art and science of beautifying and improving the skin, nails, and hair; includes the study of cosmetics and their application, 3
    license, 15
    state, boards, 10–11

co-washing, using conditioner rather than shampoo to cleanse the hair, 172

cradle cap, an oily, yellow scaling or crusting on a baby's scalp. It is common in babies and is easily treated. Cradle cap is not a part of any illness and does not imply that a baby is not being well cared for, 120

cranium, an oval, bony case that protects the brain, 138

cream rinses, 191

credit, good, 65

criticism, 60, 70

crochet weave, 252–254

crown, the soft center of the head, 155

cultural aesthetic, the styles and trends that are specific to a culture, 20

curl configuration, the natural external form of a hair fiber; refers to the straight, wave, curl, coil, kinky, or wiry shape of the hair shaft, 99, 107

curling iron, 7

curls, 7, 10, 101, 207. *See also specific curls*
    enhancing natural, 259–261
    haircut for, 275–278
    shampooing, 156–159, 198–200

cuticle, the outer layer of the hair shaft; it is made up of dead protein cells (keratin) as well as amino acids such as cystine and is arranged in overlapping scales, like shingles on a roof, 95–96, 183

ethics, a set of standards, moral judgments, and compliances determined by the state board for the practice and licensing of natural hair care and braiding, 64

code of conduct, 65, 71, 73

professional, 66

work, 59

ethmoid bone, light, spongy bone between the eye sockets; forms part of the nasal cavities, 138

eucalyptus, 128, 176, 182

evening primrose oil, 176, 182

excretory system, body system that includes the kidneys, liver, skin, large intestines, and lungs. The excretory system purifies the body by eliminating waste matter, 143

exercise, 64, 67

exocrine glands (duct glands), glands that produce a substance that travels through small, tube-like ducts; sweat glands and oil glands of the skin belong to this group, 142

exposure incident, contact with nonintact (broken) skin, blood, body fluid, or other potentially infectious materials that results from the performance of an employee's duties, 34, 44, 49–50

eye contact, 78, 79

F

facial skeleton, the framework of the face that is composed of 14 bones, 138

facial structure, 81–82

FDA. See Food and Drug Administration

fennel, 176, 182

Ferrell, Pamela, 15, 127

finasteride, 128–129

finger combing, the technique of evenly distributing a product throughout each strand of hair while it is still wet, using the fingers on both of your hands like a comb. This technique creates more definition of the client's natural curl pattern, 209

flagella, slender, hairlike extensions used by bacilli and spirilla for locomotion (moving about), 32

flat iron, 87, 88

use and care of, 216

flat twist-out, styling technique using a flat twist as a set to enhance and define a client's texture. Hair is flat twisted wet or dry and then opened to enhance and define a client's texture, 206

flexi-rod set, perm rods are used to spirally set hair, 208, 209, 225, 241–244, 262–264

folliculitis keloidalis, 129–130

Food and Drug Administration (FDA), 43, 128, 161

fragilitas crinium, technical term for brittle hair, 116

frankincense, 176, 182

free radicals, 146–147

friendships, 59

frontal bone, bone that forms the forehead, 138

frontalis, the front (anterior) portion of the epicranius; the muscle of the scalp that raises the eyebrows, draws the scalp forward, and causes wrinkles across the forehead, 139

fungi, microscopic plant parasites, including molds, mildews, and yeasts; fungi can produce contagious diseases, such as ringworm, 37–38, 119–120, 176, 183, 187, 190

G

G. A. Morgan Hair Refining Company, 10

game plan, the conscious act of planning your life for any future endeavors, 60, 61

garlic, 176, 183

ginseng, 176, 183

glycerine, 176, 183, 194

goal setting, the identification of long- and short-term goals that help you decide what you want out of your life, 59, 61–62, 78

goldenseal, 176, 183

gossip, 60

grapeseed oil, 176, 183

Grateau, Marcel, 7

green beauty, 145

grooming, the process by which the natural stylist nurtures the client's hair by cleansing, conditioning, and styling in order to enhance or improve the client's personal appearance, 204–205

Afro, 13

locks, 210–211

locks for men, 279–282

locks for women, 283–286

guanidine hydroxide (GH) relaxer, products using GH are known as no-lye relaxers; although they are technically not no-lye, the active ingredient is the hydroxide ion. GH contains two components that must be mixed immediately before using, 117

H

hair, 10. See also damaged hair; hair texture; natural hair care; natural hair textures

chemical composition of, 97–98

diameter of, 100, 101, 102, 103–104, 105

health reflected in, 144

length, 72, 205, 208

myth about natural, 88

pressed, myth, 73

ringed, 116

spiritual significance of, 155

structure, 3, 92–94, 107–108, 217

terminal, 93, 106

vellus, 93, 105–106

virgin, 18

hair analysis, 87, 103–105, 214–215

hair bulb, the almost transparent, round structure at the very bottom of the hair root. The base of the bulb is a hollowed-out or concave ball that fits over and covers the papilla, 94, 106, 107, 144

hair coloring, 184

botanical, 192–193

hair disorders, 115–116. See also specific hair disorders

hair elasticity, the hair's ability to stretch and return to its original size and shape without breaking, 105

hair extensions, 3, 86, 88, 126, 157, 158, 225, 226

for Afro, 227, 233–236, 237–240

for coils, 255–258

for crochet weave, 252–254

for sculpted cornrows, 245–248

for transitional haircut, 287–290

for twists, 249–251

hair follicle, a deep, angular, pocket-like depression in the scalp; contains the hair root, 3, 93, 99, 106, 107, 144, 179, 183, 185

hair growth, 7, 105, 131, 182, 185

phases of, 106–107

hair loss, 3, 68, 71, 108, 112, 156, 182, 185. See also alopecia

caring for client with, 114–115

medicated shampoo, contains special ingredients that are effective in reducing dandruff or relieving other scalp conditions, 168–169

medulla, the innermost core of the shaft, consisting of sponge-like, baggy cells. In very thin, light-colored hair, it may be hollow or not exist at all. For the most part, the medulla does not require any hair care services, 95, 96

melanin, 115, 116

men
    groomed lock style for, 279–282
    haircut for, 275–278

methicillin-resistant staphylococcus aureus (MRSA), a type of infectious bacteria that is highly resistant to conventional treatments such as antibiotics, 32, 33

Metropolitan Museum of Art, 4

microorganisms, any organism of microscopic or sub-microscopic size, 30. See also specific microorganisms

mildew, a type of fungus that affects plants or grows on inanimate objects but does not cause human infections in the salon, 37

mind, peaceful, 67

minerals, 148, 150–151
    in herbs, 177–190

miniaturization, a condition of the hair follicle when long, thick, and pigmented (terminal) hair strands are replaced by short, thin, and unpigmented hair, 124

minoxidil, 128

moisture, 119, 168, 169, 173, 176, 183, 184, 187

moisturizer, a product formulated to add moisture to dry hair or promote the retention of moisture, 164, 165, 170, 177, 180, 181, 182, 189, 190
    natural, 194–195
    types of, 195

monilethrix, technical term for a condition known as beaded hair, 116

monionics, detergents that emulsify well and usually have a mild cleansing action. They are gentle to the skin and cause little irritation to the scalp or eyes, 165

Morgan, Garrett Augustus, Sr., 9

Morgan, Rose, 10–11

Moroccan oil. See argan oil

MRSA. See methicillin-resistant staphylococcus aureus

multiuse (reusable), items that can be cleaned, disinfected, and used on more than one person even if the item is accidentally exposed to blood or body fluid, 47

muscular system, muscles are fibrous tissues. This body system shapes and supports the skeletal system. Its function is to produce all movements of the body. It consists of more than 500 muscles, large and small, and comprises about 50 percent of the body's weight, 136, 138–140. See also specific muscles

myrrh, 176, 186–187

nails, 3

National Braider's Guild, 16

National Negro Business League, 7

National Student Loan Data System (NSLDS), 66

natural hair care, is under the umbrella of cosmetology. Natural hair care is the study and practice of chemically free hair styling that includes working with textured hair-braiding, extensions, twists, locks, and weaves, 3, 194, 205
    history, 3–17
    holistic approach to, 19–20, 67, 72, 79, 95, 204, 291
    list of herbs used in, 175–176
    products, 17, 19, 27, 28, 162, 170

    regimens, 19
    services, 71

natural hair care license, state-recognized regulations for natural hair care and braiding. Not all states require licensing, 18–19, 53, 62

natural hair stylist, a person who advocates for the proper care of natural hair, 3, 21
    client relationship, 68–69, 72–73
    regulations, 18–19, 53

natural hair textures, virgin hair that is a non-chemical curly hair pattern described as wavy, curly, coily and highly textured hair, 17, 21. See also hair texture
    reference guide to, 100–102

natural hairstyles, chemically free hairstyles that include naturally curly hair and textured styles, like braids, extensions, twists, locks, coils, and weaves, 12, 13, 16–17. See also protective styles; specific hairstyles
    neo, 205–206
    techniques for, 207–210, 229–290
    tools for specific, 229–290

Natural Organic Hair and Skin Care (Hampton), 194

Natural Roots Magazine, 17

naturally acquired immunity, an immunity that is partly inherited and partly developed through healthy living, 39

naturallycurly.com, 17

neo-natural hairstyles, 205–206

neroli oil, 187

nervous system, body system that has three main subdivisions: the central, the peripheral, and the automatic nervous system, 136, 140–141

nettle, 121, 176, 187

New Black Esthetic, 14–17

The New Psy-Cosmetologist: Blending the Sciences of Psychology and Cosmetology, 80

Newsweek, 13

no-lye perm/ammonium thioglycolate, a chemical compound with the salt of a weak acid and weak base; ammonium thioglycolate exists in solution as an equilibrium mixture of the salt itself. Ammonium thioglycolate, also known as perm salt, is used to create permanent waves or curls, 115, 117, 118

nonpathogenic bacteria, harmless microorganisms that may perform useful functions and are safe to come in contact with because they do not cause disease or harm, 31

nonporous surfaces, surfaces that are made or constructed of a material that has no pores or openings and cannot absorb liquids, 29

nonstriated muscles, also known as smooth muscles; muscles that are involuntary and function automatically, without conscious will. These muscles are found in the internal organs of the body, such as the digestive or respiratory systems, 139

NSLDS. See National Student Loan Data System

Nubian coils, 268–270

Nubian knots, 209. See also Bantu knots

nutriceuticals, combination of the terms nutrition and pharmaceuticals; refers to food and food products that provide health as well as beauty and medical benefits, 145

nutricosmetics, refers to nutritional supplements that can support the function and structure of the skin, 145

nutrition, 19, 67, 73, 144, 146, 148–149

occipital bone, hindmost bone of the skull, below the parietal bones; forms the back of the skull above the nape, 138

occipitalis, the back (posterior) portion of the epicranius; the muscle that draws the scalp backward, 139

Occupational Safety and Health Administration (OSHA), a federal agency created as part of the U.S. Department of Labor to regulate and enforce safety and health standards to protect employees in the workplace, 27, 49

oil, 168, 175. *See also* base oils; *specific oils*

    hair, preparation, 217–218

    hot, treatment, 187

    saturated and unsaturated compounds of organic, 195

olive oil, 176, 187, 196

On Her Own Ground: The Life and Times of Madame C. J. Walker (Bundles), 8

organic

    foods, 149

    shampoos, 169–171, 194

organs, structures composed of specialized tissues designed to perform specific functions in plants and animals, 136, 137, 143

OSHA. *See* Occupational Safety and Health Administration

sodium hydroxide relaxer (lye perm; NaOH), a strongly alkaline white deliquescent compound with a high pH. It is the most caustic and reactive because of its high pH levels, which range from about 12 to 14 on the pH scale, making it potentially dangerous to the hair and scalp. When this type of chemical touches the scalp, forehead, ear, or neck, burning irritation may occur. Before applying this type of relaxer, a pre-application of petroleum is required to protect the skin and scalp. It is also used in many industrial processes such as the manufacturing of soap and paper, 117

Soft Sheen, 13

soft water, rainwater or chemically softened water; contains only small amounts of minerals and thus allows soap and shampoo to lather freely, 166

Soul Train, 13

speech, 67, 69

Spencer, Sarah, 8–9

sphenoid bone, bone that joins all the bones of the cranium together, 138

spinal cord, portion of the central nervous system that originates in the brain, extends down to the lower extremity of the trunk, and is protected by the spinal column, 140–141

spirilla, a bacterium with a rigid spiral structure, found in stagnant water and sometimes causing disease, 32

split ends, 116, 178, 184

spore, a tiny, typically one-celled reproductive unit capable of giving rise to a new individual without sexual fusion; characteristic of lower plants, fungi, and protozoans, 32, 41, 42

staphylococci, pus-forming bacteria that grow in clusters like a bunch of grapes. They cause abscesses, pustules, and boils, 32, 33

state cosmetology boards, 10–11

sterilization, the process that completely destroys all microbial life, including spores, 30, 40, 42

strand test, 99–100

straw set, plastic straws are cut for the appropriate length of hair and used to spirally set hair, 208–209

streptococci, pus-forming bacteria arranged in curved lines resembling a string of beads. They cause infections such as strep throat and blood poisoning, 32

stress, 66, 68, 105

related hair loss, 73

striated muscles, also known as skeletal muscles. Muscles that are attached to the bones and are voluntary, consciously controlled, 138

student loans, 65, 66

sub-occipital, the area underneath or below the occipital bone, 118

success, 64

principles for, 59–61

sulfur, 121, 150–151, 181

surfactants, chemical compounds designed to create the wetting, emulsifying, dispersing, and liquefying properties of a shampoo, 163, 164

sustainability, 145

Tatum, Cheryl, 16

tea tree oil, 43, 128, 176, 190

television, 13

telogen phase, during this phase of hair development, the bulb is totally separate from the root; new hair cells divide and multiply, creating a new shaft. New hair sprouts to the surface of the scalp, pushing out the old strands, or remains until the original hair returns to the next phase (anagen). This stage begins the new cycle, and it lasts two to four months, 94, 107

temporal bones, bones that form the sides of the head in the ear region. There are two temporal bones, 138

terminal hair, pigmented hair found on the scalp, arms, legs, nose, and ears. This hair is coarser than vellus hair, although it varies in texture, color, and length, 93, 106

texture on texture, a general term used to describe the set of styling techniques on naturally textured hair that alter, elongate, or enhance the original curl patterns. Hair is set or manipulated. Then it is dried and the curl opened to create a uniformed textured finish. These set styling techniques include twistout, braid-out, flat twist-out and knot-out, 206

techniques, 207–210

thermal iron. *See* flat iron

thioglycolate perm/no-lye perm, a chemical compound with the salt of a weak acid and weak base; ammonium thioglycolate exists in solution as an equilibrium mixture of the salt itself. Ammonium thioglycolate, also known as perm salt, is used to create permanent waves, 115, 117, 118

thread-wrapping, 14, 16

thyme, 176, 190

tignon, a head scarf worn by Creole women, 6

time management, 62–64, 80

tinea, technical term for ringworm, a contagious condition caused by fungal infection and not a parasite, characterized by itching, scales, and sometimes painful lesions, 37, 38, 130

tinea barbae, the most frequently encountered fungal infection resulting from hair services; also known as barber's itch. Tinea barbae is a superficial fungal infection that commonly affects the skin. It is primarily limited to the bearded areas of the face and neck or around the scalp, 38

tinea capitis, a fungal infection of the scalp characterized by red papules, or spots, at the openings of the hair follicles, 38

tinea favosa (tinea favus), an infection characterized by dry, sulfur-yellow, cuplike crusts, called scutula, on the scalp, 38

tissue, collection of similar cells that perform a particular function, 136

Tolliver, Melba, 13

touch, 68–69, 155, 209

toxins, 31, 45

in disinfectants, 41

traction alopecia, hair loss that occurs due to traction placed on hair. Traction alopecia is commonly seen with braids, ponytails, and other hairstyles that create traction on the scalp, 114

braids and, 125–127

transitional textures, occur when the hair has two textures on one strand. The hair is allowed to grow without chemically "retouching" the new growth. This is the first step toward growing out natural hair. The new growth or natural portion is strong and vital while the relaxed portion of the hair is weak, thin, and breaks easily, 224

transitioning (going natural), process that involves growing out the hair while going from chemically relaxed hair to natural. It is a conscious approach to stop relaxing or refrain from using harsh chemicals or extreme heat to reduce or modify the client's natural, virgin hair texture, 16–17, 71, 72, 73, 224, 249

haircut for, 287–290

long-term, 225–226

texture and, 224

transmission, direct and indirect, 31

treatment

alopecia areata, 128

damaged hair, 15, 178

dandruff, 121

hair loss medical, 128–129

hot-oil, 187

keratine, 115

trichoptilosis, technical term for split ends, 116. *See also* split ends

trichorrhexis nodosa, technical term for the condition known as knotted hair; it is characterized by brittleness and the formation of nodular swellings along the hair shaft, 116

trust, 78

    building, 80

    client, 68–69

tuberculoidal disinfectants, disinfectants that kill the bacteria that causes tuberculosis, 29

Tubman, Harriet, 6

Tuskegee Institute, 7

twist-outs, the technique of using a double-strand twist as a set to enhance and define a client's current texture. A setting solution or curl enhancer is applied. Hair is twisted wet and dried until set; then each twist is unraveled or opened to create a defined textured pattern, 211, 225, 226

    flat, 206

twists, 3, 157, 159, 229

    Afro, 227, 233–236

    chubby, 208

    comb, 208

    creating large, with extensions, 249–251

    removing, 160–161

two-strand twist, created by overlapping equal sections over one another, 206, 207

Ultra Wave, 10

United States Department of Agriculture (USDA), federal organization that provides a certification program with strict guidelines for all organic foods to meet government standards. If the food bears a USDA label, that means it is 95 to 100 percent organic, 149, 162

Universal Precautions, A set of guidelines published by OSHA that require the employer and the employee to assume that all human blood and body fluids are infectious for bloodborne pathogens, 44, 49–50

Uqdah, Talib-Din, 15

Urban Legend, 9

USDA. *See* United States Department of Agriculture

vellus hair, short, fine, white and downy hair, usually without a medulla. Vellus hair is found on any area of the body except the palms of hands and soles of feet, 93, 105–106

vinegar, 121

virus, a parasitic, sub-microscopic particle that infects and resides in cells of biological organisms. A virus can replicate only by taking over the host cell's reproductive functions, 31, 33, 35. *See also specific viruses*

visualize success, the practice of imagining or creating a mental picture of your dream salon, career, life, and so on, 59–60

vitamins, 19, 67, 72, 144, 145, 147, 151

    B-Complex, 121, 149–150

    in herbs, 177–190

Walker, Charles Joseph, 7

water, 147

    chemistry of, 166

    cold, 173

    deionized, 163

    hard and soft, 166

waves, 7, 101, 107

weave, 3, 225, 226

    Afro, 237–240

    crochet, 252–254

Web resources, 7, 8, 16, 17, 99, 291

Where Beauty Touches Me (Ferrell), 127

whole foods, 148–149

wigs, 5, 114, 225, 226

    Afro, 12

    making and applying, 271–274

Wilborn, Wesley, 118

witch hazel, 43, 176, 190

Woman's Voice, 8

work ethics, 59

yarn braids, 265–267

ylang-ylang, 176, 190